ACLS Scenarios:

CORE CONCEPTS FOR CASE-BASED LEARNING

To the providers of ACLS
By practicing your daily heroics
You teach us the value of knowledge and skill . . .

Good job

To the survivors of sudden cardiac death
By celebrating your renewed existence
You teach us the preciousness of life . . .

Welcome back

Richard O. Cummins

Judy Reid Graves

ACLS Scenarios:

CORE CONCEPTS FOR CASE-BASED LEARNING

Richard O. Cummins, MD, MPH, MSc

Professor of Medicine
Emergency Medicine Service
University of Washington Medical Center
Seattle, Washington

Judy Reid Graves, RN, MA, EMT–P

Clinical Research Coordinator
King County EMS
Seattle/King County Department of Public Health
Seattle, Washington

with 146 illustrations

Illustrations (except ECGs) by Kimberly Battista

Photography by Vincent Knaus

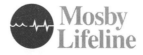

St. Louis   Baltimore   Boston   Carlsbad   Chicago   Naples   New York   Philadelphia   Portland
London   Madrid   Mexico City   Singapore   Sydney   Tokyo   Toronto   Wiesbaden

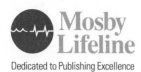

Mosby Lifeline

Dedicated to Publishing Excellence

A Times Mirror Company

Publisher: **David Dusthimer**

Editor in Chief: **Richard A. Weimer**

Executive Editor: **Claire Merrick**

Editor: **Julie Scardiglia**

Assistant Editor: **Kay E. Beard**

Editorial Assistant: **Paula Willey**

Book Design: **DesignConcept**, Hanover, Md.

Mosby-Year Book, Inc.
11830 Westline Industrial Drive
St. Louis, Missouri 63146

International Standard Book Number: 0-8151-1517-2

9 8 7 6 5 4 3 2 1 / 95 96 97 98 99

Acknowledgments

Reviewers:

Mary Fran Hazinski, RN; **Kathee Littrell**, RN, MSN; **Corey Slovis**, MD; **Frederick M. Burkle Jr.**, MD, MPH; **Barbara Aehlert**, RN; **Jon Auricchio**, PharmD; **Jim Haner**, Paramedic; **Scott Kennard**, MD; **Tim Phalen**, BS, NREMT-P; **Gary Rushworth**, BS, RRT; **Mary Alice Witzel**, RN.

Photo shoot models, locations, and consultants:

Washington Adventist Hospital, Takoma Park MD -- Pam Bowman; Lawrence Simon, MD, FACEP; Sergio Ramos, RN; Kerry Larkin, RN, CEN; Barbara Azurée, RN; Carol Ann Sperry, RN, MS, CEN.

Northern Virginia Regional Park Authority, Fairfax Station VA -- Ranger Frank T. Ryan, Kelly Stock, Megan Child.

Sterling Volunteer Rescue Squad, Inc., Sterling VA -- Byron Andrews, Jeff Johnson, James Harvey, Kevin Barnes, Jacquiline Smith, Don Freudenthal, Stuart MacKenzie.

Harrisonburg Electric Commission.

David J. Taminger, ACLS Instructor, Charlottesville, VA.

Central Shenandoah EMS Council -- Andy Funkhouser, NREMT-P, ACLS Coordinator; Eve Loudermilk, RN, Training Coordinator; Mark Adams, NREMT-P, Executive Director; Bill Downs, NREMT-P, BLS Coordinator.

Harrisonburg Fire Department, Harrisonburg VA -- Jeff A. Morris; Captain Jim LaPrevotte, Lieutenant Bill Stickley, Chief Larry Shifflett.

Rockingham Memorial Hospital -- Kathy Hill, RN, Nurse Manager; Frieda R. King, RN; Tina Howell, RN; Debra Simmons, RN; Sherry Doyle, RRT; Janna Steiner, HT; Jeffrey Gibbons, MD.

Harrisonburg Rescue Squad -- Chief Ronnie Hensley, EMT-CT; Phil Neff, EMT-CT; Janet Smith, EMT-ST; Jessica Kahn, EMT; Meg Sanders, EMT; Nancy Gottheimer, EMT; Justin Witt, EMT-CT; Wanda Driver, EMT-CT; Keith Johnson, EMT; Warren Knicely, EMT-ST; Bill Porter, EMT; Brian Moore, EMT; Tim Barb, EMT; Todd Barb, EMT.

Equipment loaners:

Jim Springer of Physio-Control Corporation; **Jim Cardwell** of Marquette; also the folks at Laerdal Medical Corp, Armonk, NY; and First Medic, Redmond, WA.

Art & Design:

Vincent Knaus, photographer; **Kimberly Battista**, illustrations; **Jim Fanzone & Jay Harrison**, DesignConcept, Hanover MD, cover and text design.

Contents

Introduction

We have written this book to introduce advanced cardiac life support (ACLS) providers to case-based learning in ACLS. This book presents ACLS through the use of clinical vignettes, cases, scenarios, and clinical challenges. This case-based approach represents a change in the way emergency care providers traditionally have learned ACLS. How did this new way of learning ACLS come about, and why we have prepared another ACLS book?

The American Heart Association (AHA) and its emergency cardiac care committees and subcommittees have done an outstanding job developing guidelines for ACLS. Advanced cardiac life support instructors present these ACLS guidelines in thousands of courses each year across the United States and around the world. In 1994 the AHA published the *Textbook of ACLS* and a companion *ACLS Instructors Manual*. The ACLS textbook's chapters have continued to be divided into traditional subjects of emergency cardiac care with each chapter providing a detailed presentation from topic experts.

In its 1994 edition, however, the *ACLS Instructors Manual* recommends a major change in the way ACLS courses are taught—from the traditional subject-based format to a much more clinically relevant case-based or problem-based approach. Numerous studies of adult learning and adult education have confirmed that adults learn best when material is presented in ways that resemble how they will actually use the information. In fact, the majority of medical schools in the United States have now adopted a case-based or problem-based learning curriculum.

Since ACLS providers will use the ACLS guidelines to care for and treat patients, it makes sense to present the ACLS in a patient-based format. Pediatric advanced life support courses have confirmed the success of a case-based learning approach. The ACLS subcommittee adopted this approach in the new *ACLS Instructors Manual*. All the core and supplemental ACLS topics contained in the ACLS textbook have been distributed among a series of cases found in the *ACLS Instructors Manual*. The AHA's goal is for ACLS instructors everywhere to use the case-based teaching material in the instructor's manual. The majority of ACLS courses have presented the material in a traditional subject-based format but also through the use of clinical questions and scenarios.

No Case-based ACLS Textbook (Until Now)

A problem exists. Advanced cardiac life support courses present the ACLS material in a case-based format, while the ACLS textbook presents the material in a subject-based format. What is missing is a study guide for ACLS students that is case-based, just like the 1994 ACLS course. To fill this gap, we produced a case-based ACLS book in which the patient becomes the vehicle for learning. Each set of cases teaches particular themes and then summarizes the material. The end of this book includes an ACLS drug formulary, which synthesizes critical information about each ACLS medication. Since the ACLS course will be case-based, there should be a student textbook that is case-based. After all, that is how we approach problems in our professional environment—one case at a time.

Case-based Teaching: The Basic Principles

Subject-based teaching falls short in helping students "synthesize" clinical information. Patient management requires complex thinking at many levels. We must possess a basic core memory of knowledge and facts. Case-based teaching delivers these facts in the context of an actual patient. Subject-based teaching simply delivers facts but does not ask the students to display their comprehension, analytic abilities, and ability to synthesize. Examples of this concept follow:

- Subject-based memory: If you are asked, "What is the most critical drug to give for people in ventricular fibrillation?" you would answer "epinephrine." You must recall a specific fact.

- Subject-based comprehension: If you are asked, "Why is epinephrine the most critical drug to give for ventricular fibrillation?" you would comment on the vasoconstrictive effects of epinephrine and how those effects lead to increased coronary and carotid artery flow during cardiopulmonary resuscitation (CPR). This demonstrates why epinephrine is the most critical agent.

- Case-based analysis: Case-based analysis requires you to bring together more subject-based facts, but to think about the facts in a different way. For example, if you are asked, "What is the most important action to take for a person who suddenly collapses?" you would have to think deeper because the answer depends on the exact mechanism of the sudden cardiac collapse in that particular patient. This question is much more clinically relevant because it illustrates a patient problem that we are likely to confront in our professional role. After some analysis, you would respond, "Assuming the most common cause of collapse is ventricular fibrillation, I would want to perform the Primary ABC Survey and look for ventricular fibrillation and defibrillate it if present." This time there is no mention of epinephrine. You are not recalling a specific fact but are analyzing a particular clinical scenario.

- Case-based synthesis: Suppose, however, you were confronted with this specific clinical scenario: In the emergency department you are examining a patient with suspected renal stones. The patient is in severe pain. You give an injection of a strong pain medication and send the patient to the radiology department for an intravenous pyelogram (IVP). Ten minutes later you hear the overhead paging system state that there has been a sudden collapse in the radiology department. Someone shouts out that "they are doing CPR for the person you just sent to x-ray." Here the question would be a synthesis of multiple pieces of information: "What could have happened? What is going on? What is the rhythm? What should I do?"

The preceding case challenges you to think about why the person collapsed and to begin thinking of a differential diagnosis before you arrive at the scene. If you discover that the rhythm is "some sort of pulseless electrical activity (PEA)," you must think about the differential diagnosis and how to modify the usual algorithms to accommodate this particular patient. You have to think further than just, "The rhythm is PEA: that means give epinephrine and maybe atropine." You will have to think: "Is this a ventricular fibrillation (VF) arrest that has deteriorated to PEA? Is this a vasovagal reaction to the injected medication? Is this a pseudoallergic reaction to the IVP contrast medium? Is this true anaphylaxis? Does the patient really have a kidney stone? Could it have been a dissecting abdominal aneurysm or an atypical presentation for an acute myocardial infarction?" Case-based learning forces you to think further and in more depth about your patients—this is what you are going to have to do as an emergency cardiac care provider.

In this book we present a series of cases which require that you know many facts. We do not, however, neglect the facts and their importance. We present them in our comments and critical action lists. We still present the "first principles" around which you must organize your learning and your case management. At its center this is a reference handbook—around each case we present the core information you need to know to think about and manage patients you might encounter. However, you must still take that all-important ACLS course and bring together the appropriate information (memory) and facts (comprehension). This book will help you with the synthesis and analysis and the more in-depth learning required for successful completion of the ACLS course.

The Organization of Our Case-based Book

We have organized the ACLS material into a series of cases followed by our ACLS Formulary, which summarizes all medications introduced in the various cases. The cases fall into the following general areas:

- People in full cardiac arrest (respiratory arrest, VF arrest, PEA, and asystole)

- People not in full cardiac arrest (bradycardias, tachycardias, acute myocardial infarction, hypotension, shock, and acute pulmonary edema)

- Special resuscitation situations (toxicologic conditions and electrolyte abnormalities, drowning, electrical shock and lightning stroke, hypothermia, traumatic cardiac arrest, and arrest associated with pregnancy)

The following sections may be found within each of the cases and contain the core ACLS material:

- Overview

- Major concepts to master (learning objectives)

- Critical actions (what you should always do when managing such cases)

- Skills to learn (reading electrocardiograms and using equipment)

- Rhythms to learn

- Medications to learn

- Case scenarios

- Comments on the case scenarios

- Major points to remember about similar cases

- Summary comments

How To Use This Book

There is a lot of information contained in this study guide. We suggest that you initially skim through each case and notice the numerous tables, figures, and summary comments. We have attempted to make the Comments sections broad and applicable to a wide range of patients, not just the particular patient in that scenario. An in-depth review of each case will give you a strong sense of how you can approach patients with similar problems in clinical practice. For a complete understanding of each medication's role, try looking up each drug in the Formulary as you encounter it in the body of the text. You can use this book as a true handbook—referring to the summary tables, Formulary, and figures as many times as necessary until you have mastered the material.

Who Should Use This Book?

This book is designed to help both the student and the instructor of ACLS. The case-based concept of learning will be new for many of you and will be a different way of learning for many of you, including experienced ACLS practitioners as well as the novice. Once you have mastered the major principles in this book, your ability to manage the immense variety of emergency situations seen daily will be enhanced. This is the beauty of case-based learning.
Have fun!

Richard O. Cummins, MD

Judy Graves, RN, EMT-P

Cardiac Arrest!
General Approaches to Cardiopulmonary Emergencies

OVERVIEW

The Five Quadrads Approach

The purpose of this chapter is to give you the major, generic tools to manage most types of cardiopulmonary emergencies. We think that one major approach—the "Five Quadrads" —will give advanced cardiac life support (ACLS) providers a powerful conceptual tool. With this tool ACLS providers will be able to systematically approach all cardiopulmonary emergencies. This approach covers both cardiac arrest patients and "peri-cardiac arrest" patients—those patients "on their way to a cardiac arrest."

The Five Quadrads approach is simply five sets of four items to remember. Apply the Five Quadrads whenever you walk into an emergency setting, whether in-hospital, in the emergency department, or in the prehospital setting. The Five Quadrads are a layered approach to guide action and to stimulate thinking, not just a list of things to remember. The items of the Five Quadrads approach include assessment actions, intervention actions, and stimulants to thinking.

The following cases present typical clinical challenges and demonstrate the power of the Five Quadrads approach to help ACLS providers access, diagnose, and treat a wide variety of cardiopulmonary emergencies. Consider how you would approach each of these challenges.

Case 1: Bystander witnesses a sudden collapse

While attending your daughter's soccer game, you notice a young woman run up to the spectators standing on the sidelines shouting "Somebody please help! A man just collapsed over here on the jogging trail!"

Case 2: Emergency Medical Technician equipped only with an automated external defibrillator

You are a firefighter on duty when a 65-year-old man comes in with dizzy spells and chest tightness. While you are taking his blood pressure, he breaks out in a heavy sweat, becomes agitated, complains of severe chest pain, and suddenly falls back in the chair.

Case 3: Single rescuer with an automated external defibrillator

You are the head nurse for the night shift at a senior citizens' home. On your rounds you find one of the elderly residents sprawled unconscious on the floor. You know how to use an automated external defibrillator (AED), and one is available down the hall.

Case 4: Responding late to a complicated code already in progress

You are the code resident at a large academic medical center when you hear announced a "code" in the radiology department. You find a 50-year-old woman lying on the floor, surrounded by at least 20 people. Everyone is yelling out commands, but no one seems to be in charge.

Case 5: Witnessed collapse of patient short of breath, with tachycardia

You are a family medicine resident on rotation in the Emergency Department. A nurse suddenly calls you to Room 3. You find an elderly woman sitting upright with marked respiratory distress. During your assessment she slumps over, unresponsive.

Case 6: Complicated medical problems with failure to respond to usual measures

You are supervising a code in Room 1 of the emergency department. The patient is a 22-year-old woman with lupus and renal failure that requires dialysis. Depressed, she tried to commit suicide with cyclic antidepressants earlier. She was unresponsive, hypoventilating with a systolic blood pressure of 80 mm Hg, but then she went into a full cardiac arrest.

Case 7: Patient intubated despite "EMS–No CPR" order and terminal lung cancer

You are on duty in the emergency department. You receive a call from the Medic One doctor stating that the medics have just intubated a patient after he was choking at home. After medics intubated the patient's trachea, the wife produced a signed emergency medical service (EMS)—no CPR form for the patient. It seems the patient has metastatic lung cancer and did not wish CPR to be attempted should he suffer a cardiac arrest.

The Five Quadrads Approach

DEVELOPING A POWERFUL CONCEPTUAL TOOL TO USE WITH CARDIAC EMERGENCIES

The cases just presented are varied and complex. Two critical variables for decision making are whether you are alone or with others and the amount and types of equipment you have available. Nevertheless, regardless of available people or equipment, you should approach every cardiopulmonary emergency in the same systematic manner—*the Five Quadrads approach.* With this powerful conceptual tool rescuers can effectively and confidently deal with the following:

- Patients with full cardiac arrests
- Patients with full cardiac arrests who are not responding to therapy
- Patients "on their way to a cardiac arrest"—patients who, if you fail to identify their problem and start appropriate treatments, will progress to full cardiac arrest
- Patients who have responded to resuscitation efforts and are in the post-resuscitation period
- Any major clinical challenge or decision-making point

Through the chapters of this book you will learn how to apply the Five Quadrads approach to each of these challenging situations. What are the elements of the Five Quadrads approach? To make it simple, here is a quick summary list, without details:

CARDIAC ARREST
1. Primary ABCD Survey
2. Secondary ABCD Survey

PERI-CARDIAC ARREST
3. Oxygen/IV/Monitor/Fluids
4. Temperature/Blood Pressure/Heart Rate/Respirations
5. Tank (Volume)/Resistance/ Pump/Rate

Important points to note here include the following:

- The first two quadrads, the Primary and Secondary Surveys, apply to people in full cardiac arrest and not necessarily to people who are conscious, are breathing, and have a pulse. The Primary-Secondary Survey Approach is adapted from the specialty of emergency medicine. All emergency personnel learn to perform, first, a primary survey to identify immediate, life-threatening problems and then a secondary survey to initiate more advanced interventions and to think further about the differential diagnosis. This approach has also been recommended by the ACLS subcommittee of the American Heart Association (AHA) in the 1994 *Textbook of ACLS of Advanced Cardiac Life Support* and in the *ACLS Instructors Manual.*

- The third, fourth, and fifth quadrads apply, in general, to people who are having a cardiopulmonary emergency but have not yet gone into full cardiac arrest.

- We recommend, however, that you always apply the full Five Quadrads to every patient in whom you suspect a cardiopulmonary emergency. Just because a patient appears to be conscious and making eye contact does not mean he or she would successfully complete the Primary and Secondary Surveys. For example, assessing and treating the Primary Survey's A, that is, Airway, has saved many patients from deteriorating to a full cardiac arrest.

- We will, in the cases throughout this book, use the full Five Quadrads for virtually every patient, often quickly passing through the Primary and Secondary Surveys but never omitting those quadrads completely.

- We will modify the elements of the Five Quadrads in later chapters of the book, depending on the specific problems discussed. For example, you will learn that cervical spine immobilization must be added to the Five Quadrads when you are dealing with patients suffering from cardiac arrest associated with trauma, drowning, electrical shock, and often hypothermia. Modifications will be necessary in dealing with hypothermic cardiac arrest and in handling cardiac arrest associated with pregnancy. Despite the necessity to make modifications, the essential framework of the Five Quadrads is always applicable. You will

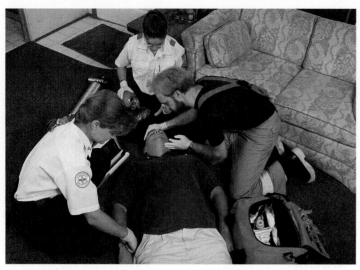

Fig. 1-1: Patient surrounded by personnel and items of the Primary Survey: gloves, airway barrier devices, and automated external defibrillator.

simply learn where the framework supports slightly different elements.

- Notice that there are overlaps among the Five Quadrads. This is because the Five Quadrads approach attempts to cover both cardiac arrest patients and peri-cardiac arrest patients. For example, the pulse and breathing check in the Primary ABCD Survey accomplishes the same assessments as the blood pressure, heart rate, and respirations in the fourth quadrad (Temperature/Blood Pressure/Heart Rate/ Respirations). Also, the Secondary Survey's C includes the "IV/Monitor/Fluids" of the third quadrad's "Oxygen/IV/Monitor/Fluids."

The Five Quadrads approach involves elements that can be either an *assessment* of the patient or a *treatment* of the patient.

CARDIAC ARREST PATIENTS

1. THE PRIMARY ABCD SURVEY. This easily remembered series of assessments and interventions covers basic CPR and defibrillation (Fig. 1-1).

- **Airway:** Open the airway (a treatment).
- **Breathing:** Check for breathing (an assessment); if not breathing, provide two ventilations (a treatment). If you cannot provide the two ventilations, (an assessment) then correct a possible obstructed airway (a treatment).
- **Circulation:** Check for a pulse (an assessment); if no pulse, provide chest compressions (a treatment).
- **Defibrillation:** Check the rhythm for the presence of ventricular fibrillation or ventricular tachycardia (VF/VT) (an assessment); if VF/VT is present, provide direct-current shocks (a treatment).

2. THE SECONDARY ABCD SURVEY. This series of assessments and treatments covers more advanced interventions of airway management and rhythm-appropriate intravenous (IV) medications and moves the ACLS code leader toward thinking about the cause of the emergency, differential diagnoses, and alternative treatment approaches (Fig. 1-2).

- **Airway:** Determine whether initial airway techniques and ventilations are adequate (an assessment). If not adequate, perform endotracheal intubation (a treatment).
- **Breathing:** Check adequacy of tube placement and ventilations (an assessment); provide positive-pressure ventilations through the endotracheal tube (a treatment).
- **Circulation:** Attach monitor leads to determine the rhythm (an assessment); obtain IV access to administer fluids and medications (treatments); administer rhythm-appropriate medications (assessment and treatment).
- **Differential diagnoses:** This part of the treatment of a cardiopulmonary emergency is critical. This is the part where you think. Most other steps involve dichotomous, yes-no decision making. Here, however, the Five Quadrads approach requires you to pause a moment and think specifically and carefully about why the person went into cardiac arrest. As you consider various causes, you must consider the treatment associated with each cause. Consideration of the differential diagnoses becomes of paramount importance when dealing with asystolic and pulseless electrical activity (PEA) cardiac arrest. In addition, you will learn that "differential diagnoses" play a major role in the many special resuscitation situations, in particular, toxicologic conditions and electrolyte abnormalities.

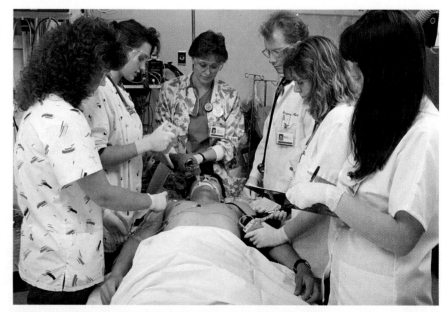

Fig. 1-2: Patient surrounded by personnel and items of the Secondary Survey: IV fluid bags and bottles, defibrillator and monitor, and endotracheal intubation equipment.

PERI-CARDIAC ARREST PATIENTS

3. OXYGEN/IV/MONITOR/FLUIDS

Many experienced ACLS instructors teach "Oxygen/IV/Monitor/Fluids" as one word. These assessment or treatment actions are required on virtually every cardiopulmonary emergency. These should become ingrained in every ACLS provider as early actions to take for every patient. We think making these actions a core part of the Five Quadrads will help ACLS providers become systematic and will help them avoid unfortunate delays or omissions of these actions.

4. TEMPERATURE/BLOOD PRESSURE/ HEART RATE/RESPIRATIONS

The vital signs are probably one of the most neglected areas in ACLS training. Nevertheless, the vital signs provide critical information that ACLS providers need to manage patients with cardiopulmonary emergencies.

5. TANK (VOLUME)/RESISTANCE/PUMP/RATE

These terms introduce the concept of the "cardiovascular quadrad," the fifth of the Five Quadrads. The cardiovascular quadrad provides a useful analytic tool to approach problems of shock, hypotension, and acute pulmonary edema. This quadrad directs ACLS providers to consider whether patients with abnormal blood pressure, perfusion, and possible pulmonary edema have a clinical problem dominated by the following:

- Inadequate or excessive vascular volume
- Profoundly increased or decreased peripheral vascular resistance
- Problems with cardiac performance as a pump
- Inadequate perfusion due to heart rates that are too fast or too slow

KEY PRINCIPLES TO UNDERSTAND WHEN APPLYING THE PRIMARY AND SECONDARY SURVEYS

- The survey sequence looks for problems in their order of importance. Fortunately, the alphabet supplies a helpful memory aid.

- If at any point you identify a problem, you go no further with the survey but treat that identified problem. For example, the inability to move air through an endotracheal tube (B of the Secondary Survey) must be solved before starting an IV and administering medications.

- Follow the survey sequence as far as personnel and equipment allow. For example, a single rescuer would be limited to basic CPR and, if available, automated defibrillation until other help arrived.

- When other help does arrive, the survey sequence tells them exactly where to insert themselves. For example, additional personnel would take on responsibility for defibrillation, endotracheal intubation, IV access, medications—and in that order.

- Of course, if personnel are available, they can proceed with the survey parts simultaneously, but the surveys supply useful reviews to make sure that someone has responsibility for all tasks.

- Finally, the Secondary Survey ends with a reminder to stop and think. The D (for differential diagnoses) directs the rescuers, especially the team leader, to think about why the arrest occurred in the first place and why the person remains in arrest or remains in an unstable condition.

MAJOR CONCEPTS TO MASTER

- *The Five Quadrads approach (including the Primary-Secondary Surveys) to Emergency Cardiac Care.* This will be the conceptual tool used to approach all cardiopulmonary emergencies, both full cardiac arrest and peri-cardiac arrest.

- *Calling 911 or other EMS number.* An essential step, no resuscitation will succeed unless someone recognizes an emergency early and calls for help.

- *Chain of Survival concept.* Emergency cardiac care, in both prehospital and in-hospital settings, will fail unless a series of actions and interventions falls into place—early access, early CPR, early defibrillation, and early advanced life support.

- *Community-based early defibrillation with automated external defibrillators.* This is the most important link in the out-of-hospital Chain of Survival, because most patients who can be resuscitated are those in ventricular fibrillation who are defibrillated early.

- *Post-resuscitation support.* Once resuscitation efforts succeed in returning a pulse, the patient must continue to receive constant vigilance and care, again following the Five Quadrads approach.

- *The Universal Algorithm.* The Universal Algorithm of the AHA incorporates the major elements of the Five Quadrads and is another way of conceptualizing the same important principles.

- *Resuscitation-stopping criteria.* There comes a moment in every resuscitation attempt beyond which successful resuscitation, with meaningful survival, becomes impossible. While no stopping criteria apply to every patient, all ACLS providers must learn to consider when resuscitation attempts should be terminated.

- *Telling the living: conveying news of a death to survivors.* At the moment when a resuscitation attempt ends with pronouncement of death, the resuscitation team acquires another set of patients—the family, friends, and loved ones who must go on living.

- *Recommendations for critical incident debriefing.* Every resuscitation attempt represents a critical incident for the personnel who participated. Critical incident debriefing provides a moment to review what went right and what went wrong and to consider how the staff reacted emotionally to the events and the outcome.

- *How to assume command of a resuscitation scene.* Many resuscitation attempts proceed clumsily and in a disorganized manner because no one asserts himself or herself and assumes a leadership role.

- *Code organization: assigning tasks, assigning priorities.* Many resuscitation attempts start in a tiered fashion with different numbers of personnel and with personnel who possess different skill levels. The code leader must become skillful at identifying the resources available and the tasks that need to be accomplished and matching the two effectively.

- *Phased-response format for resuscitations.* This provides a helpful model for achieving effective code organization.

- *Using the Primary-Secondary Survey Approach to "troubleshoot" difficult codes.* The Primary-Secondary Survey Approach can also be applied in a systematic manner to those resuscitation attempts that are not going well and those in which the patient is not responding, or when the patient's condition remains unstable.

- *Assessment-based versus diagnosis-based emergency care.* This concept represents a subtle, but critical distinction that is gaining wider acceptance in emergency care—do not base all of your therapeutic approach in some suspected diagnosis, but rather proceed based on the clinical assessment of the patient.

- *Ethical issues of starting (or not starting) and stopping CPR attempts.* ACLS concentrates on learning to perform effective resuscitation of patients who have lost their cardiac output and stopped breathing. Often, however, these events represent the natural end of someone's life, and resuscitation efforts are inappropriate. These issues need to receive greater attention from ACLS providers.

- *Criteria for organ and tissue donation.* Emergency care providers need to become more aware of the critical national shortage of donated tissues and solid organs.

Antonio Loera

CASE 1

You are a fairly well-behaved spectator at your daughter's soccer game. With great agitation a young woman runs shouting up to the spectators standing on the sidelines. "Somebody please help! A man just collapsed over here on the jogging trail!" You run over to the man, where several other spectators are standing around. You gently shake the man and realize that he is not responding. What is the first thing you would do?

COMMENTS

- According to the AHA, the first action here should be to call for help. In a crowded, public cardiac arrest someone should think to call 911. Cellular phones might be readily available. To make sure, however, identify someone directly, look them in the eyes and tell them "Go call 911. Tell the operator that a man has collapsed at the Montlake Play Field on the jogging track. Tell them that we may have to start CPR."

- Note that this "Call First" recommendation of the AHA means you must call before starting CPR and even before verifying that the victim has lost his or her pulse. The 911 call activates the EMS system; in particular, the call gets a defibrillator on the way to those victims who may be in ventricular fibrillation.

- Everyone should know how to report an emergency. The key element is to know the address of the emergency and the nature of the problem. Identify yourself and make sure the *address* is understood. Offer to stay on the phone if the dispatcher is unclear of the address.

- In most communities the 911 dispatchers are trained to offer "prearrival" emergency instructions, including advice on how to do CPR. Using *priority dispatching*, the 911 dispatcher will automatically dispatch an emergency vehicle as soon as you state that the problem involves a collapsed, unconscious, and unresponsive person. With *enhanced 911 systems* the dispatcher will automatically see the address of the telephone you are calling from displayed on the dispatcher terminal.

- Trained dispatchers most often will ask the following questions:
  - What is your address and phone number?
  - What's the problem?
  - Is the person conscious?
  - Is the person breathing normally?
  - Do you want to do CPR? I can help you.

Antonio Loera

CASE 1 Continued

You remember your training in basic life support. From a small packet attached to your key ring you remove a plastic CPR barrier device handed out at a recent EMS Conference. You kneel down beside the man, place the barrier device on his mouth, and follow the steps for basic CPR:

- *A—Open the airway by lifting the chin up and tilting the head back.*
- *B—Check for breathing by looking, listening, and feeling; there are no breaths.*
- *B—Provide two breaths through mouth-to-barrier ventilations; the air moves easily in and the chest rises gently.*
- *C—Check for a pulse at the carotid artery on the side of the neck; there is no pulse.*

At this point you know you have a full cardiac arrest, since the man is unconscious, without breathing, and without a pulse. You need to start CPR. "This man is in full cardiac arrest! I'm starting CPR. Did anyone call 911?"

What would you do now? What is the next step?

COMMENTS

- You started your emergency care by following the first of the Five Quadrads, the Primary Survey: ABCD. The Primary Survey led you to initiate CPR. The call to 911 gets D—the defibrillator—on the way to the cardiac arrest.

- At this point you are taking all actions available to you in this setting. Until the emergency response team arrives you have few options other than to continue CPR.

- You could get someone else to help with CPR by taking over chest compressions. Often bystanders will

hesitate to become the person who does ventilations. Surveys have observed that chest compressions are performed more often in citizen CPR events than are mouth-to-mouth ventilations. Basic CPR classes in most communities now teach the use of barrier devices to help overcome this reluctance to perform CPR. While there are no data to confirm actual disease transmission of hepatitis or human immunodeficiency virus (HIV) during CPR, several studies have confirmed that fear of disease is common among people trained in CPR.

Antonio Loera

CASE 1 Continued

Two minutes later the person you instructed to call 911 returns saying "The AID car ambulance staffed with EMTs is on its way!" You are already tiring with the CPR efforts. Two people have taken over chest compressions, but you must continue to perform ventilations. At first the man took several agonal, gasping respirations and you thought briefly that you might get this man back with just CPR alone. However, as the minutes go by, the agonal respirations disappear and the man appears progressively more cyanotic.

You hear the sound of the fire truck siren, and soon three uniformed firefighters rush up to the patient. One firefighter carries an automated external defibrillator (AED). She places the AED next to the patient's left ear, turns on the device, and begins to open the adhesive defibrillator pads. One firefighter takes over chest compressions. The other places an oropharyngeal airway in the victim's mouth, attaches an oxygen tank to a bag valve mask, and takes over ventilations.

The woman who is the lead firefighter has attached the AED and directs everyone to stand back. She delivers two shocks, each one making the man jerk suddenly. After the second shock she presses the button labeled "analyze" and the voice prompt on the device responds, "No shock indicated. Check patient." She quickly puts her fingers on the man's neck and after 5 seconds states, "No pulse. Resume CPR."

They perform CPR for 60 seconds, and then the defibrillator-firefighter checks the pulse again.

Antonio Loera

CASE 1 Continued

"Hey, I think I feel a pulse. Let's check a blood pressure." In the background you can hear the siren of the ambulance carrying the paramedic crew. The blood pressure is "90 over 60" mm Hg, and the man is beginning to make spontaneous, gasping respirations.

What is special about this community? Why did the defibrillation work and save this man when he seemed to be getting steadily worse during your CPR?

COMMENTS

THE COMMUNITY'S CHAIN OF SURVIVAL.

This community displayed strength in all four links of the Chain of Survival, as follows:

• **Early access:** The arrest was witnessed, allowing someone to call 911 quickly and get the EMS system started rolling toward the patient.

• **Early CPR:** The bystanders knew CPR and initiated ventilations and chest compressions without hesitation. This man received basic CPR, which slowed his process of dying. All cardiac arrests possess a very narrow window of opportunity, and the window closes rapidly with each passing minute. Early CPR slows the rate at which this window closes, preserving and prolonging VF and making VF more likely to be present when the defibrillator arrives.

• **Early defibrillation:** This community has implemented an early defibrillation program. In such programs the first responding EMS personnel (in this city that would be firefighters) are trained and equipped to perform early defibrillation using automated external defibrillators.

• **Early ACLS:** The paramedic teams displayed a rapid response time. They arrive with the ability to stabilize the patient with endotracheal intubation (if needed) and intravenous medications.

Fritz Langendorf

CASE 2

You are a firefighter on duty at Station 10. Fritz Langendorf, a 65-year-old retired real estate agent, comes in for a blood pressure check because of dizzy spells and chest tightness. While you are taking his blood pressure he breaks out in a heavy sweat, becomes agitated, complains of severe chest pain, and suddenly falls back in the chair.

What would you do? How would you approach this man?

COMMENTS

• First, you would apply the Primary ABCD Survey, as follows:

• The man is unresponsive and unconscious, so shout out a local call for help in the fire station.

  • **A**—Open the airway with the head tilt–chin lift method: no respirations observed.

  • **B**—Look, listen, and feel for breathing: no respirations observed; give two breaths and check that they enter the man's lungs easily and that the chest wall rises.

  • **C**—Check the pulse: there is no pulse. Faced now with a full cardiac arrest, you would need to confirm that 911 had been called. and that an advanced life support unit was on the way; then begin compressions.

  • **D**—Hunt for VF with the defibrillator: to fulfill this step you would need to retrieve the AED that is stored on the fire engine. Apply this device, and use it to assess for VF rhythm and deliver shocks. (The use of AEDs is presented in Chapter 3.)

• Second, you are not able to proceed further with the Secondary Survey because in this state a basic EMT is not authorized to perform the advanced interventions of endotracheal intubation, IV access, and intravenous medications.

Fritz Langendorf

CASE 2 Continued

Your partner on duty with you today responded to your initial call for help. He called 911 to start an ACLS response. He also retrieved the AED from its rack in the engine bay, plus an oxygen tank and ventilation equipment. He takes over CPR efforts while you attach the AED.

Following the AED protocols, you deliver three shocks to this man. After a brief period of post-shock CPR the man begins to move without purpose and to mumble incoherently. His heart rate is 85 beats per minute and his blood pressure is 110/78 mm Hg.

What would you do? How would you approach this man?

POST-RESUSCITATION SUPPORT

- Since this patient has been converted out of VF to a spontaneous pulse and blood pressure, you need to provide basic post-resuscitation support.

- The Primary Survey provides us with a useful memory aid for the actions to take in the post-resuscitation period, as follows:

  - *Airway:* Pay close attention to maintaining an open airway. Mr. Langendorf will be slowly recovering from his period of unconsciousness, and airway compromise is still possible. In addition, he may easily revert to the rhythm (presumably VF) that caused his original arrest.

- *Breathing:* Attach the oxygen tank to the inlet port on the bag-valve-mask assembly. Insert an oral pharyngeal airway (if he will tolerate it), and deliver oxygen initially at 15 L/min. As an alternative, you can supply oxygen through the inlet port on pocket face masks.

- *Circulation:* Continue to check the pulse and blood pressure regularly (every 30 to 60 seconds in the post-resuscitation period).

- *Defibrillation:* Leave the AED adhesive pads attached. He may refibrillate. In addition, many models of AEDs have a rhythm display screen, which will be valuable to the advanced life support (ALS) unit when it arrives.

Fritz Langendorf

CASE 2 Continued

Mr. Langendorf continues to recover following the shocks from the AED. He continues to make garbled sounds, pushing you away with his hands in a somewhat purposeful manner. He tries to sit up. You pay careful attention to holding the oxygen mask on his face and speak reassuringly toward him even though he does not appear to hear what you are saying. In the distance you hear the siren of the ALS unit. In 2 minutes the paramedics rush into the station. "This man just walked in here for a blood pressure check and suddenly collapsed. We started CPR, attached the AED, and delivered three shocks. He seems to have recovered: BP=110/80; pulse=90. I think the screen shows an organized rhythm."

You have successfully resuscitated this man by following the Primary Survey through assessment, CPR, and early defibrillation. The American Heart Association has a Universal Algorithm for cardiopulmonary emergencies. Why did you not follow the AHA Universal Algorithm guidelines instead of this Primary-Secondary Survey Approach?

THE UNIVERSAL ALGORITHM

- The Primary Survey is consistent with the AHA Universal Algorithm. In fact, the 1994 ACLS textbook discusses both techniques and prefers the Primary-Secondary Survey Approach as the more comprehensive method to follow in emergency cardiac care:

  The Primary ABCD Survey and the Secondary ABCD Survey described in the first part of this chapter incorporate all the steps and actions of the Universal Algorithm. Some people may find it easier to remember the steps of the Universal Algorithm; some may prefer the steps of the Primary or Secondary ABCD Surveys. Whatever works best for each learner is acceptable (AHA, Textbook of ACLS, Dallas, 1994, pp. 1-11).

- Fig. 1-3 presents the Universal Algorithm for adult emergency cardiac care.

- Notice how this algorithm is useful as a teaching aid for it directs the rescuer through the major steps of the Primary and Secondary Surveys as follows:

- Assess responsiveness
  - If not responsive:
    - Activate EMS
    - Call for defibrillator
- Assess breathing *(A of Primary Survey)*
  - If not breathing:
    - Give two slow breaths *(B of Primary Survey)*
- Assess circulation *(C of Primary Survey)*
  - If no pulse, start CPR *(C of Primary Survey)*
  - If VF/VT present on defibrillator/monitor, attach defibrillator and deliver shocks *(D of Primary Survey)*
  - If VF/VT not present on the defibrillator, go to the Secondary Survey:
- Intubate *(A of Secondary Survey)*
- Confirm tube placement *(B of Secondary Survey)*
- Confirm ventilations *(B of Secondary Survey)*
- Determine rhythm and cause *(C and D of Secondary Survey)*

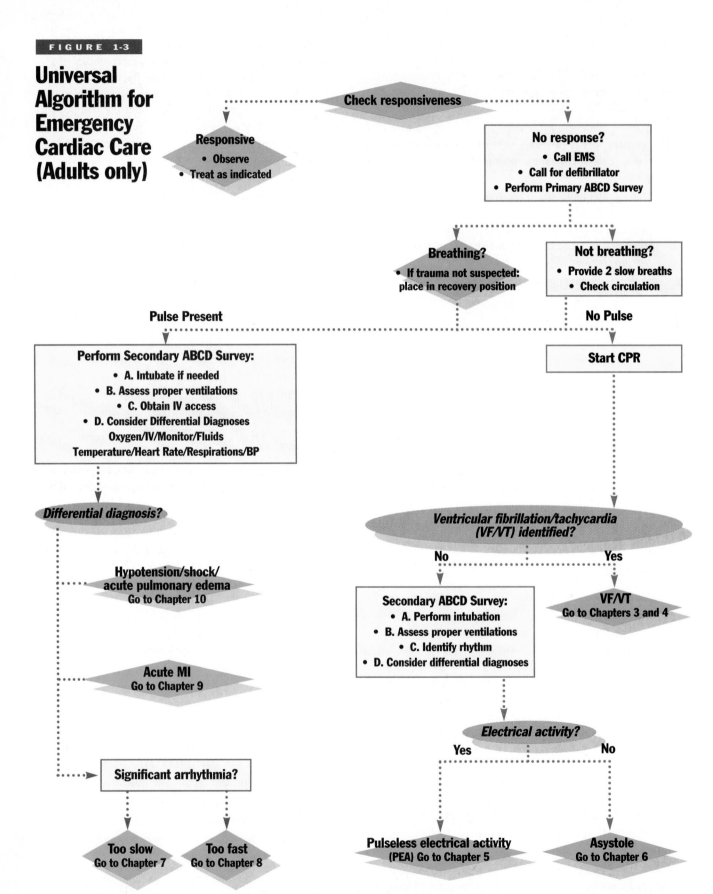

FIGURE 1-3

Universal Algorithm for Emergency Cardiac Care (Adults only)

Check responsiveness

Responsive
- Observe
- Treat as indicated

No response?
- Call EMS
- Call for defibrillator
- Perform Primary ABCD Survey

Breathing?
- If trauma not suspected: place in recovery position

Not breathing?
- Provide 2 slow breaths
- Check circulation

Pulse Present

No Pulse

Perform Secondary ABCD Survey:
- A. Intubate if needed
- B. Assess proper ventilations
- C. Obtain IV access
- D. Consider Differential Diagnoses
  Oxygen/IV/Monitor/Fluids
  Temperature/Heart Rate/Respirations/BP

Start CPR

Differential diagnosis?

Ventricular fibrillation/tachycardia (VF/VT) identified?

No   Yes

Hypotension/shock/ acute pulmonary edema
Go to Chapter 10

Secondary ABCD Survey:
- A. Perform intubation
- B. Assess proper ventilations
- C. Identify rhythm
- D. Consider differential diagnoses

VF/VT
Go to Chapters 3 and 4

Acute MI
Go to Chapter 9

Electrical activity?

Yes   No

Significant arrhythmia?

Too slow
Go to Chapter 7

Too fast
Go to Chapter 8

Pulseless electrical activity
(PEA) Go to Chapter 5

Asystole
Go to Chapter 6

Adapted with permission, Journal of the American Medical Association, 1992, Volume 268, *Guidlines for Cardiopulmonary Resuscitation and Emergency Cardiac Care*, page 2216, copyright © 1992, American Medical Association.

- There is not complete overlap between the Universal Algorithm and the Primary and Secondary Surveys. This is because the Universal Algorithm branches into several subalgorithms (too slow, too fast, PEA, asystole, acute myocardial infarction, and hypotension/shock/acute pulmonary edema).

- You will learn, however, that each of these other algorithms incorporates the Primary and Secondary Surveys.

For cardiac arrest, we recommend use of the Primary and Secondary Surveys of the Five Quadrads as the major conceptual approach to cardiopulmonary emergencies. This powerful tool is easy to remember. When you combine the Primary and Secondary Surveys approach with the Five Quadrads, you will have an extremely robust approach to deal with almost all cardiopulmonary emergencies. Using this tool will be a major theme throughout this book.

Sophie Leibowitz

CASE 3

You are the head nurse for the night shift at a senior citizens' home. While making your rounds you hear the noise of a person falling in the TV room. You enter the room to find one of the women residents sprawled on the floor. You have just completed a course on the use of an automated external defibrillator (AED), one of which has been purchased recently by the home. What should you do? Start CPR? Go get the AED? Call for help? Call 911?

COMMENTS

The scenario in Case 3 presents "the lone rescuer" who knows CPR and who knows how to operate an AED. The rescuer does not have immediate help, and the AED is located a short distance away. There is no ideal answer to this scenario, since Mrs. Leibowitz needs multiple things done simultaneously and you are by yourself. The AHA recommends the following actions:

- Verify unconsciousness.

- Call for help. In this scenario you should shout loudly down the hall, since you know someone will most likely hear you and come to help.

- Initiate the Primary Survey up to the point of starting chest compressions, as follows:

  - *Airway:* Open the airway with head tilt and chin lift. (Some people would argue that cervical spine trauma is possible here, given that the woman was heard to fall. With a high suspicion of cervical trauma use the jaw-thrust technique to open the airway.)

  - *Breathing:* Check for breathing. Respirations are absent. You therefore provide two ventilations through the mouth with a pocket face mask. As a health care worker you always carry a pocket face mask with you when you are on duty so that you do not need to perform mouth-to-mouth ventilations. Your hospital makes a pocket face mask available in each room.

  - *Circulation:* Check for a carotid pulse. Since there is no pulse, you move immediately to retrieve the AED.

  - *Defibrillation:* Go and get the AED once you have confirmed (1) absence of an obstructed airway (with the two breaths) and (2) full cardiac arrest. NOTE: the AHA Guidelines do *not* recommend a period of chest compressions before retrieving the defibrillator. Many experts think that 1 minute or more of CPR would be useful before departing to get the AED. This is a tough call. The AHA rationale is that the person in VF will continue to deteriorate during the 1 minute or more of CPR and would be better off foregoing the CPR and receiving defibrillation as soon as possible.

- This particular scenario, of a lone rescuer with access to an AED, is becoming common. Early defibrillation programs, driven by the new technology of AEDs, are developing everywhere and are being implemented in many settings. Nursing or chronic care facilities are starting AED programs for the staff within their facilities. Many acute care hospitals have also developed in-hospital AED response teams, mainly to reduce the time intervals between the patient's collapse and the time of first defibrillation.

- The well-trained, competent ACLS provider must know and understand this new technology of automated defibrillation to be an effective member of the ACLS team.

Sophie Leibowitz

CASE 3 Continued

You bend over Mrs. Leibowitz and speak her name loudly, touching her shoulder. She does not respond and is clearly unconscious. You yell down the hall for help as you turn back to perform the Primary Survey. You deliver two ventilations through your pocket face mask. The ventilations enter the lungs easily and cause the chest to rise. After a rapid carotid pulse check you turn to retrieve the defibrillator located at the nurses' station.

You encounter one of your co-workers and tell her to call 911. It appears Mrs. Leibowitz has had a sudden collapse and possible cardiac arrest. You locate the AED and return with it to Mrs. Leibowitz's side. You follow the correct procedures, checking the pulse and respirations. After attaching the AED and delivering two shocks, the device's voice synthesizer states, "No shock indicated." You check for a pulse and fail to locate one. You perform several more cycles of CPR–pulse check–AED analyze mode. The device never delivers a subsequent shock.

The medics arrive and take over CPR. They initiate the Secondary Survey with intubation, IV access, medications, and further rhythm monitoring. They comment that Mrs. Leibowitz was in asystole when they arrived and that 10 minutes after intubation they were going to radio for permission to stop the resuscitation efforts.

Why did the AED fail to save Mrs. Leibowitz? Why did the medics stop resuscitation efforts so soon and not transport Mrs. Leibowitz to the Emergency Department?

COMMENTS

- We know that most resuscitation attempts do not succeed. The best prehospital resuscitation rates, even for witnessed ventricular fibrillation, are no better than one of four persons surviving to hospital discharge.

- Here at an extended care facility, you are faced with older patients and with a high frequency of associated chronic illnesses. The elderly, unless "do not attempt resuscitation" (DNAR) orders exist, deserve every effort at resuscitation and, once resuscitated, do as well as younger patients.

- The medics stopped the resuscitation attempt in the field rather than transporting the patient back to the Emergency Department. This was because we now accept that the Emergency Department offers virtually no advantage over skilled paramedics in the field. There are very few effective interventions available in Emergency Departments that the medics cannot initiate in the field. (Exceptions do exist, for example, in hypothermic arrests and arrests due to trauma, drug overdoses, and electrolyte abnormalities. In such cases Emergency

Department physicians can provide therapy not available in the prehospital setting. These will be discussed in later chapters.)

- The question of how soon to stop the resuscitation efforts is a complex one and will be covered in Chapter 6. No valid "stopping rules" exist for all situations. Here the medics reached a point at which the AHA recommends that serious thought be given to stopping the efforts, as follows:

  - Successful intubation achieved

  - IV access achieved

  - Rhythm-appropriate medications administered

  - Documented asystole (no cardiac electrical activity) for 10 minutes *after* above interventions

- Note that no EMS system authorizes medics to make such decisions independent of a physician. Medics always call their medical control physician at their base hospital. From a medicolegal perspective it is the medical control physician who makes the decision to stop the efforts.

Sophie Leibowitz

CASE 3 Continued

Later that night Mrs. Leibowitz's attending physician comes in to the nursing home. The family is contacted about Mrs. Leibowitz's death, and her daughter requests permission to come view her mother one last time. You begin to anticipate what to say when the daughter arrives. The funeral home representatives are scheduled to pick up the body in 1 hour.

The attending physician asks you to describe the attempt to revive Mrs. Leibowitz. As you begin to tell him about putting the defibrillator on and the jerks from the defibrillation shocks, you start to cry. You are still bothered by why the AED did not work. In addition you were puzzled by what appeared to be the hurried manner in which the medics packed up their equipment and left after they stopped their efforts. They received another call toward the end of the resuscitation, and as they started to leave you asked them, "Are you just going to leave her body here on the floor?" Though they seemed genuinely sympathetic and concerned, their reply, that local laws prevent them from moving a person who has died outside the hospital, upset you even more.

What are some recommended techniques for "telling the living," and conveying the news of a death to family members? What is "critical incident debriefing," and what are the basic elements? Do you think such a debriefing is needed here?

COMMENTS

• All ACLS providers must learn to deal with many unsuccessful resuscitations. The reality speaks for itself—sudden cardiac death often represents the end of someone's life, and resuscitation may be impossible and even inappropriate. Most resuscitations will end with a dead person, not a living, thinking survivor.

• Therefore you must learn how to convey the bad news of death to the survivors—to the friends, family members, and loved ones of the person you have just worked so hard to save.

• In the long run, this is perhaps one of the most important skills an ACLS provider can learn. In all candor, this is the skill that will be used most frequently.

• The 1992 AHA, ECC and CPR Guidelines and the 1994 *Textbook of ACLS* provided recommendations for conveying news of a sudden death to family members. A revised list of these suggestions appears in Table 1-1.

• This situation, described in the case of Sophie Leibowitz, provides an excellent example of when a *critical incident debriefing session* will be helpful.

• The nurse who attempted defibrillation is emotionally upset and concerned about the events she witnessed. She has a growing sense that she may have failed or may be at fault for the failure to resuscitate Mrs. Leibowitz.

• Critical incident debriefings can be conducted formally or informally. "Routine" resuscitations by experienced personnel do not require the formal, Critical Incident Stress Debriefing (CISD). However, even the most experienced emergency care providers can benefit from a brief conversation asking how things went, and whether they could have gone better or at least differently and asking how they feel about the "code."

• Table 1-3 provides recommendations for a modified critical incident debriefing.

TABLE 1-1

Suggestions for Conveying News of a Death to Concerned Survivors

- *It is critical to remember that the moment you stop resuscitation efforts on one patient, you immediately acquire new patients—the family and friends who now must go on living without their loved one.*

- *Call the family if they have not been notified. Explain that their loved one has been admitted to the Emergency Department, hospital, or critical care unit and that the situation is serious. In general, survivors should not be told of the death over the telephone; however, many circumstances, such as great travel distance, will affect the decision to inform the survivors.*

- *Ask if there is someone else who can be with them, or help drive them to the hospital. Encourage them not to rush in an unsafe manner to the hospital.*

- *Learn as much information as possible about the patient and the circumstances surrounding the death. Carefully go over the events as they happened in the Emergency Department to make sure you can explain the events to the family and friends.*

- *Ask someone to take family members to a private area. Walk in, introduce yourself, and sit down. Address the closest relative.*

- *Briefly describe the circumstances leading to the death. Go over the sequence of events in the Emergency Department. Avoid euphemisms such as "he's passed on," "she is no longer with us," or "he's left us." Instead use the words "death," "dying," and "dead."*

- *Allow time for the shock to be absorbed. Make eye contact, touch, and share. Convey your feelings with a phrase such as "You have my (our) sincere sympathy" rather that "I (we) am sorry." "Sorry" sounds like an apology for how the code went rather than an expression of sympathy for the family.*

- *Allow as much time as necessary for questions and discussion. Go over the events several times to make sure everything is understood and to facilitate further questions.*

- *Allow the family the opportunity to see their relative. If equipment items are still connected, prepare the family for what they will see.*

- *Know in advance what happens next with regard to the body and who will sign the death certificate. Physicians may impose burdens on staff and family if they fail to understand policies about death certification and disposition of the body. One of the survivors will surely ask, "What do we do next?" Be prepared with a proper answer.*

- *Remember to consider tissue donation from people who have died. State and federal laws require hospital personnel to offer the option of donation to the next of kin when a death occurs. Consult your hospital's transplant services for their advice. For patients who may be resuscitated but experience brain death consider solid organ donation (also called "beating heart" or "vascular organ" donation). (See Table 1-2 for points to consider in organ and tissue donation.)*

- *Remember to consider the need for an autopsy. There are legal criteria for autopsies on people who die in Emergency Departments or for people brought in with continuing CPR who are not resuscitated. Consult the medical center's autopsy service or medical examiner's office for further information.*

- *Enlist the aid of a social worker or the clergy if a representative is not already present.*

- *Offer to contact the patient's attending or family physician and be available if there are further questions. Arrange for follow-up and continued support during the grieving period.*

TABLE 1-2

Tissue and Solid Organ Donation: Points To Consider

Emergency cardiac care providers need to become well informed about organ and tissue donation. Organ and tissue transplantation has begun a medical revolution that saves lives and improves the quality of life for millions.

Requests for tissue and organ donation should be separated in time from discussions that inform the survivors of the death or the determination of brain death. This "uncouples" the request for tissue and organ donation from the pronouncement that death has occurred or that the patient has been declared brain dead. Families should not link the request for organ/tissue donation with care withdrawal.

TISSUE DONATION

- *Tissue donations come from patients who have recently died (within 24 hours of death). Consider tissue donation when cardiopulmonary function ceases or resuscitation efforts have failed.*

- *Tissue transplants make possible skin grafts, corneal transplants, heart valve replacements, and bone, cartilage, and tendon reconstructions.*

- *There are relatively few exclusion criteria for tissue donation. These include IV drug abuse, acquired immunodeficiency syndrome (AIDS), or hepatitis or high-risk factors for these; viral meningitis; systemic infection; transmissible disease; malignancy; and other medical conditions.*

- *Time limits are, maximum, 24 hours but preferably less than 6 hours, since death. Ideally the donor should be refrigerated soon after death.*

- *Consult the local tissue donation center regarding specific patients. Most tissue donation centers have 24-hour answering services to answer any questions.*

SOLID ORGAN DONATION ("BEATING HEART" OR "VASCULAR ORGAN" DONATION)

- *Solid organ donation requires that the donor have a beating heart and be declared brain dead. The donor will be maintained on a ventilator.*

- *All ACLS providers should be aware of the criteria for solid organ donation.*

  - *They will often be able to identify potential donors following certain clinical resuscitations (for example, resuscitation from traumatic cardiac arrest following massive head injuries).*

  - *ACLS providers will also often care for possibly*

brain dead patients who are nearing the need for cardiac resuscitation. Maintenance of adequate organ perfusion and initiation of organ procurement procedures will frequently become the responsibility of ACLS providers.

- *There are few donor contraindications to solid organ donation. Always consult the local federally funded organ procurement agency before any potential organ donor is rejected. If in doubt, call! Common relative contraindications are the following:*

  - *Untreated sepsis or transmissible disease*

  - *Inadequate resuscitation with prolonged organ ischemia*

  - *Significant organ dysfunction*

  - *Most malignancies*

  - *Evidence of IV drug abuse*

- *Solid/vascular organ donation may take 6 to 12 hours from brain death pronouncement to organ recovery. Therefore, maintenance of adequate ventilation and perfusion becomes critical.*

  - *However, high doses of vasoactive agents (for example, dopamine, epinephrine, or norepinephrine) may compromise cardiac, renal, and hepatic function and should be weaned if possible. Inability to taper these agents raises the question of the adequacy of cardiac function.*

  - *Recently, thyroid hormone has been used to help restore or maintain blood pressure and organ perfusion in organ donors and may enable a reduction in vasoactive therapy (levothyroxine dose: 200 ug in 500 ml normal saline; give 100 ml for 1 hour, then 50 ml per hour as needed).*

  - *The psychology and vocabulary surrounding brain death are important to remember:*

  - *A patient is considered "dead" from the moment he or she is pronounced "brain dead." From that moment refer to the patient as the "donor," not the patient. This will help the family and staff accept the death of the patient, even though support of ventilation and perfusion (do not use the term "life support") will continue for several more hours.*

  - *Most hospitals will consider the patient "discharged" from the moment he or she is pronounced dead; the patient is then readmitted as "a donor." This ensures that charges associated with vital organ maintenance are transferred from the donor's family to the organ procurement agency.*

- *Solid organ donation should not delay normal funeral arrangements. Although incisions are made in the body, they are not visible, even during an open-casket funeral.*

TABLE 1-3

Recommendations for Critical Incident Debriefing

- *The debriefing should occur as soon as possible after the event, with all team members present.*

- *Call the group together, preferably in the room where the resuscitation attempt occurred. In the prehospital setting the group can come together when they return to quarters.*

- *State that you want to have a "code debriefing" to review how things went.*

- *Review the events and conduct of the code. With certain personnel, review the contributory pathophysiology leading to the code, the decision tree followed, and why there were any variations.*

- *Make sure everyone understands that once you understand the rules and recommendations in ACLS, it is acceptable to break those rules as long as there is a good reason.*

- *Ask if any of the personnel thought errors were made or skills performed incorrectly. Discuss the topics that come up as having been wrong. Discuss especially the things that were done right. Allow free discussion.*

- *Ask for recommendations/suggestions for future resuscitative attempts.*

- *Ask the team members (all of them, even the new clinical assistant who just stood in the corner and watched) to share their feelings, anxieties, anger, and possible guilt.*

- *Team members unable to attend the debriefing should be informed of the process followed, the discussion generated, and the recommendations made.*

- *The team leader should encourage team members to contact him or her if questions arise later.*

Modified with permission from © *Textbook of Advanced Cardiac Life Support*, 1994, pp. 1-71. Copyright American Heart Association.

Lisa Slater

CASE 4

You are the on-call senior medical resident in a large academic medical center when you hear the overhead page announce a "code" four floors down in the radiology department. Upon your arrival 3 minutes later you find Lisa Slater, a 50-year-old woman, lying on the floor. She had open heart surgery 3 days previously and is in the radiology department for a chest computed tomography scan. Her cardiovascular surgeon, the medicine chief resident, and the surgery chief resident, as well as the radiologist and the Emergency Department attending physician have all arrived to "help out" in the code. A burly x-ray technician is doing chest compressions. The woman appears to be intubated. A code cart has been pushed into the room, and a man stands by it with unconnected monitor cables in his hand. Mrs. Slater is surrounded by at least 20 people. Everyone is yelling out one command or another, and no one seems to be in charge.

As you catch your breath, you realize that someone has to try and make sense out of this mess. Suddenly, one of the nurses calls out in a firm voice, "OK, you guys, someone needs to take charge of this code." That "someone" is you, since the on-call senior medical resident is supposed to run all the codes. How do you assume leadership and control of the scene?

COMMENTS

- First of all, this scene never should happen. In hospitals that institute a hospital-wide code response, issues of leadership always should be settled in advance.

- Unfortunately, reality seldom cooperates with our plans, and in this scenario all the ingredients for confusion are present. Multiple people have arrived on-scene perceiving that they have some responsibility for the patient (her surgery attending physician, the radiologist in the area where the arrest occurred, the code anesthesiologist, and the emergency attending physician, who always responds to codes in care areas not designated for patient care).

- Again, the Primary-Secondary Survey Approach serves as an excellent way of getting control of the situation and assessing where things stand and what needs to be done. You can use the Primary-Secondary Survey Approach in multiple situations such as the following:

  - When you arrive very early on the scene of an emergency and all equipment and personnel are available

  - When you arrive early on the scene and the additional personnel are arriving "in response layers"

  - When you arrive late and things have already started, as in the scenario in Case 4.

- The first action to take is to establish control of the scene. Prehospital care personnel, whose daily work requires that they arrive late at confused scenes, are taught to use "the voice."

- "The voice" is simply speaking in a firm, confident voice, making a forceful statement: that you are now in charge, that everyone else should speak only if absolutely necessary, and that you will be giving directions for what happens next. Announce that you are going to review the ABCs.

Lisa Slater	
CASE 4 Continued	

You stand quietly at the foot of the patient and announce, "I am Doctor Mosby and I am the physician in charge of directing codes in this area. Would everyone please be quiet and listen to my directions? If you have nothing immediate to do for this patient, please leave at once. We need more room, and we need to hear the orders."

"First, I'm going to do a Primary Survey and review the ABCs. Who is in charge of the airway? How are you ventilating this patient? Is she breathing at all? Is she being ventilated well?" (You learn the patient has been intubated by the anesthesiologist, that there are no spontaneous respirations, and that bag-valve-mask ventilation produces good, bilateral breath sounds.) "Stop CPR and check for a pulse." (There is no pulse.) "Okay, start CPR."

"What about the CPR? Are the chest compressions producing a pulse?" (Someone responds that a carotid pulse is palpable with CPR.)

"What about defibrillation? Has anyone done a 'quick-look' to see if she is in VF?" (You learn that the radiology code cart carries an old-model defibrillator without a quick-look feature and that no one has been able to get to the patient to attach the monitor cables to the patient's chest. In addition, you can see that people are trying to start an IV in each antecubitial space and that they have not yet succeeded.)

Now that the room is more quiet and people are listening to you, how would you proceed?

COMMENTS

- You can see that the ABCD approach of the Primary and Secondary Surveys allows the ACLS team leader to review a great deal more quickly and effectively and gives a greater sense of order to the scene.

- For the Primary Survey, A, B, and C have been accomplished. D, however, has been omitted because the initial responders could not assess the rhythm with quick-look paddles. In addition, they did not move quickly to attach the monitor leads to the patient because of the tumult caused by chest compressions, the intubation, and the attempts to start the IVs.

- One principle for using the Primary Survey Approach tells you to immediately address any identified problem at the moment you recognize it. In the scenario in Case 4 you must now place the highest priority on determining whether the patient is in VF/VT.

- Note that two major problems have been encountered here already: first, the obsolete defibrillator on the code cart and second, people not sure how to operate their code defibrillator. These are major sources of errors and delays in codes. Surveys have demonstrated that many locations maintain defibrillators on code carts far beyond their expected life. While budget restraints are a reality, everyone should recognize the false economy of out-of-date equipment that does not work.

- Of the Secondary Survey, A and B have been accomplished effectively but C is incomplete, since no one has yet obtained IV access and because the rhythm remains unidentified.

- You know enough, however, to direct the endotracheal administration of epinephrine. This patient is in confirmed cardiac arrest and will need epinephrine. Since the endotracheal tube is in place, use that route.

Lisa Slater
CASE 4 Continued

"Julie, would you please attach the monitor leads and make sure the lead selector switch is set on lead II? We need to check the rhythm quickly. In the meantime, would the anesthesiologist please administer 3 mg of epinephrine mixed in 10 mL of normal saline down the endotracheal tube and hyperventilate several times after injection. Let me know every 3 minutes and then inject an additional dose of EPI 3 mg down the tube. Stop CPR please and let's check the monitor." (The rhythm is VF.) "Gary, please start with immediate defibrillation at 200 J. Everybody clear the patient!" (After three consecutive shocks [200 J, 300 J, and 360 J] the rhythm converts to a slow junctional escape rhythm.)

"May we please have a check for a pulse and a BP if there is a pulse." (Heart rate is 55 beats per minute; blood pressure is 100/60 mm Hg.) "Please let me know when the IV is started. The first drug should be lidocaine 60 mg IV push.

"Now, who knows the situation with this patient? Does anyone have any information on why she might have arrested?"

COMMENTS

- Notice here that the team leader still follows the Primary-Secondary Survey Approach. The leader first catches up with the earlier omission of the Primary D of defibrillation and continues with the Secondary C of circulation with medications (epinephrine and lidocaine). The leader ends with the Secondary D of differential diagnoses, in which attention is paid to why the arrest occurred.

CODE ORGANIZATION

- The code team leader has four major responsibilities:
  - To assign the four critical resuscitation tasks (listed later in this section)
  - To ensure that each rescuer performs his or her tasks safely and effectively
  - To order interventions according to protocols
  - To think about why the person arrested and possible reversible causes

- Note that none of these four responsibilities are performed by the team leader. The team leader should avoid doing procedures, if possible. The most effective team leader spends his or her time thinking. The leader should stand with arms folded on his or her chest in a position suited to view the monitor and the patient.

- The team leader is observing, directing, and, most important, thinking. Once the team leader establishes control, one effective approach "street smart" leaders use is to progressively lower the voice volume. This brings even more quiet to the scene as the other personnel attempt to hear every word.

- The leader of the resuscitation team must assign the four critical tasks of resuscitation. These tasks are as follows:
  - Airway patency and intubation
  - Chest compressions
  - Monitoring and defibrillation
  - Intravenous access and medications, including endotracheal drug administration

- The preceeding list reflects the priority of the tasks. As more and more personnel become available, assign more and more of the tasks. If less than four team members are present, follow this order of priorities:

- *One person:* Do basic CPR (airway, breathing, and chest compressions).

- *Two people:* Person A does basic CPR; person B does monitoring and defibrillation.

- *Three people:* Person A does basic CPR; person B does defibrillation; person C does airway management including endotracheal intubation (the defibrillator moves to IV access when able).

- *Four people:* Person A does basic CPR; person B does defibrillation; person C does airway management including endotracheal intubation; person D does IV access and medications.

- *Five people:* Same as with four people, with the fifth person assuming role of leader.

- Videotape and audiotape reviews of Emergency Department and out-of-hospital resuscitations reveal that the most effective and well-run codes are those that are the most quiet. In recordings of prehospital resuscitations using well-trained EMTs and paramedics, almost no talking is heard. Team members know their tasks so well that they seldom even have to speak other than to announce the accomplishment of their assigned task. This should be a model for all ACLS providers. A resuscitation marked by loud voices, anger, confusion, and rushed, clumsy movements indicates an inexperienced and possibly incompetent code team.

Mildred Perkins

CASE 5

You are a family medicine resident rotating through a month of Emergency Department work. A nurse rushes from Room 3 and catches your attention. "Doctor, could you please come in here at once. She is short of breath and her heart rate is more than 150!" You walk into the room to find an elderly woman sitting upright with marked respiratory distress. She meets your eyes with an intensity you will long remember, for they convey profound panic and fear. "Please, doctor, help me. I can't breathe!"

Your ACLS training has taught you what to do for a person in full cardiac arrest, but this patient is not in cardiac arrest. She looks desperately ill, however, as if she might soon collapse in arrest. How would you approach someone in whom the Primary-Secondary Survey Approach does not seem to apply?

COMMENTS

- In fact, the Primary-Secondary Survey Approach should be used for people in cardiopulmonary emergencies even when they are conscious and alert.

- It takes only seconds to visually inspect the patient with the Primary Survey to verify the following:
    - A—That there does appear to be an open airway
    - B—That the patient is breathing
    - C—That there is a pulse
    - D—That VF is not present

- Modify the Secondary Survey somewhat in the conscious, peri-cardiac arrest patient (in fact, this is part of the third quadrad—Oxygen/IV/Monitor/Fluids—but this makes the point that you should apply all parts of the Five Quadrads, even to patients without full cardiac arrest), as follows:
    - A—Listen for stridor; observe how hard the patient is working to move air.
    - B—Listen to the lungs for wheezing and signs of pulmonary edema.
    - C—Check the pulse, rhythm, and blood pressure and start an IV line.
    - D—Start thinking about the differential diagnosis and what might be wrong.

- Apply the third quadrad: Oxygen/IV/Monitor/Fluids. We recommend that "oxygen-IV-monitor-fluids" always be considered as one word, based on the following:

- You are always correct to administer oxygen, start an IV, and attach the monitor to a person with possible cardiorespiratory emergency.

- In fact, one axiom in emergency medicine holds that you can judge the quality of an Emergency Department, a critical care unit, or prehospital providers simply by how soon they begin oxygen, start an IV, and attach the monitor on seriously ill patients.

- Continue to apply the Five Quadrads, as follows:
    - Primary ABCD Survey
    - Secondary ABCD Survey
    - Oxygen/IV/Monitor/Fluids
    - Temperature/Blood/Pressure/Respirations/Pulse
    - Tank (Volume)/Resistance/Pump/Rate

- With these Five Quadrads you have 20 easily remembered items to consider and initiate on all cardiopulmonary emergencies, in particular, the following:
    - "Fluids" reviews the type and rate of IV infusion to start.
    - "Temperature" reviews the core body temperature, either too high or too low, and this factor becomes critical in many emergencies.
    - "Vascular resistance" is an important factor to consider in emergencies resulting from shock, hypotension, and acute pulmonary edema. (These emergencies will be presented in more detail in Chapter 10.)

Mildred Perkins	*You have completed your quick Primary and Secondary Surveys and identified marked bilateral wheezing and rales. You mentally review the other elements of the Five Quadrads. You ask the nurses to start oxygen delivery by nasal cannula at 4 L/min, start an IV with normal*
CASE 5 Continued	

saline at 125 mL/hour, and attach the monitor. The monitor shows a rapid, narrow complex tachycardia of 180 beats per minute; blood pressure is 80 mm Hg systolic; temperature is 37.2° C; respiration rate is 28 breaths per minute. Her fingers feel cool and clammy, and her fingers and lips are cyanotic. How do you assess this information?

COMMENTS

- You can see how the systematic approach to the emergency in Case 5 using the Five Quadrads packs a lot of information into a quick review. You have reviewed 20 aspects of this woman's presentation by an easily remembered list, identified major problems, and embarked on important interventions.

- Although you do not yet have "a diagnosis," you know the following:

  - This woman is in severe respiratory distress, with rapid breathing, pulmonary rales and wheezing, and peripheral cyanosis.

  - She also has an extremely rapid heart rate and symptomatic hypotension.

  - The low blood pressure appears to be associated with early signs of shock.

- As you will learn later in Chapters 8 and 10, you now know enough to initiate treatment. The recommended approach is to treat heart rate problems first, then tank problems, then pump problems. In acute pulmonary edema you need to raise the hypotensive blood pressure before you can initiate the first-line actions for treatment of pulmonary edema.

Mildred Perkins	*Suddenly she slumps over and becomes unresponsive. You cannot feel a pulse. Now what do you do?*
CASE 5 Continued	

COMMENTS

- It is surprising that many ACLS providers will now feel more comfortable managing this woman. She has gone into cardiac arrest, which we know how to respond to, using the first two quadrads that focus on cardiac arrest, the Primary and Secondary Surveys.

- The challenge is to have recognized from the moment you first walked into the room that this patient is a person "on her way to a cardiac arrest." You have the responsibility to rapidly assess your patients and initiate aggressive "peri-cardiac arrest" interventions in order to actually prevent the arrest.

- You will need to initiate the full Five Quadrads and start the treatments indicated in the surveys. These are discussed in later chapters; in particular, the cases in Chapter 10—of hypertension, shock, and acute pulmonary edema—that demonstrate the use of the cardiovascular quadrad of Tank (Volume)/Resistance/Pump/Rate.

- We will leave Mrs. Perkins now: the details of her treatment will come in later chapters.

- However, the case of Mrs. Perkins demonstrates the power of the Five Quadrads, showing how you can apply the Primary and Secondary Surveys to both full cardiac arrest and peri-cardiac arrest patients.

TABLE 1-4

Using the Primary and Secondary Survey Approach to Troubleshoot a Difficult Code

STEP ONE

Troubleshoot by checking to see that A, B, C, and D are proceeding correctly.

AIRWAY

- *Patient is receiving 100% oxygen.*
- *Airway is open and air is moving easily.*
- *Endotracheal tube is open and unobstructed.*

BREATHING

- *Bag-valve-mask ventilation is provided at correct rate and force.*
- *Bilateral, symmetric chest expansions occur with each ventilation.*
- *Order arterial blood gas levels.*

CIRCULATION

- *CPR chest compressions are adequate in rate, force, depth, and location.*
- *IV access is established correctly.*
- *Medications are administered properly: no infiltration. Line is flushed after each drug; arm is elevated with drug administration.*
- *Monitor is used correctly (leads connected, correct control settings).*
- *Medications are selected appropriately according to indications.*

DEFIBRILLATION

- *Numerous defibrillator errors, most resulting from operator errors, are possible.*
- *Failure of muscle contractions during shock does not mean current failed to be delivered.*

STEP TWO

Review D (differential diagnoses) by asking, "What else could be causing this lack of response?" Again use the following ABC model to review the diagnostic possibilities.

AIRWAY

- *One useful mnemonic, as follows, for the potential causes of acute deterioration of the intubated patient is DOPE:*
  - *Displacement of the tube*
  - *Obstruction of the tube*
  - *Pneumothorax and other leaks*
  - *Equipment failures*
- *Tube obstructed or kinked*
- *Foreign body aspiration*
- *Anaphylaxis (angioedema)*
- *Inflammation of the hypopharynx (epiglottis, retropharyngeal abscess)*
- *Craniofacial trauma, laryngeal or tracheal disruption*

BREATHING

- *Preexisting chest wall mechanical abnormalities (scoliosis, emphysema)*
- *Tension pneumothorax from resuscitation efforts*
- *Subcutaneous emphysema*

CIRCULATION

- *Pericardial tamponade from resuscitation efforts*
- *Occult trauma: cardiac tamponade, hypovolemia, exsanguination*
- *Pulmonary embolus*
- *Massive acute myocardial infarction*
- *Carbon monoxide poisoning*
- *Prolonged hypoxia*
- *Drug overdoses of many types: tricyclic antidepressants, aspirin, beta blocker or calcium channel blocker overdoses*
- *Illicit drugs: cocaine, heroin, cyanide poisoning (after fires with synthetic materials)*
- *Inhaled aerosols (glue, fabric protector, cleaning products)*
- *Electrolyte disturbances (potassium, calcium, magnesium)*
- *Acidosis or alkalosis*
- *Occult pseudoallergic drug reaction leading to cardiovascular collapse (e.g., radiographic contrast agents, vitamin K infusion)*
- *Occult drug intoxication (e.g., theophylline intoxication in persons taking erythromycin or ciprofloxacin)*

Meredith Knopp

CASE 6

You are the chief resident in emergency medicine. As you start your 7 AM shift you notice the familiar signs of a code in progress in Room 1. The tired intern doing chest compressions looks in your direction. "This 22-year-old college student has lupus and renal failure and is on dialysis. She has been depressed and OD'd on 20 Amitriptyline capsules earlier this morning. Her friends brought her in unresponsive, hypoventilating with a BP of 80 systolic. About 25 minutes ago she went into a full cardiac arrest and we have been doing CPR off and on ever since. We get her going for a few minutes and then she goes back into some weird rhythm without a pulse."

How would you approach this extremely complicated resuscitation effort in a systematic manner?

COMMENTS

- In Case 6 you have a difficult code that is not going well, one in which the patient is not responding. Once again the Primary and Secondary Surveys can be used to troubleshoot a difficult code. Miss Knopp has pulseless electrical activity (PEA—a slow, idioventricular rhythm without a pulse). You will learn that PEA has a large differential diag-

nosis. Without identifying treatable causes of PEA the resuscitation attempt will not be successful.

- Systematically review with the code team each item of the Primary–Secondary Survey Approach, focusing on the differential diagnosis. Table 1-4 demonstrates using the Primary and Secondary Surveys to troubleshoot a difficult code.

Meredith Knopp

CASE 6 Continued

You review the ABCDs of the Primary and Secondary Surveys and identify no immediate cause for the persistence of PEA. You focus on the C of the Secondary Survey and consider the following possibilities: electrolyte abnormalities and acidosis from the renal failure, volume problems from the recent dialysis, and the cardiotoxicity of tricyclic antidepressant overdose. You learn that the initial potassium level obtained 10 minutes after the arrest was 5.8 and the pH was 7.1. When asked how much sodium bicarbonate the intern had administered, he replies, "Well, I haven't given any sodium bicarbonate. The K is not really that high, we intubated her immediately, and ventilation is the best treatment for acidosis. Besides, you always said sodium bicarbonate is not a good drug to give in cardiac arrest."

What would be your response to the bicarbonate question?

COMMENTS

- The immediate answer is that sodium bicarbonate is a drug just like any other—there are clear indications for the use of bicarbonate in a resuscitation attempt, and there are definite contraindications. The intern failed to adjust the usual approach. Here there is a unique patient with unique clinical problems. Adjustments are necessary.

- This case also displays the need for someone to possess a wide range of specific information. For example, more experienced clinicians will know that aggressive use of sodium bicarbonate is the mainstay of treating the cardiotoxic effect of severe tricyclic antidepressant overdoses. Sodium bicarbonate 1 mEq/kg should be administered at once.

- In addition, the more knowledgeable ACLS provider will know that patients with renal failure may have the cardiac morbidity of hyperkalemia without extremely high potassi-

um levels. Therefore this patient needs to be treated with a regimen that addresses the possibility that hyperkalemia is contributing to the refractory nature of this emergency. Hyperkalemia is treated with the following approaches:

- Block the site of action of excessive potassium (with calcium gluconate).

- Shift the excess potassium from one body compartment to another (with sodium bicarbonate and insulin plus glucose).

- Remove potassium from the body (with cation exchange resin, peritoneal dialysis or hemodialysis, or diuretics).

- Case 6 illustrates another simple but critical point: you have got to know what you are doing. No matter how clever some systematic approach might be—for example, the Five Quadrads—there is no substitute for facts and knowledge. The ACLS course provides the core basics for people who might occasionally encounter a cardiac arrest in their professional lives. The advanced ACLS provider, however, needs to conscientiously learn, through reading, continuing medical education, and clinical experience, as

much as possible about emergency cardiac care. Your patients deserve it.

• See Chapter 11 for further management of cardiac arrest associated with electrolyte abnormalities.

Wilson Brewer

CASE 7

While on duty in the Emergency Department, you receive a call from the "Medic One" doctor. She tells you the medics have intubated a 65-year-old man after a choking episode at home. His pulse is 120 beats per minute and his blood pressure is 130/90 mm Hg. They estimate arriving in the Emergency Depatrment in 5 minutes. The medics said that after they intubated the patient the wife produced an EMS-No CPR form that the patient had signed. The patient has metastatic lung cancer and did not wish CPR to be attempted should he suffer a cardiac arrest.

How would you prepare the Emergency Department for the arrival of this patient? What are your first thoughts about the "No Code" status of this patient whose trachea had just been intubated?

COMMENTS

• The scenario in Case 7 provides an excellent example of the use of the "phased-response format." The 1994 *Textbook of ACLS* recommends adoption of this planned, mul-

tistage approach to resuscitations and cardiopulmonary emergencies.

• Table 1-5 presents the phases of the phased-response format and the actions to perform within each phase.

SIDEBAR

Assessment-based Versus Diagnosis-based Emergency Care

• The conceptual power of the Five Quadrads with the Primary-Secondary Survey Approach emerges from how it combines two separate philosophies about emergency training and education: the assessment-based approach and the diagnosis-based approach.

• The assessment-based approach follows a series of assessment steps, completely independent of the diagnosis. Once you encounter a problem in the assessment, you then implement an intervention, again independent of the diagnosis. For example, if, during the assessment of B (respirations) you observe that the patient is not breathing (for whatever reason), you immediately initiate ventilations.

• A diagnosis-based approach, on the other hand, requires that emergency personnel establish a tentative diagnosis and then initiate their interventions based on that diagnosis. For example, shortness of breath can only be treated once you make a "diagnosis" of presumed acute pulmonary edema. From that diagnosis follows a series of prescribed interventions.

• The Primary-Secondary Survey Approach uses an assessment-based approach all the way to the last D of the Secondary Survey. This D (differential diagnosis) directs the ACLS provider to now consider the causes for the arrest. Why did this person experience this cardiopulmonary emergency? The focus here must be even further defined: search not just for the cause but for *reversible* causes. Often the only hope of successful resuscitation lies with searching for, finding, and treating reversible causes.

TABLE 1-5
Phased-Response Format

PHASE I: ANTICIPATION

As rescuers await the arrival of a possible cardiac emergency from a prehospital setting, they should do the following:

- *Analyze available clinical data*
- *Gather the personnel of the code team*
- *State leadership responsibilities*
- *Prepare and check equipment*
- *Assume positions*

PHASE II: ENTRY

When the patient arrives, the team leader should introduce himself or herself to the prehospital or floor resuscitation team, and then do the following:

- *Obtain entry vital signs*
- *Perform orderly transfer*
- *Evaluate baseline arterial blood gas levels and other laboratory values if necessary*
- *Gather concise history*
- *Repeat vital signs*

PHASE III: RESUSCITATION

Keep to the Primary-Secondary Survey Approach, and keep the resuscitation room quiet so that all personnel can hear.

*The **team members** should:*

- *State the vital signs every 5 minutes or with any change in the monitored parameters*
- *State when procedures and medications are completed*
- *Request clarification on any orders*
- *Provide primary and secondary assessment information*

*The **team leader** should:*

- *Appear decisive, professional, calm, and composed*
- *Assume control with "the voice"*
- *Communicate her or his observations*
- *Always be open to and actively seek team member suggestions*

PHASE IV: MAINTENANCE

In this phase either the patient has regained a spontaneous pulse or the immediate emergency has started to stabilize. This is a vulnerable period.

- *Continue to secure the patient and stay ahead.*
- *Maintain attention by repeatedly returning to the Primary and Secondary Surveys.*

PHASE V: FAMILY NOTIFICATION

Remember that concerned family members and loved ones are desperate for information on the patient. "Telling the living"—either good news or bad news—must be done promptly, and with honesty and sensitivity (see Table 1-1 for more details).

- *Ask to be notified whenever relatives arrive.*
- *Respect the privacy of the family members.*
- *Offer to let them see their relative as soon as possible, but realize what the effect of seeing their relative in an extreme emergency might have. Discuss this with them.*
- *Realize you will have to repeat information several times because their concentration on medical details at such a time will be divided.*

(Note that a number of hospitals and emergency departments are adopting the practice of allowing family members or loved ones to be present at resuscitation attempts. Pediatric resuscitation centers are leading the way in this activity, and initial family responses have been very positive.)

PHASE VI: TRANSFER

Medical professionalism requires the resuscitation team to transfer the patient to a team of equal or greater expertise. Perform this transfer and deliver this information in a manner that is respectful, complete, concise, and well organized.

PHASE VII: CRITIQUE PROCESS

Every team should perform a code critique, no matter how brief. This activity provides feedback to prehospital and in-hospital personnel, an avenue to express grieving, and an opportunity for education. Critical incident stress debriefing is summarized in Table 1-3.

Modified with permission. © *Textbook of Advanced Cardiac Life Support*, 1994, p.1-69. Copyright American Heart Association.

Wilson Brewer

CASE 7 Continued

Soon the medics arrive with Mr. Brewer. Every member of the Emergency Department team moves swiftly into action for the transfer. He is intubated but is not spontaneously breathing. His blood pressure has dropped to 80/60 mm Hg, and his heart rate is 50 beats per minute. His medical chart and his wife arrive simultaneously. You learn a complicated history. He has metastatic lung cancer and has signed a Do Not Resuscitate form. His respiratory status has been marginal at best. Tonight he appeared to have a respiratory arrest while choking on a piece of ice his wife gave him. She called 911, and when emergency personnel arrived they immediately reacted to the respiratory difficulty and intubated his trachea.

What are your thoughts about the "No Code" status of this patient who had just been intubated?

COMMENTS

• In Case 7 you have an example of a core ethical issue in emergency cardiac care—the issue of starting and stopping resuscitation efforts. More and more EMSs are developing programs that will allow patients to experience death with dignity. Eventually everyone reaches the end of life on Earth. Cardiac arrest at the end of a life simply represents a death—not the requirement for immediate resuscitation.

• "No CPR" or "Do Not Attempt Resuscitation" (DNAR) programs allow patients to call for comfort care at the end of their life. These programs allow EMS personnel to provide this comfort care but allow the personnel to withhold resuscitation in the event of a full cardiac arrest.

• In the scenario in Case 7 one could argue that several judgment errors were made. If Mr. Brewer and his wife did not want resuscitation efforts, why did she call 911?

Once the EMS personnel arrived, why did they proceed with endotracheal intubation? Here Mrs. Brewer panicked when she observed the frightening choking episode. She did not know that the choking really represented an acute deterioration in Mr. Brewer's respiratory status—a deterioration that will prove fatal.

• Similarly the EMS personnel responded as they were trained to do. They did not have immediate access to the formal "No CPR" order, which was folded in an envelope inside the bedside table. Some states have adopted a "No CPR" bracelet program that helps solve this problem for EMS response teams. The bracelet signals that they should not start resuscitation efforts but that they should provide support and comfort.

• This is not a time for blame, however. You now have responsibility for Mr. Brewer.

Wilson Brewer

CASE 7 Continued

You confirm the diagnosis and the poor prognosis. In your discussion with Mrs. Brewer you learn that she and her husband are firmly committed to their decisions to "have no heroics" at the end and their strong desire "for a dignified death not hooked up to those breathing machines." The nurses determine that Mr. Brewer takes only brief, infrequent breaths. He needs a ventilator, and his blood pressure and heart rate are declining rapidly. They look at you and ask, "Do you want us to call respiratory therapy for the ventilator and arrange an ICU bed?"

How would you respond?

COMMENTS

• Here resuscitation has been started, and with hindsight this appears inappropriate. Are you obligated to continue with these efforts? While few people have objections to withholding CPR, withdrawing CPR, once started, seems more difficult.

• The contemporary ethical viewpoint is that there is no difference, ethically, between withholding life support and

withdrawing life support. You decide to withdraw positive-pressure ventilations and discuss your recommendations with Mrs. Brewer.

• The chapter "Ethical Aspects of CPR and Emergency Cardiac Care" in the *ACLS Textbook* provides an ethical framework for considering issues of starting and stopping CPR. We strongly recommend review and discussion of these issues by all resuscitation teams.

Wilson Brewer

CASE 7 Continued

You tell Mrs. Brewer, "I would recommend that we leave the tube in place for now and see whether he can breathe on his own. If he does not, I think we should not put him on the ventilator. What do you think?"

Mrs. Brewer remains emphatic that her husband wanted a dignified death and no life support efforts. You ask if she wants to be in the room while you see how he does on his own. She comes in the room and sits by the gurney, holding his hand. You ask if she wants family members or a chaplain called.

You direct the respiratory therapist to stop ventilating Mr. Brewer's lungs. He takes deep agonal breaths about 4 times per minute. The oxygen saturation level begins to fall, and the heart rate slows steadily. You explain to the nurses, "If Mr. Brewer cannot breathe on his own with the tube in place, we are going to let him go. We are going to let him die."

After 10 minutes the agonal respirations cease completely, but organized cardiac complexes remain on the monitor screen at 12 beats per minute. Mr. Brewer's skin becomes mottled and cyanotic. It is clear that the persistent beats on the monitor make everyone uncomfortable. "Please turn off the monitor screen," you ask the clinic assistant. Two minutes later you place your hand gently on Mrs. Brewer's shoulder and say, "Mrs. Brewer, he has just this moment died." She bends her head over and begins to cry softly.

COMMENTS

- There are now many details to consider and take care of: social service for Mrs. Brewer, calling other family members, tissue donations, autopsy consideration, disposition of the body, helping with the funeral home arrangements, and completion of the death certificate. All of these matters are as important for the ACLS provider to learn as the operation of a defibrillator. Do not neglect these areas (see Table 1-2).

- Later, you should call together the personnel who were involved in the care of Mr. Brewer and conduct an informal critical incident debriefing. Do not let the "busy-ness" of the typical acute care setting prevent this review.

Allowing someone to die as in this scenario will always be a challenge to emergency care providers—it contradicts the major goals of emergency training. Be sensitive to these tensions and conflicts.

- A sensitive, dignified approach to situations like this requires the maximum skill from the ACLS provider. There is no greater challenge to emergency providers than to help provide a dignified end to someone's life.

- Developing your abilities to know when to start and when to stop CPR, how to tell the living, how to talk to your colleagues—these are skills that are more important and more challenging than any others in emergency cardiac care.

KEY POINTS

S U M M A R Y

This chapter introduces the basic tools you need to approach all adult cardiopulmonary emergencies. Once you have mastered these general approaches, you have the framework for dealing with a wide range of resuscitation challenges.

This chapter provides major review points for the following:

- **The Five Quadrads Approach to Emergency Cardiac Care**

- **Calling 911 or EMS number**

- **Chain of Survival concept**

- **Community-based early defibrillation with automated external defibrillators**

- **Post-resuscitation support**

- **The Universal Algorithm**

- **Resuscitation-stopping criteria**

- **Telling the living: conveying news of a death to survivors**

- **Recommendations for critical incident debriefing**

- **How to assume command of a resuscitation scene**

- **Code organization: assigning tasks, assigning priorities**

- **The Five Quadrads**

- **Using the Five Quadrads and the Primary-Secondary Survey Approach to troubleshoot difficult codes**

- **Assessment-based versus diagnosis-based emergency care**

- **Phased-response format for resuscitations**

- **Ethical issues of starting and stopping cardiopulmonary resuscitation**

- **Criteria for organ and tissue donation**

The other chapters in this book apply these core approaches to more detailed case scenarios and present more treatment details. Never forget, however, the value of a systematic, routine approach to all emergencies. While treatment details can always be looked up and reviewed, a systematic approach will give you the confidence to handle virtually every cardiopulmonary emergency.

FILE
02.

Code Blue
Respiratory Arrest, Airway Management, and IV Access

O V E R V I E W

• *This chapter teaches you to assess and care for persons with respiratory compromise. Airway management is the first priority in the care of any seriously ill or injured person.*

• *Airway management skills are critical components of the Five Quadrads concept, in particular, the Primary and Secondary ABCD Surveys:*

  • *Primary ABCD Survey: Use noninvasive airway adjuncts to maintain oxygenation and ventilation.*

  • *Secondary ABCD Survey: Perform endotracheal intubation, provide positive-pressure ventilation, verify effectiveness.*

• *The Primary and Secondary ABCD Surveys place the actions of airway management and ventilation into a logical scheme. Using the Universal Algorithm and the Five Quadrads, you can make decisions that lead to correct and rapid management of a patient's breathing.*

• *Several critical manipulative skills must be coupled with decisions in a limited time frame if you are to reverse cerebral anoxia.*

• *You are not expected to make a differential diagnosis of respiratory failure. Just search for the possible causes as you treat the patient's hypoxia, then arrange for transfer to an area where mechanical ventilation can be provided.*

MAJOR CONCEPTS TO MASTER

• Learn the decision sequence in the Five Quadrads, the Primary and Secondary ABCD Surveys, and the Universal Algorithm.

• Learn to recognize a patient with respiratory compromise.

• Learn to manage an airway with noninvasive techniques with and without devices.

• Learn the "Why?" "When?" "How?" and "Watch out!" for oxygen, the first drug of choice in emergency cardiac care.

• Learn to manage an airway with invasive techniques.

• Learn to alter airway and ventilation techniques as the person's needs change.

• Know when and how to initiate IV access.

Critical Actions

The most critical respiratory action in any successful cardiac emergency is to meet the challenges of the following:

- Airway control (the airway is kept open and protected from obstruction)
- Oxygenation (oxygen supplied to the blood)
- Ventilation (carbon dioxide removed from the blood)

The following actions are critical:

- Follow the Universal Algorithm.
- Perform the Five Quadrads as follows:
  - Primary ABCD Survey
  - Secondary ABCD Survey
  - Temperature/Heart Rate/Blood Pressure/Respiratory Rate (Vital signs)
  - Oxygen/IV/Monitor/Fluids
  - Tank/Resistance/Pump/Rate
- Take immediate corrective action for problems identified in the Primary Survey.
- Recognize a patient with respiratory compromise.
- Learn noninvasive airway techniques that do not utilize devices.
- Know the "How?" "When?" "Why?" and "Watch out!" for the common tools used for noninvasive airway maintenance and ventilation.
- Learn invasive airway techniques: endotracheal intubation remains the gold standard for definitive control of the airway.
- Know the complications associated with orotracheal intubation.
- Learn where, when, and how to achieve intravenous (IV) access.
- Properly ventilate a patient's lungs.
- Alter airway management techniques as the person's needs change.

Skills To Learn

- You should know basic airway management without devices, which includes the following:
  - Assessment of breathlessness (look, listen, and feel)
  - Head tilt–chin lift (easy to perform and produces maximum airway patency)
  - Mouth-to-mouth ventilation
  - Mouth-to-barrier ventilation
  - Abdominal thrust
- You should know how to operate common noninvasive airway adjuncts. Be familiar with the devices you might use in your professional work, including the following:
  - Barrier devices and face shields
  - Oropharyngeal airway
  - Nasal trumpet (nasopharyngeal airway)
  - Pocket face masks
  - Suction devices
  - Administration of oxygen using various masks (Oxygen/IV/Monitor)
  - Pulse oximetry (the fifth vital sign!)
  - Bag-valve-mask (BVM) ventilation
- Demonstrate knowledge and skills required for endotracheal intubation.
- Be familiar with the following alternative advanced airway control techniques in case you might be called to assist:
  - Guided digital intubation or intubation using a lighted stylette
  - Nasotracheal intubation
- You should know the equipment and skills for establishing peripheral venous access.
- We do not cover the operation and use of ventilators here. You must know when a patient will require such measures and how to get your patient to a facility that provides such care.

Rhythms To Learn

- Bradycardia is the rhythm most commonly associated with respiratory compromise.
- Always attach hypoxic patients to an ECG monitor, since hypoxia will adversely affect their heart rate and ECG.
- The treatment for hypoxic arrhythmias is to manage the airway and ventilate the patient's lungs.

Medications To Learn

- Oxygen

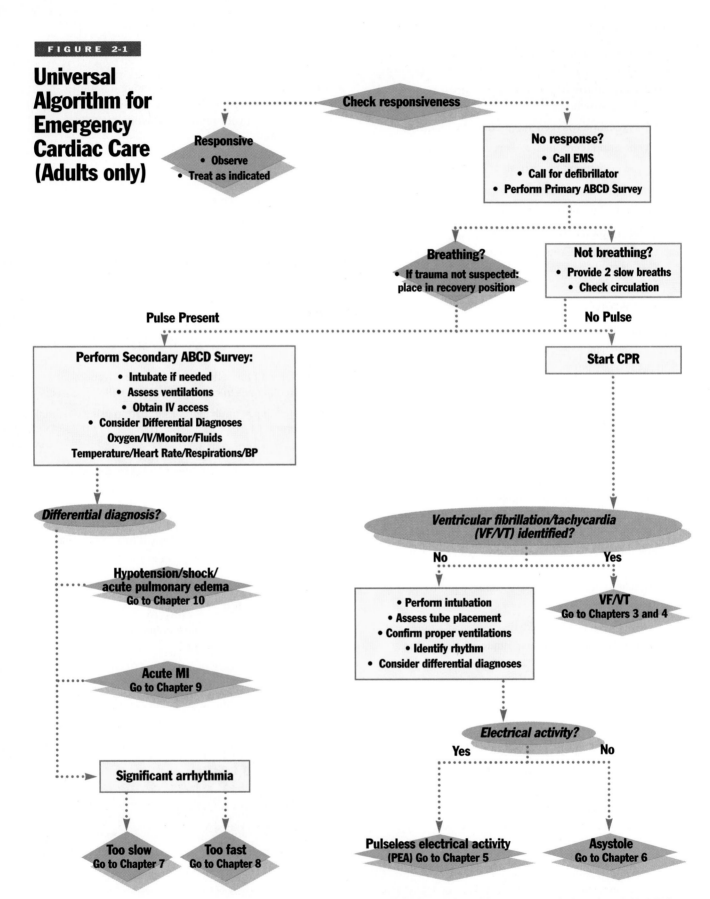

FIGURE 2-1

Universal Algorithm for Emergency Cardiac Care (Adults only)

Check responsiveness

Responsive
- Observe
- Treat as indicated

No response?
- Call EMS
- Call for defibrillator
- Perform Primary ABCD Survey

Breathing?
- If trauma not suspected: place in recovery position

Not breathing?
- Provide 2 slow breaths
- Check circulation

Pulse Present

No Pulse

Perform Secondary ABCD Survey:
- Intubate if needed
- Assess ventilations
- Obtain IV access
- Consider Differential Diagnoses
Oxygen/IV/Monitor/Fluids
Temperature/Heart Rate/Respirations/BP

Start CPR

Differential diagnosis?

Ventricular fibrillation/tachycardia (VF/VT) identified?

No   **Yes**

Hypotension/shock/ acute pulmonary edema
Go to Chapter 10

- Perform intubation
- Assess tube placement
- Confirm proper ventilations
- Identify rhythm
- Consider differential diagnoses

VF/VT
Go to Chapters 3 and 4

Acute MI
Go to Chapter 9

Electrical activity?

Yes   **No**

Significant arrhythmia

Too slow
Go to Chapter 7

Too fast
Go to Chapter 8

Pulseless electrical activity
(PEA) Go to Chapter 5

Asystole
Go to Chapter 6

Adapted with permission, Journal of the American Medical Association, 1992, Volume 268, *Guidlines for Cardiopulmonary Resuscitation and Emergency Cardiac Care*, p. 2216 Copyright © 1992, American Medical Association.

Craig Dorn	You are an off-duty paramedic eating in a cafeteria at a mall. Craig Dorn, a 34-year-old construction worker, is found in the men's bathroom by his friends. They had been having lunch at the cafeteria and grew tired of waiting for him. They found him slumped in the bathroom.
CASE 1	

room. He is unconscious and unresponsive, without respirations, but he has a strong pulse. His friends call for help. You respond to the scene while a security guard runs to call EMS.
How would you approach Mr. Dorn?

COMMENTS

- Always begin with the Five Quadrads, in particular, the Primary ABCD Survey, which covers noninvasive airway techniques, and the Secondary ABCD Survey, which covers invasive airway techniques.

- The Universal Algorithm (Fig. 2-1) incorporates the major components of the Primary and Secondary ABCD Surveys.

- The Primary ABCD Survey must be performed for all patients in arrest as well as nonarrested unresponsive patients.

- Your concerns, as you approach this patient, revolve around these airway and ventilation questions:

  - Is his airway patent?

  - Are ventilations present and adequate?

  - How long has he been hypoxic?

  - How relaxed is his jaw?

  - Is a cervical spine injury possible?

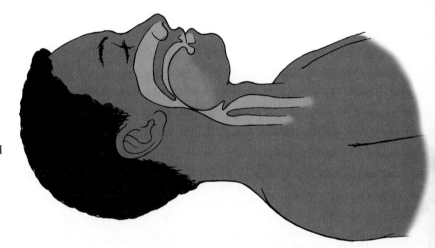

Fig. 2-2: Tongue obstructing the airway.

PRIMARY ABCD SURVEY:
DOES HE HAVE AN AIRWAY (A)? (Fig. 2-2)

- Partial airway obstruction in someone who has decreased level of consciousness is most often due to a tongue sagging against the posterior pharynx, or an epiglottis acting as a valve to occlude the airway. This is often accompanied by snoring sounds and can go undetected in the quiet apneic person who is not moving air. Other signs of airway obstruction are the following:

  - Faint or absent breath sounds

  - Use of accessory muscles for respiration

  - Cyanosis

- Try this demonstration on yourself: Tilt your head forward with your chin on your chest and try to swallow. It is easy to do. Now lift your head back as far as you can and try to swallow— it's very difficult. The difference is that in tilting the head back you move the tongue away from the back of the throat. The same thing happens when you tilt the chin back on an unconscious patient.

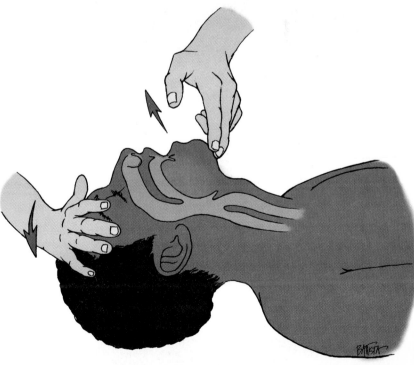

Fig. 2-3: Opening the airway.

OPENING THE AIRWAY USING THE HEAD TILT–CHIN LIFT (A)

- This will usually relieve the anatomic airway obstructions (Fig. 2-3).

  - Place the tips of your fingers beneath the person's chin.

  - Gently lift the jaw forward.

  - Open the mouth by pulling down on the lower lip with the thumb of the same hand lifting the chin.

- **Provide two breaths (B)**. If it is properly equipped, use a noninvasive airway adjunct (pocket face mask or barrier devices [discussed later]) (Figs. 2-4 and 2-5).

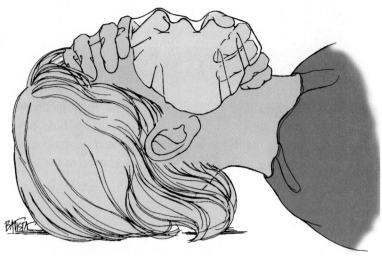

Fig. 2-4: Airway barrier device being used.

Craig Dorn

CASE 1 Continued

Your open the airway using the head tilt–chin lift. Mr. Dorn, unlike many unconscious patients, still cannot breathe on his own. You must provide two breaths to confirm an open airway and then venti-late using a mouth-to-barrier method. You reach in your pocket for your simple barrier device. This device eliminates direct contact of your mouth with the patient's nose and mouth but permits ventilations. It is a small sheet of plastic with a filter in the center of the plastic. You pinch Craig's nose and continue the chin lift while placing the barrier over your hands. You then put your lips over the filter that is over his mouth and give two slow breaths (1 ½ to 2 seconds per breath). The air enters easily and the chest rises symmetrically.

Was he unconscious from choking?

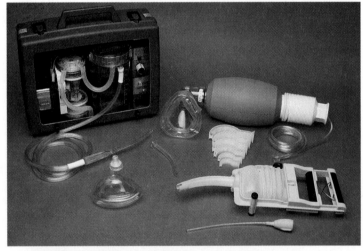

Fig. 2-5: Noninvasive airway devices.

COMMENTS

- Certainly choking is something to consider for this man, since his collapse occurred near an eating area. Clearing the airway of foreign objects requires more than a sim-ple chin lift. If you had been unable to ventilate, you would reposition his head and try again.

- If this is unsuccessful, give as many as five abdominal thrusts, as follows:

  - The patient must be supine.

  - Kneel next to the patient's hips, facing his head.

  - Place your overlapping palms on his epigastrium (above the umbilicus but below his ribs).

  - Give inward and upward thrusts.

Craig Dorn

CASE 1 Continued

You are able to ventilate Mr. Dorn's lungs. His chest rises bilaterally with each breath. Since he is still not breathing, you continue to per-form rescue ventilations for him. His pulse remains strong.

An emergency medical technician (EMT)–firefighter responds to the site with an airway box and an automated external defibrillator (AED). "Can you tell me what is going on?" she asks. "Advanced Life Support is on the way!"

What airway adjunct would you select from the EMS airway box?

COMMENTS

- Start with protective gloves whenever possible.

- Select an *oropharyngeal airway* (Fig. 2-6) as the initial noninvasive airway device to use as follows:

  - Insert it, curved side up.

  - Rotate it into position against the posterior wall of the patient's pharynx.

  - Sometimes it helps to use a tongue blade to push down the tongue and then slide the airway device, curved side down, into place.

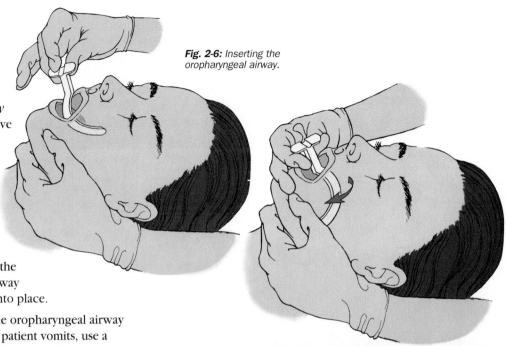

Fig. 2-6: Inserting the oropharyngeal airway.

- If the patient has a gag reflex, the oropharyngeal airway could make the patient vomit. If patient vomits, use a hand-operated or battery-powered suction device (Fig. 2-7) as follows to clear away any debris.

  - A working suction is a marvelous thing to have.

  - Commonly available suction devices for field use include battery-powered and hand-operated units.

  - You can also improvise with what is around you.

  - Turn the patient on his side and clear his airway with a gauze-, cloth-, or tissue-wrapped finger.

  - Use a bulb syringe attached to some IV extension tubing, or even a standard *baster* from the kitchen.

  - Unorthodox methods and creative thinking can save lives.

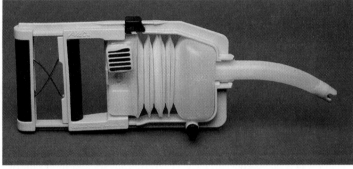

Fig 2-7: Hand-powered suction device.

- Use the "*nasal trumpet*" or the *nasopharyngeal airway* (Fig. 2-8) as follows for semiconscious patients (for example, severe intoxication) still ventilating spontaneously:

  - Conscious or obtunded patients who cannot tolerate an oropharyngeal airway may benefit from this soft, flexible tube inserted down one nostril and passed behind the tongue.

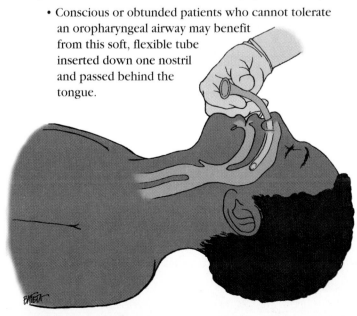

Fig. 2-8: Inserting the nasal trumpet.

This keeps a clear air passage from the nose to the lower airway.

- The nasal airway is less likely to stimulate vomiting than an oropharyngeal airway.

- Use an anesthetic jelly or lubricant on the tube before insertion to avoid nasal passage trauma. If you meet an obstruction, don't force it.

- Check your angle of insertion, and twist the tube slowly.

- If it won't progress, try the other nostril.

- You can use the trumpet to ventilate the patient's lungs, or to pass a suction catheter to clear the airways.

- If you want to use a bag to ventilate through the nasal trumpet, put an endotracheal tube connector into the nasal flange opening. Make sure it is of a size that fits with no leaks.

- Next, connect your ventilation bag to the connector and perform ventilations.

- If the patient continues to need artificial ventilation, use a *simple "pocket" face mask* (Fig. 2-9). This mask also has a filter between the mouthpiece and the patient.

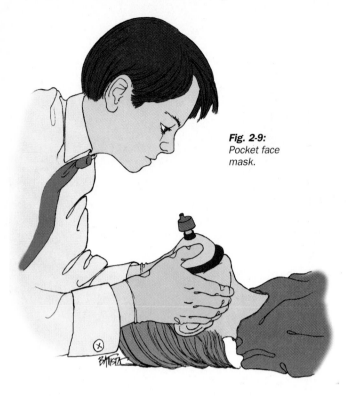

Fig. 2-9: *Pocket face mask.*

- Some of these masks also have an oxygen inlet valve that connects to standard bag connectors on a bag-valve-mask device.
- The mask is clamped firmly to the face using both hands.
- Use the fingers to grasp the jaw just beneath the angles, and pull upward, maintaining a patent airway.
- Blow intermittently into the mask.
- It is possible to attach oxygen tubing, set at a high rate of flow, and to deliver a mix of your own breath enriched with oxygen to this person.
- This is an effective device for one person to use during a field resuscitation.

Oxygen

WHY ?

- Oxygen is essential for life (cellular metabolism and survival).
- Oxygen is the first agent to use for respiratory compromise, cardiorespiratory distress, or cardiac arrest.

WHEN?

- Use in any suspected cardiopulmonary emergency.
- Use with any complaints of shortness of breath.
- Use for any patient complaining of chest pain.
- Use any time you suspect hypoxemia.

HOW?

- Deliver oxygen to the patient as a gas at 100% concentration from portable tanks or installed wall-mounted sources.
- Other delivery devices (Fig. 2-10) give the following percentages of oxygen:

DEVICE	FLOW RATE	OXYGEN DELIVERED (%)
Bag-valve-mask	*15 L/min*	*100*
Non-rebreather mask	*8-12 L/min*	*80-95*
Partial rebreather mask	*6-10 L/min*	*35-60*
Venturi mask	*4-8 L/min*	*24-40*
Nasal cannula	*1-6 L/min*	*24-44*

Watch Out!

- Never withhold oxygen from any patient who needs it. (One measure of the efficiency of emergency care is the length of time required to get a patient on oxygen.)
- Observe closely when giving oxygen to spontaneously ventilating pulmonary patients who are dependent on a hypoxic respiratory drive. This is very rare, however. Never withhold oxygen from such patients—you simply must watch them closely to see if they begin to hypoventilate. Assisted ventilations may then be necessary.

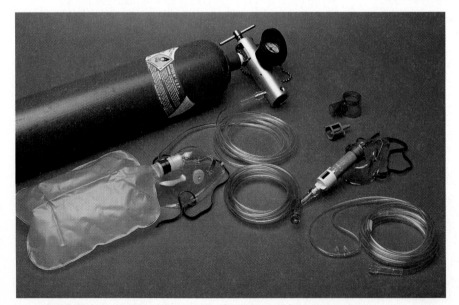

Fig. 2-10: *Oxygen delivery techniques: oxygen tank with (from left to right) non-rebreather mask, Venturi mask, and nasal cannula.*

Cralg Dorn

CASE 1 Continued

The EMT calls out "He's got a great BP of 132 over 88. I'll hook up the pulse oximeter, and you bag him."

The EMT sets up and connects an oxygen tank with regulator and tubing to a bag-valve-mask device with attached reservoir. She sets the flowmeter to 15 L/min, which can deliver close to 100% oxygen. Why pulse oximetry?

COMMENTS

- Pulse oximetry assesses both peripheral perfusion and oxygen saturation.

- When someone is hypoxic, small changes in arterial O_2 pressure (Pao_2) can mean a large change in oxygen saturation.

- Pulse oximetry gives a simple, easy-to-use method to "dose" oxygen.

- A probe is attached to the patient's skin, often on the finger (Fig. 2-11). This probe measures oxygen saturation of hemoglobin in the circulating blood.

- Many clinicians consider pulse oximetry a fifth vital sign. This technology assesses the adequacy of oxygenation with either continuous or intermittent readings.

- Many modern EMSs have made pulse oximetry mandatory for anyone receiving oxygen. Leave the device in place as a monitoring tool, not for a single reading.

WHAT DO THESE NUMBERS MEAN?

- When the oximeter shows a saturation level of 97% to 100%, the person has adequate oxygen in the blood. (Note that pulse oximetry tells you nothing about how well the patient is ventilating. Nor do you learn anything about the acid-base status of the patient. This information comes from arterial blood gas measurement of the pH and carbon dioxide (CO_2) level.

- Aim to keep the patient's O_2 saturation level above 96% or 97%.

- When the saturation level falls below 95%, hypoxemia is present.

- Remember: Someone who lives with chronic lung disease may have a low saturation level as a norm. High-flow oxygen may result in increased CO_2 as ventilations slow.

- As the saturation percentage goes down, administer oxygen more aggressively.

- Saturation levels below 90% indicate severe hypoxemia.

Watch Out!

This new technology has a few disadvantages. The devices have difficulty giving accurate readings in the following circumstances:

- Hypoperfusion (e.g., hypothermia or the hypotension present during resuscitation. Readings can be obtained during effective CPR, but always suspect their accuracy.)

- Anemia

- Nail polish or acrylic nails on the patient

- Dark pigmentation or bruising

- High bilirubin concentration

- Carbon monoxide poisoning (smoke inhalation and so forth)

BAG-VALVE-MASK DEVICE

- Ventilating with a bag-valve-mask device (BVM) with oxygen attached appears to be simple and effective. The BVM's major advantage is that it can administer close to 100% oxygen when it is hooked up to a tank flowing at a rate of at least 10 L/min and the reservoir bag is properly attached.

- Because there are many pitfalls to ventilating with a BVM effectively, manual ventilation takes practice, coordination, and a certain amount of strength.

- Bag-valve-mask devices are best used with an oropharyngeal airway in place.

- Get a good seal between the mask and the patient's face to prevent the air from escaping around the edges.

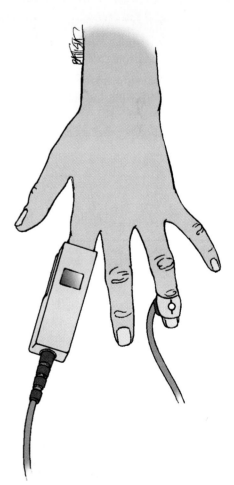

Fig. 2-11: *Pulse oximeter attached to the patient.*

ONE-PERSON BAG-VALVE-MASK TECHNIQUE (Fig. 2-12)

Face and Thigh Smash Technique

• Choose a size of mask that fits snugly about the person's mouth and nose.

• Press down with the palm while simultaneously pulling upward on the jaw with the same fingers. (Ventilation will be successful only if you have the correct size of mask and the patient is in the optimal position.)

• The rescuer should kneel at the patient's head. Backward head tilt can be maintained by applying gentle pressure with the knees.

• Squeeze the resuscitation bag flat against your thigh. Try to empty the bag. Use the thigh to provide counter-resistance to the hand squeeze. One-handed squeezing often fails to deliver adequate tidal volumes.

• Watch for chest rise and listen to the chest. If you don't have a stethoscope, have a bystander put an ear to the patient's chest directly over each lung and listen for breath sounds.

• Abruptly release the bag for patient exhalation.

TWO-PERSON BAG-VALVE-MASK TECHNIQUE (Fig. 2-12)

• Use a two-person method for operating the BVM, when space and people are available to assist.

• One person presses the mask firmly against the face with both hands while holding the head in head tilt–chin lift position.

• The second person squeezes the bag with both hands.

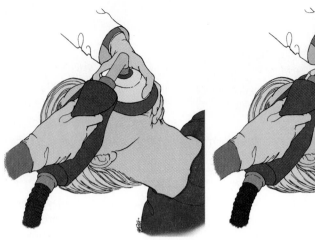
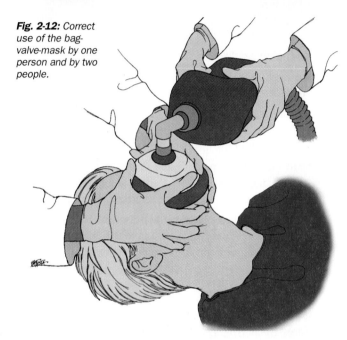

Fig. 2-12: Correct use of the bag-valve-mask by one person and by two people.

Craig Dorn
CASE 1 Continued

As you press the bag, the EMT reads out the numbers from the pulse oximeter. "His O₂ saturation is 92! When the medics get here he will need a tube."

This man has had a respiratory arrest. He has no gag reflex to protect his airway against aspiration. He needs the best airway support available. He needs endotracheal intubation. When the ALS personnel arrive you give a brief history while continuing to ventilate Mr. Dorn's lungs. One of the paramedics prepares to intubate Mr. Dorn where he lies. The paramedic kneels next to you and opens his ventilation equipment box.

Where are you now in the Five Quadrads? Apply the Primary and Secondary Surveys to this resuscitation attempt.

COMMENTS

Remember the elements of the Primary and Secondary ABCD Surveys:

PRIMARY SURVEY

• **Airway:** Yes, he has an open airway.

• **Breathing:** Yes, you are supplying ventilations using the oropharyngeal airway and BVM ventilations.

• **Circulation-defibrillation:** A pulse is present. Therefore CPR and defibrillation are not indicated.

SECONDARY SURVEY

• **Airway:** With continued absence of spontaneous respirations you need to perform endotracheal intubation.

• **Breathing:** Verify that the endotracheal intubation is effective.

- **Circulation:** Start IV line, monitor the cardiac rhythm, provide rhythm-appropriate medications.
- **Differential diagnosis:** Consider what has caused the patient to have the respiratory arrest.

Endotracheal intubation: What are the critical actions regarding equipment, positioning, technique, and tube placement? (See Figs. 2-13 to 2-16)

RESCUER POSITIONING

- One option is for the rescuer to sprawl prone on the floor lying at the patient's head.
- Lean onto the elbows for balance and the best anatomic view (Figs. 2-13 and 2-14).
- An alternate position for a tight space is lying supine on your back next to and superior to the patient's head.
- Recline next to the patient with your head elevated in semi-"sit up" position, which leaves your hands free to perform the procedure above the patient's face.

OPTIMAL EQUIPMENT (Fig. 2-15)

- Disposable gloves
- A BVM with oxygen connected
- An oral airway
- Stethoscope for checking proper tube placement
- Magill forceps
- An end-tidal CO_2 detector to check for tube placement
- Laryngoscope with curved and straight blades (when possible) and a light that works (Fig. 2-16)
- Several sizes of endotracheal tubes with an intact inflatable balloon
- Stylet for endotracheal tube
- A working suction device with rigid and flexible catheters

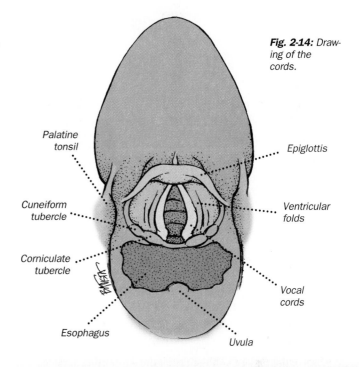

Fig. 2-14: Drawing of the cords.

Palatine tonsil
Epiglottis
Cuneiform tubercle
Ventricular folds
Corniculate tubercle
Vocal cords
Esophagus
Uvula

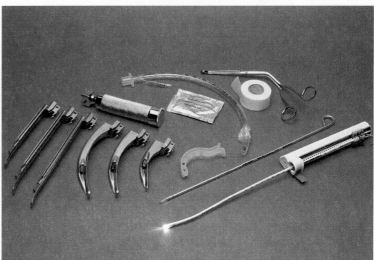

Fig. 2-15: Invasive airway technique: layout of endotracheal intubation equipment.

- 10-mL syringe
- A water-soluble, sterile lubricant
- Adhesive tape

PATIENT POSITIONING (NON-TRAUMATIC INJURY)

- Align the airway by placing the person (if no cervical trauma suspected) in the "sniffing position" (Fig. 2-13). This position requires flexion of the neck and extension of the head. Try leaning over as if sniffing food in front of you—you will flex your neck—and then tilt your head back to sniff. This aligns the airway passages in the most direct manner.

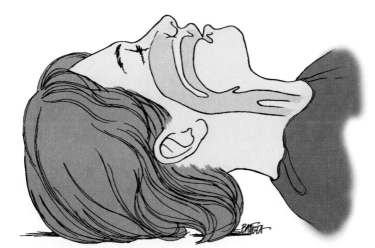

Fig. 2-13: Anatomy of the airway.

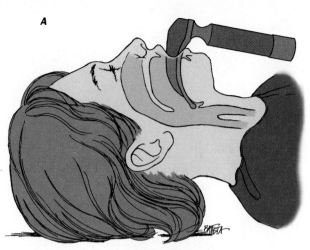

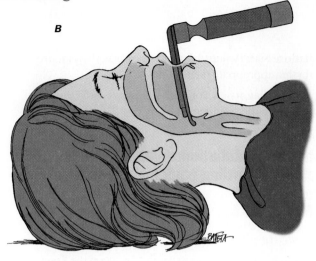

Fig. 2-16: A, Curved and **B**, Straight blades.

- Flex the neck by lifting the patient's head about 3 to 4 inches off the surface using a folded towel or sheet.
- Extend the head by tilting the head back. Maintain this position.
- Leave the patient's shoulders on the supporting surface.

TECHNIQUE FOR ENDOTRACHEAL INTUBATION

(Figs. 2-16 and 2-17)

1. Lubricate the tube with a water-soluble lubricant. (Do not use petroleum lubricants! They can deteriorate the tube.)

2. Insert the stylet to within 1 cm of the tip of the endotracheal tube. Bend it into a slight angle. (Stylet positioned at or past the tip of the endotracheal tube can lacerate the tracheal mucosa.)

3. Hyperventilate the patient's lungs several times before beginning. Take no longer than 30 seconds on any attempt between ventilations. (Get a bystander to time you, or try holding your breath during the intubation attempt. When you have to breathe, stop the intubation attempt and "bag" the patient again.)

4. Tilt the head into extension with your right hand, and remove the oropharyngeal airway and dentures if not already removed. Use suction to clean out vomit, mucus, blood, or other materials if necessary.

5. Hold the laryngoscope in your left hand, and open the mouth using your right hand. Insert the blade to the right of the tongue, and sweep the tongue to the left while inserting the blade further into the hypopharynx. Advance the blade until you see the tip of the epiglottis. (The blade will be at the base of the tongue-epiglottis junction) (Fig. 2-16, *A and B*).

6. Lift the laryngoscope both upward and forward without twisting the blade. You should be able to see the vocal cords. Do not use the teeth as a fulcrum. Lift "up and away."

7. If another rescuer is available, ask him or her to apply cricoid pressure (see Fig. 2-18) while you slide the tube to the right of the blade, through the cords, and into the

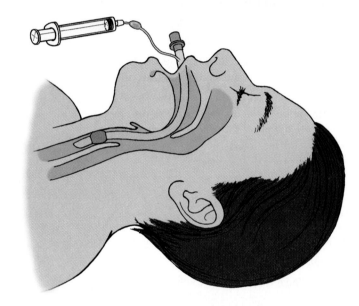

Fig. 2-17: Final position for endotracheal tube.

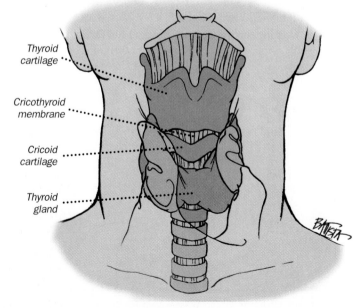

Thyroid cartilage

Cricothyroid membrane

Cricoid cartilage

Thyroid gland

Fig. 2-18: Landmarks of cricoid cartilage.

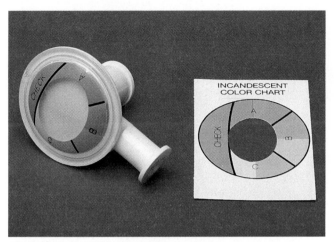

Fig. 2-19: End-tidal CO₂ detectors.

9. Prehospital care providers have learned that a bulb aspiration syringe (used to suction the mouths of newborns) can be used to detect esophageal intubations. Compress the syringe bulb, attach it to the end of the endotracheal tube, and release it. If the tube lies in the esophagus, the bulb syringe will not re-expand fully because it collapses the pliant esophagus. If the endotracheal tube is in the trachea, the bulb will immediately re-expand. Toomey aspiration syringes can be used for the same purpose.

10. *Esophageal detection devices* based on the preceding principle are now available. As a makeshift equivalent, the rescuer can use his or her mouth over the end of the endotracheal tube, supplying a gentle suction—inability to draw back air indicates esophageal intubation.

trachea. Stop when you see the deflated balloon just past the cords.

8. Carefully hold the tube in place to the right side of the mouth as you remove the laryngoscope blade and then the stylet. Inflate the cuff.

9. Ventilate and listen for equal breath sounds over both lung fields. Listen specifically over the left and right midaxillary lines. Listen for the absence of gurgling over the stomach.

10. Insert an oral airway as a bite block, and secure the tube with tape.

CONFIRM TUBE PLACEMENT

1. Listen over the abdomen for gurgling with ventilation. This indicates esophageal intubation. If esophageal intubation is suspected, deflate the cuff, remove the tube, and reattempt the intubation.

2. Listen for lung sounds over the epigastrium, then move up to each lung field and listen bilaterally over the midaxillary areas. A tube too deep in the trachea will block one mainstem bronchus and allow ventilation sounds in only one lung.

3. Listen again after you move the patient to the stretcher.

4. Constantly watch the chest rise and fall with each ventilation.

5. If the person is breathing spontaneously, you can feel air movement against your skin if you put your arm or cheek next to the tube.

6. When an end-tidal CO₂ detector is available (Fig. 2-19), attach it to the tube and watch for the color change that indicates CO₂. Carbon dioxide will not be present if the tube is in the esophagus.

7. Do not fix the tube in place firmly until correct placement is confirmed.

8. As soon as is feasible, obtain a chest x-ray as an additional confirmation of proper tube placement. Follow this with arterial blood gas measurements in the in-hospital setting.

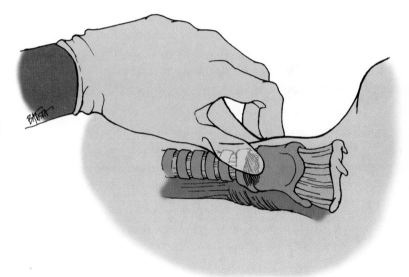

Fig. 2-20: Hand applying cricoid pressure.

DIFFERENCES IN INTUBATION: PERSON VERSUS MANIKIN

- Manikin practice is a fundamental part of intubation training. A manikin can help you become familiar with anatomy and technique and gain a great deal of confidence. This psychomotor skill requires effective, coordinated use of both hands.

- There are, obviously, differences between a manikin and a warm-blooded human being. The first time you intubate a real person's trachea, you will notice that the flesh is more pliant and limp. Tissues will sag and cast shadows exactly where you want to look.

- Human heads are heavy and not easy to move around or prop up. The heads of unconscious people tend to displace easily, and it takes more physical strength to hold them in the desired position.

- Human tongues are wet, floppy, and difficult to control and to direct.

- Be prepared for people to feel different from manikins.

CRICOID PRESSURE (Fig. 2-20)

• Cricoid pressure achieves two goals:

   • First, you force the ring of the cricoid cartilage down against the vertebra, thus pinching the esophagus shut. If stomach contents are regurgitated, you block them in the esophagus and prevent aspiration.

   • Second, during intubation attempts, cricoid pressure displaces the trachea downward so that a better view of the tracheal opening is obtained.

• Grab the cricoid ring with your thumb on one side and first (or third) finger on the other side.

• Press firmly, to seal off the esophagus and to push the vocal cords down into view for the person attempting intubation.

• If the patient vomits with great force, stop the cricoid pressure and prepare to suction and clear the airway. Cricoid pressure against forceful vomiting can rupture the esophagus.

• Maintain the cricoid pressure until the patient's trachea is successfully intubated and the airway is protected.

COMPLICATIONS OF ENDOTRACHEAL INTUBATION

Common misadventures associated with intubation are the following:

   • Trauma to the neck, teeth, eyes, and soft tissue

   • Inadvertent esophageal intubation

   • Severe hemorrhage in the airway or esophagus

   • Adverse physiologic reactions such as hypertension, arrhythmias, laryngospasm, or bronchospasm

   • Aspiration of vomitus, blood, or oral secretions

ALTERNATIVE ACLS AIRWAY TECHNIQUES

• You should be familiar with two alternative ACLS advanced airway techniques, in case you might be called to assist.

• Two intubation techniques you may use, digital intubation and lighted stylet, do not directly visualize the trachea.

DIGITAL INTUBATION (Fig. 2-21)

• Digital intubation is used with an unconscious patient when the larynx cannot be seen and in cases of hemorrhage in the airway or cervical spine injury.

• The intubator does need to have fairly long digits. Use good surgical gloves; there is a risk that the patient may bite down or "seize" during this procedure.

• Technique is as follows:

   • Position yourself to the side of the patient, facing the head.

   • Check all equipment, lubricate the tube well, and insert the stylet. Then bend it into the shape of a J.

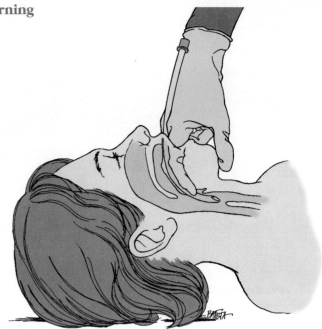

Fig. 2-21: *Digital intubation.*

• Put the first two digits into the side of the mouth, pushing the tongue down.

• Insert the tube between the two fingers in the patient's mouth toward the epiglottis, and guide it beneath the epiglottis. Then move it anteriorly toward the larynx.

• After the tip is secured in the larynx, withdraw the stylet, inflate the cuff, ventilate, and check tube placement.

LIGHTED STYLET (Fig. 2-22)

• A second method, becoming more common, is the use of a lighted stylet to transilluminate the larynx when the tube is placed correctly.

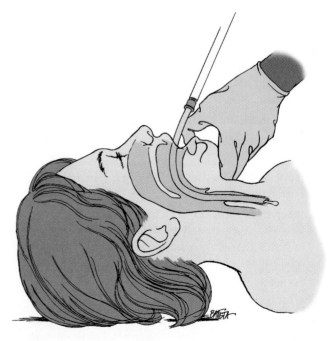

Fig. 2-22: *Lighted stylet intubation.*

- The light produces only a dull glow if the endotracheal tube has been inserted into the esophagus. The stylet can be used blindly, digitally, or in conjunction with a traditional laryngoscope.

- Technique is as follows:
  - Assemble and check all equipment.
  - Place the lighted stylet into the tube with a right-angle "hockey stick" angulation about 1½ inches from the tip.
  - The intubator stands at the patient's side, facing the head, and grasps the lubricated tube as if holding a pen.
  - Advance the tube into the trachea until a more intense light appears in the middle of the neck, over the midline of the trachea.
  - Hold the tube in place, remove the stylet, inflate the cuff, and ventilate.

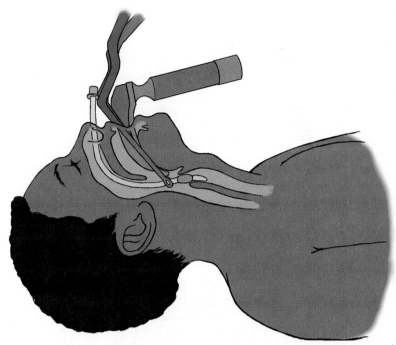

Fig. 2-23: *Nasotracheal intubation.*

NASOTRACHEAL INTUBATION (Fig. 2-23)
Use this technique with breathing patients.

Nasotracheal intubation is indicated as follows:
- When the victim is awake and cooperative
- When cervical spine trauma is suspected
- When acute epiglottitis is suspected
- After facial trauma or surgery involving the jaw
- When prolonged intubation is anticipated
- This approach is dangerous if people have nasal or skull fractures, since intracranial intubation can occur. Avoid this airway in patients with a history of nosebleeds or in patients taking anticoagulants.

TECHNIQUE FOR NASOTRACHEAL INTUBATION
- Assemble and check adequacy of equipment.
- Select the most patent nostril.
- Lubricate the tube with an appropriate lubricant, such as 2% viscous lidocaine. Prelubricate the nostril with lidocaine on progressively larger nasal airways for 5 minutes if you have extra time. As an alternative, you can instill a mixture of 1 mL phenylephrine with 4 mL viscous lidocaine into the nares while the person inhales.
- Gently slide the tube straight back into the nose until the tube turns the corner into the posterior pharynx. This is usually the most uncomfortable part of the procedure.
- Slowly advance the tube and listen to the sounds of breathing through the endotracheal tube. You will hear loud breath sounds and see condensed matter inside the tube as long as the tube is placed in line with the trachea. Advance the tube during inspiration and expiration.

- Inflate the cuff and check for tube placement. If you have advanced the tube too far, pull back. The patient will no longer be able to speak after cuff inflation. Breath sounds vanish if the tube is in the esophagus, and the patient may gag.

- If the tube does not advance smoothly, use the laryngoscope to visualize the larynx. Have an assistant push the tube down while you guide it using Magill forceps via the pharynx (Fig.2-23). Avoid grabbing the cuffed part of the tube, since this may cause a cuff leak. If you are not able to view the trachea, listen for breath sounds in the tube to guide your progress.

TRANSTRACHEAL CATHETER INSUFFLATION
Percutaneous translaryngeal ventilation

- This is a means to provide ventilation by using a large-bore needle that is inserted directly through the cricothyroid membrane.

- Use this technique for an obstructed upper airway that is unrelieved through other means. This is a dangerous, desperate procedure.

- Like the cricothyrotomy, it should be performed only by persons trained in this technique, using appropriate equipment.

- Technique is as follows:
  - Position the person supine with his or her head extended, unless you suspect spinal injury, in which case you must maintain the head in a neutral position.
  - Locate the cricothyroid membrane (Fig. 2-18), and prepare the puncture site with antiseptic.
  - Using a 12- or 14-gauge over-the-catheter needle with a

10 ml syringe attached, make a puncture over the lower half of the cricothyroid membrane. You will feel a slight pop as the needle enters the larynx. Confirm correct placement by aspirating air into the syringe.

• Advance the catheter into the larynx until the hub is next to the patient's skin.

• Check catheter placement again by aspirating through the syringe.

• Remove the needle, secure the catheter to the patient's skin, and attach a transtracheal ventilating device to the catheter and then to an oxygen source.

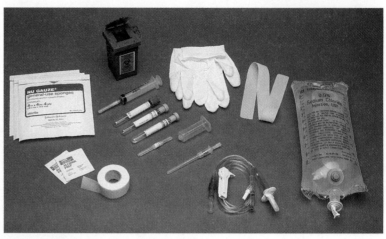

Fig. 2-24: *Equipment required to start an intravenous line.*

Craig Dorn	After intubation, Mr. Dorn's vital signs are as follows: O$_2$ saturation = 94%, blood pressure = 132/88 mm Hg, and pulse = 84 beats per minute. Anytime you move his stretcher or change people ventilating his lungs, recheck the endotracheal tube for correct placement.
CASE 1 Continued	

Now that you have completed the A and B (airway and breathing) part of the Secondary Survey, you proceed to the C (circulation) part by establishing IV access, and by attaching an ECG monitor to watch for cardiac arrhythmias.

Which fluid, vein, and needle are used to establish an IV?

Establish an intravenous "lifeline" (Fig. 2-24)

WHICH FLUID?

• The fluid of choice to keep the vein open is normal saline. Lactated Ringer's solution is acceptable; 5% dextrose in water (D$_5$W) is the least preferred solution.

• Check the bag for expiration date, leaks, and cloudiness.

• Connect an appropriate infusion set, and flush the air from the tubing.

WHICH VEIN?

• The first choice is the antecubital space of either arm (Fig. 2-25).

• If a subclavian, an internal, or an external jugular line is in place, use this for administering resuscitation medications.

WHICH SIZE OF NEEDLE?

• A large-bore 18-gauge needle is preferable for rapid volume replacement.

• For thrombolytic therapy, you would not want to use a larger size.

• In the presence of fluid replacement, choose a 16- or 14-gauge needle.

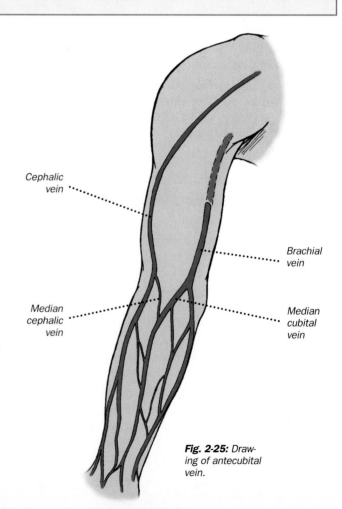

Cephalic vein

Brachial vein

Median cephalic vein

Median cubital vein

Fig. 2-25: *Drawing of antecubital vein.*

KEY POINTS SUMMARY

All ACLS providers should master these skills.

FOR THE PRIMARY ABCD SURVEY

Noninvasive airway adjuncts

- Oxygen tanks
- Barrier devices
- Pocket face masks
- Oropharyngeal airways
- Nasal cannulas
- Venturi mask
- Non-rebreathing masks
- End-tidal CO_2 volume monitors
- Oxygen saturation monitors (pulse oximeters)

FOR THE SECONDARY ABCD SURVEY

Invasive airway adjuncts

- Endotracheal intubation
- Nasotracheal intubation
- Digital intubation
- Lighted stylet intubation

INTRAVENOUS ACCESS

- In the rest of the case-based scenarios in this textbook, these skills are critical. No one can consider himself or herself a qualified and well-trained ACLS provider without mastery of the techniques and devices used to maintain an airway, ventilate a nonbreathing person's lungs, and initiate IV access.

FILE 03.

The Hunt for Ventricular Fibrillation
Automated External Defibrillators
in Advanced Cardiac Life Support

OVERVIEW

This chapter describes people with sudden, unexpected cardiac death from ventricular fibrillation(VF). In this book we recommend always using a systematic approach for treating ACLS emergencies. As noted in Chapter 1, the Five Quadrads approach provides a powerful conceptual tool that can be applied to virtually any cardiopulmonary emergency. The Five Quadrads start with the Primary ABCD Survey. For patients in VF—the cases in this chapter—you do not have to go any further than the Primary Survey.

The D of the Primary Survey stands for defibrillation. In the initial hunt for VF all you really need to know about are automated external defibrillators (AEDs). Defibrillation will always remain the major focus in adult ACLS for two simple reasons: first, most sudden cardiac arrests in adults are due to VF and, second, defibrillation is the only known sufficient treatment for VF. This focus on defibrillation must not, however, diminish the importance of basic CPR. You must continue to follow the full ABCs, providing an open airway, positive-pressure ventilations, and effective chest compressions. Otherwise, the effectiveness of defibrillation becomes markedly diminished. Defibrillation gets back the heart, CPR maintains the head. The two interventions are intertwined and essential.

The new technology of AEDs has been one of the most successful medical technologies to develop over the past decade. Therefore this chapter discusses "the hunt for VF" using only AEDs. Obviously, if conventional manual defibrillators were available it would be appropriate to employ those devices. However, because of the growing, widespread availability of AEDs the AHA ACLS course has now added hands-on experience with AEDs as a requirement for successful course completion. You must know how to apply an AED to a pulseless person and know how to follow the AED treatment algorithm, to be considered a successful and competent ACLS provider.

Ask yourself these questions as you study the cases in this chapter:

* *How fast can you eliminate VF?*

* *Can you operate any AED available wherever you find someone with this lethal reversible arrhythmia?*

* *Can you make sudden cardiac death a mere interruption in someone's life, and not "the end?"*

MAJOR CONCEPTS TO MASTER

- Learn how to activate the EMS system or code team to get an AED to the victim.
- Learn to rapidly attach an AED.
- Learn the four steps of operating any AED.
- Learn to operate an AED with minimal interruption of CPR.
- Learn to deliver shocks with an AED in less than 1 minute from arrival of the AED to the patient.
- Learn the most frequent problems that occur during defibrillation.
- Learn how to maintain the AED in a "state of readiness."
- Learn the AED decision priorities for adult cardiac arrest.

Critical actions

The major critical actions to take in treating an adult in cardiac arrest from VF are the following:

- Rapidly perform the initial steps of the Five Quadrads approach in, particularly, the Primary ABCD Survey recommended in the Universal Algorithm, as follows:
- Assess responsiveness.
- Call for AED.
- Determine lack of breathing and pulse.
- Begin basic life support (BLS) (ventilation and chest compressions).
- Get the defibrillator. (Properly attach and operate an AED.)
- Give the first shock within 1 minute of AED arrival.
- Administer shock again when indicated.
- Always use proper safety techniques.
- Provide immediate proper airway maintenance and positive-pressure ventilation using noninvasive techniques (insertion of oropharyngeal airway, use of pocket face mask, bag-valve-mask device [BVM], and various barrier protection devices).
- Recognize the presence of a pulse following shocks. (Know when in the treatment protocols to check for a pulse; if you can detect a pulse, measure blood pressure.)
- Demonstrate how additional caregivers are integrated into the management of a continuing cardiac emergency. (AED and BLS personnel help ACLS-equipped personnel begin their work smoothly and without interrupting patient care.)
- Provide clinical information to the next caregiver during transfer of someone who has been resuscitated using BLS and an AED.

Skills to learn

- Know the four steps involved in operating all AEDs.
- Know basic CPR.
- Know how to ventilate a nonbreathing patient using noninvasive airway methods.
- Know how to tell when an AED is ready for use.
- Know safety procedures related to AED use.
- Know how to restock and prepare the AED for the next resuscitation effort.
- Is there a single, best defibrillator to use? The best defibrillator to use during a cardiac arrest is immediately available, with a charged battery and correct supplies, and is the one the operator knows how to use.

Rhythms to learn

- None. The AED will detect most shockable ECG rhythms of VF and ventricular tachycardia (VT).

Medications to learn

- Other than oxygen, no pharmacologic agents are considered in these cases. Cardiopulmonary resuscitation and defibrillation are the major interventions.

Sherwin Bradley

CASE 1

You are headed home from a night shift. You work as a nurse in a busy coronary care unit (CCU). You stop for a red light. Bang! Someone rear-ends your car at a slow speed, then leaves the engine running. You burst from your bucket seat to discuss this situation. A man, however, is slumped over his steering wheel in the car lodged against your rear bumper. His ashen face is turned toward the driver's-side window. He makes one slow, gasping breath and then is still. How would you initially respond to this man?

COMMENTS

- Always begin with the **Five Quadrads.** The Primary ABCD Survey is the best way to remember the following steps of the Universal Algorithm (Fig. 3-1):

  - *Airway:* Open the airway.

  - *Breathing:* Ventilate using positive-pressure ventilation through appropriate airway adjuncts.

  - *Circulation:* Begin chest compressions.

  - *Defibrillation:* Defibrillate if VF/VT is present.

- Note that defibrillation is part of both the Universal Algorithm and the Primary Survey.

- Given the scenario in Case 1, VF is the most likely arrhythmia and early defibrillation has the highest priority.

- The widespread emphasis on early defibrillation is supported by a powerful rationale, as follows:

  - VF is the most common first ECG rhythm in sudden cardiac arrest.

  - Defibrillation is the treatment for VF.

  - VF deteriorates to asystole within a few minutes.

  - As minutes pass, the chance of defibrillating a fibrillating myocardium fades.

  - Every minute that a fibrillating heart remains in VF, the probability of survival declines by 7% to 10%. Since the maximum chance of survival with immediate defibrillation is about 70%, after 10 minutes the probability of survival approaches zero.

- What about the rest of the Five Quadrads after the Primary ABCD Survey (as follows)?

  - **Primary Survey:** What is the first major action for an unresponsive adult? Activate the EMS system.

  - **Secondary Survey:** Initate treatment of the primary ABCD requirements before moving to the Secondary Survey.

  - **Oxygen/IV/Monitor/Fluids:** These are considered after primary CPR and defibrillation.

  - **Vital signs:** None.

  - **Tank/Resistance/Pump/Rate:** There is no forward flow of blood in the cardiovascular system except that which is generated by external chest compressions.

Summary of the initial management of all cardiac arrests

- Assess responsiveness.

- Call for help to get the defibrillator moving toward you and your patient.

- Perform Primary ABCD Survey as follows:

  A—Open the airway.

  B—Breathe for the patient.

  C—Circulate blood through chest compressions. (The single rescuer should omit this step when a defibrillator is immediately available.)

  D—Defibrillate VF/VT as quickly as possible.

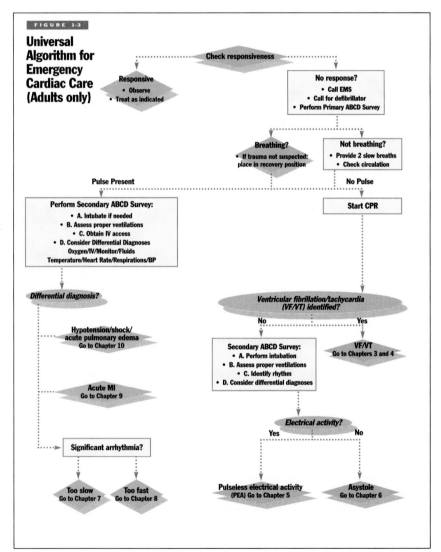

Fig. 3-1: *The Universal Algorithm.* Adapted with permission, Journal of the American Medical Association, 1992, Volume 268, *Guidelines for Cardiopulmonary Resuscitation and Emergency Cardiac Care*, p.2216, Copyright © 1992, American Medical Association.

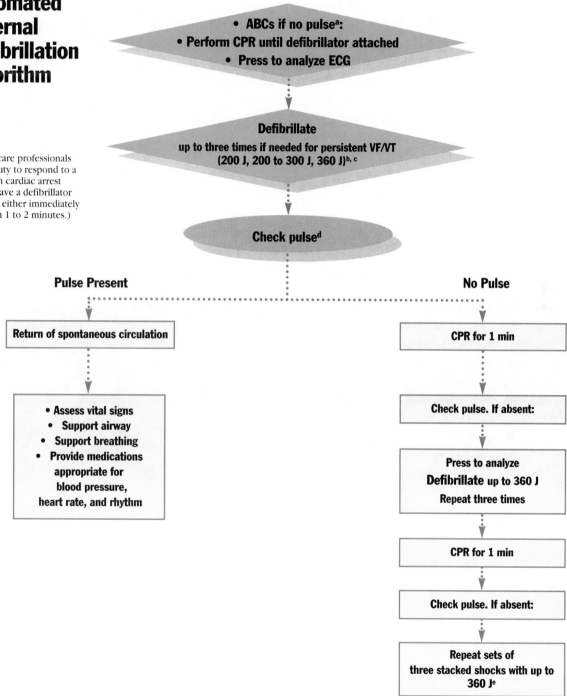

FIGURE 3-2

Automated External Defibrillation Algorithm

(Health care professionals with a duty to respond to a person in cardiac arrest should have a defibrillator available either immediately or within 1 to 2 minutes.)

- **• ABCs if no pulse[a]:**
- **• Perform CPR until defibrillator attached**
- **• Press to analyze ECG**

Defibrillate
up to three times if needed for persistent VF/VT
(200 J, 200 to 300 J, 360 J)[b, c]

Check pulse[d]

Pulse Present   **No Pulse**

Return of spontaneous circulation

- **• Assess vital signs**
- **• Support airway**
- **• Support breathing**
- **• Provide medications appropriate for blood pressure, heart rate, and rhythm**

CPR for 1 min

Check pulse. If absent:

Press to analyze
Defibrillate up to 360 J
Repeat three times

CPR for 1 min

Check pulse. If absent:

Repeat sets of three stacked shocks with up to 360 J[e]

---

[a] The single rescuer with an automated external defibrillator (AED) should verify unresponsiveness, open the airway (A), give two respirations (B), and check the pulse (C). If a full cardiac arrest is confirmed, the rescuer should attach the AED and proceed with the algorithm.

[b] Pulse checks not required after shocks 1, 2, 4, and 5 unless "no shock indicated" message is displayed.

[c] If no shock is indicated, check pulse, repeat 1 minute of CPR, check the pulse again, and then reanalyze. After three "no shock indicated" messages are received, repeat analyze period every 1 to 2 minutes.

[d] For hypothermic patients, limit to three shocks (see Hypothemia Algorithm).

[e] In the event that VF persists after nine shocks, repeat sets of three stacked shocks with 1 minute of CPR between each set, until no shock-indicated message is received.

The approach is to shock until VF is no longer present or the patient's heart converts to a perfusing rhythm.

Sherwin Bradley

CASE 1 Continued

You open the door of the man's car. He is unconscious. You switch off his engine, pull the parking brake, and feel for a pulse. He has no carotid pulse. A passing motorist stops and yells out his car window, "I have a cellular phone, do you want me to call someone?"

You respond, "Yes! Call 911. Tell the EMS dispatcher there is a man unconscious at this address. I am beginning CPR." Several bystanders run up and help you remove the man from his car and place him face up on the ground. He is pulseless and making no respiratory efforts. You are still wearing your lab coat which contains a pocket face mask. One bystander identifies himself as a firefighter. He begins compressions while you start ventilating the man's lungs.

Why is so much emphasis being placed on early defibrillation? Why did you make an effort to call 911 and get the defibrillator moving rather than doing immediate CPR?

COMMENTS

• Call for help as soon as a cardiac arrest is recognized, before performing CPR. If the man in Case 1 is in VF, the only chance for his survival is to get a defibrillator to him before the VF deteriorates into asystole. This deterioration of VF to asystole takes only minutes.

• Cardiopulmonary resuscitation buys a few extra minutes and delays irreversible brain damage and other vital organs' tissue death. This brief interval leads to a constant focus on quick

assessment and timely arrival of people able to defibrillate. Get a defibrillator moving toward the patient, and at the same time initiate basic CPR.

• Establish an open airway, and perform effective ventilations. Defibrillation will not work without an adequate airway and effective ventilations coupled with chest compressions. Cardiopulmonary resuscitation will gain some delay in this man's dying processes. Cardiopulmonary resuscitation may allow the defibrillator to arrive before irreversible damage occurs.

Sherwin Bradley

CASE 1 Continued

A city police officer arrives and removes an AED from the trunk of her vehicle. She states, "I had a class about this thing, but have not had to use it." As an ACLS provider, you know the basic steps for operating any AED. You offer to talk the officer through the AED operation.

This scenario immediately suggests the following questions:

• *Isn't this unusual to find a city police officer carrying a defibrillator?*
• *What do you, an ACLS provider, know about AEDs?*
• *Why is learning AED operation an added requirement for all ACLS providers?*
• *What are the basic steps in operating all AEDs?*

COMMENTS

• Arrival of a defibrillator and monitor presents a major decision point in emergency cardiac care (Fig. 3-2).

• Apply AEDs only to patients who are pulseless and in full cardiac arrest.

• AEDs are proven safe and effective. AEDs have consistently demonstrated a sensitivity of over 95% for VF and VT. AEDs are more accurate at detecting VF/VT than individuals who rarely see ECGs.

• AEDs do not shock fine VF of less than 1 to 2 mm in amplitude. Ventricular fibrillation this fine may more accurately be considered "coarse asystole." Ventricular fibrillation this low in amplitude has an expected survival rate as dismal as asystole, or about 1% to 3%.

• AEDs are simple to use, but hands-on practice is required to achieve proficiency. Emergency personnel have used AEDs successfully on thousands of patients and have confirmed their technical and clinical accuracy. AEDs are one of the most extensively studied interventions in prehospital emergency cardiac care (Figs. 3-3 and 3-4).

• The best way to learn to use these devices is to practice directly with a machine. By hooking the AED to a rhythm simulator and using the controls, you will see the messages and prompts it offers and how to use the AED to deliver shocks.

• AEDs have been proven effective in a variety of settings. Since AEDs are becoming commonplace equipment in many noncritical care settings, the AHA has added practical experience with AEDs as a core requirement for ACLS courses.

Clinical Operation of All Automated External Defibrillators

Several manufacturers produce a variety of models of AEDs. More than eighteen have market approval. All connect to the patient through adhesive pads and patient cables. All display three mandatory controls: power, analyze, and shock (Fig. 3-4).

FOUR STEPS TO SHOCK WITH ALL AUTOMATED EXTERNAL DEFIBRILLATORS (Fig. 3-3)

- Turn the power on.
- Attach device to patient using adhesive pads (Fig. 3-5).
- Analyze ECG rhythm.
- Deliver a shock, if indicated.

SPECIAL FEATURES (Fig. 3-6)

- Microprocessor-based circuits that detect the ECG rhythms.
- Attachment to patients by two-function (monitoring and defibrillation) adhesive pads.
- Prompting for users: operating directions given by voice or visual cues, or both.
- Some manufacturers produce conventional defibrillators that can also operate in the automated mode by means of special adapters (Fig. 3-7).

CRITICAL SOURCES OF OPERATOR ERRORS

- Never place an AED in analyze mode unless the patient is in cardiac arrest.
- Never touch the patient during analysis of the rhythm or delivery of the shock.

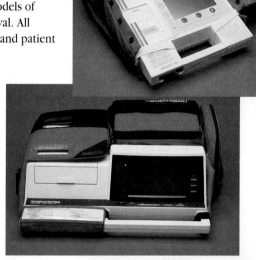
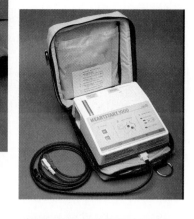
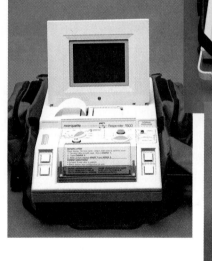
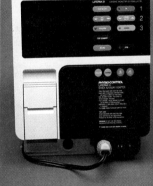
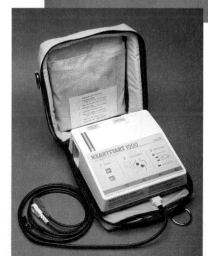

Fig. 3-4: Commercial AEDs.

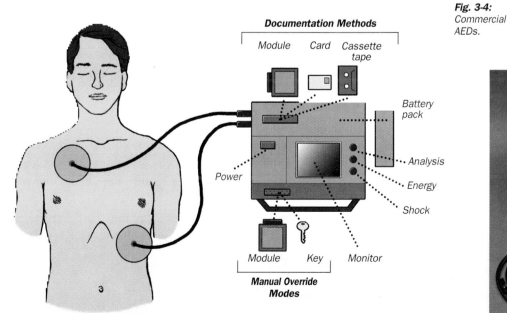

Documentation Methods

Module   Card   Cassette tape

Battery pack

Power

Analysis

Energy

Shock

Module   Key   Monitor

Manual Override Modes

Fig. 3-3: Generic automated external defibrillator (AED).

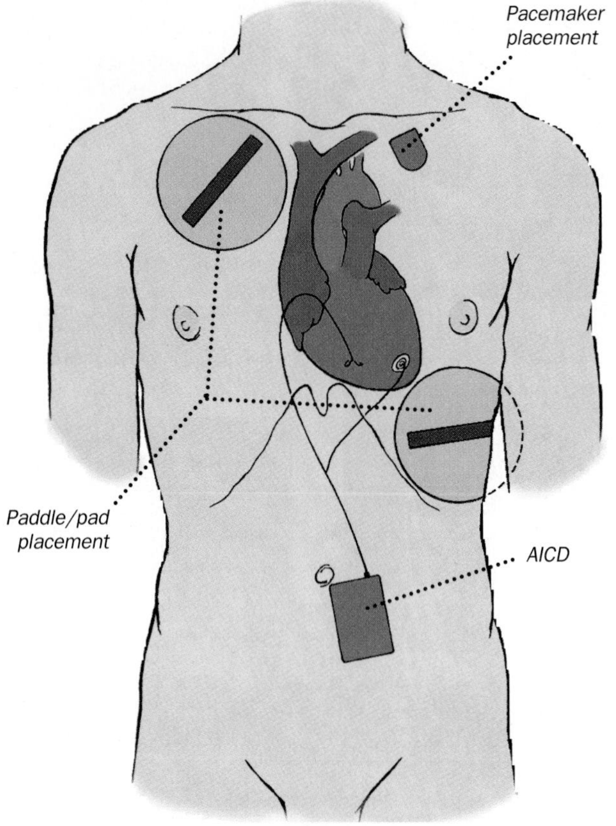

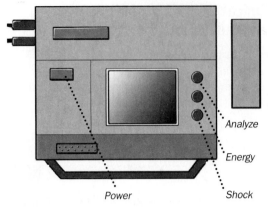

Key Defibrillator Controls

Analyze

Energy

Power

Shock

Fig. 3-6: Generic AED control panel.

Pacemaker placement

Paddle/pad placement

AICD

Fig. 3-5: Generic AED on patient's chest showing AED adhesive pad placement and typical location of implanted pacemaker. Typical location of automatic implantable cardioverter-defibrillator (AICD) is also shown.

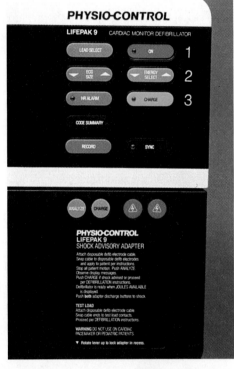

Fig. 3-7: LifePak 9 with shock advisory adapter.

Sherwin Bradley

CASE 1 Continued

The police officer places the device near the man's chest and pushes the power button (Fig. 3-8). You continue CPR, and start a verbal commentary with the police officer.

"Open that defibrillator pads package. There should be two big pads. Connect the two ends of the AED's patient cable onto the snaps on each pad. Pull off the protective pad backing and put the adhesive side on his chest—one to the right of his sternum and just below his clavicle. The other goes down over the lateral side of his heart. That's to the left of his nipple along the midaxillary line" (Fig. 3-5).

The officer gains confidence as she remembers the action sequence. She takes over directing the group. "Okay, everyone stop touching this man. Stop CPR, and get back. I'm clear, you are clear, everybody's clear." She puts the AED into analyze rhythm mode, and her eyes sweep around the group. Everyone moves back a few more inches.

How long must you stop CPR during AED analysis and shock delivery?

COMMENTS

• The time required for ECG analysis ranges from 5 to 15 seconds, with additional time required for charging (10 to 30 seconds depending on energy level and charge state of the batteries). The potential benefit of early defibrillation outweighs the harm of delaying CPR. Cardiopulmonary resuscitation will not terminate VF/VT, and even with the optimum CPR, survival possibilities decline with every passing minute.

• During ECG detection and analysis there must be *no* movement or contact with the patient (including CPR and ventilations).

• Radio and electrical signals can interfere with an AED's ability to analyze a rhythm. Unplug electric blankets, and move patients away from fluorescent lighting fixtures and radio transmitters.

• If the victim is moving at all, for example, in a vehicle, on a stretcher, or in a moving extrication basket or sled, *stop* these movements before ECG analysis. For transport ambulances this means pulling over on the side of the road and stopping the vehicle before pressing the analyze control.

• All AEDs use disposable defibrillation electrodes. These have a thin metal pad covered by a thick layer of adhesive gel. They are as effective in defibrillation as the paddles. These pads perform both monitoring and defibrillation.

• Disposable pads may be dislodged during resuscitation, especially if the patient's skin is wet, dirty, diaphoretic, or hairy.

You may need to dry or clean the chest with whatever cloth is available, and some EMS's systems even carry a surgical prep razor in case they must shave an area for electrode placement. It is a good idea to carry an extra set of these electrodes, and to replace outdated electrodes or those on which the gel is disrupted or pads are torn.

   • Do not put electrodes on top of a nitroglycerin patch. Before applying pads, remove the patch and ointment without getting any on your hands, or you may feel the drug's hypotensive effects.

• **Automated implantable cardioverter-defibrillators.** Some people at high risk for lethal arrhythmias will have automated implantable cardioverter-defibrillators (AICDs) surgically implanted in the abdomen or thorax. This AICD automatically gives shocks to VF/VT at a low energy level. Some newer devices incorporate pacemakers.

   • If someone with an AICD is unconscious, treat the situation as any other cardiac emergency. The person may require external defibrillation. Touching the person will not harm rescuers or monitoring equipment during AICD shocks.

   • Place the defibrillation pads away from the generator unit of the AICD. Automated external defibrillators perform best with the pads in anterior-anterior chest position (Fig. 3-5). Do not put adhesive defibrillation pads posteriorly unless the alternative routes appear to be consistently unsuccessful.

Sherwin Bradley

CASE 1 Continued

The AED indicates that a shock is appropriate by a voice prompt, "Press to shock!" The police officer reminds the group to "Stay back." The AED echoes her command with a similar prompt. "Stand back. Stand back!" The next tone from the machine indicates the battery is charging the capacitor for the shock. Everyone waits. Seconds seem longer than they are. You find it difficult to do nothing for this man while the AED is analyzing and charging. The officer throws out her arm in a protective gesture to keep bystanders from breaking rank and touching the patient. The man's entire body lurches with the shock. "Stay back, I'm going to try again." She switches to analyze mode a second time and gives a second shock when indicated.

What energy levels do AEDs deliver with their shocks? Why was there no pulse check between shocks?

COMMENTS

• Modern AEDs deliver standard amounts of electricity. Energy levels are programmed into the device and are usually set at the following levels:

   • 200 J for the first shock

   • 200 to 300 J for the second shock

   • 360 J for the third shock and all subsequent shocks until the device is turned off

• AEDs have to detect an ECG, charge, and shock. People must not touch the person in cardiac arrest. Operators must keep the patient clear during a 10 to 30-second interval while the devices analyzes, charges, and delivers a shock.

• There are no pulse checks between shocks for persistent VF/VT. The AED will signal if another shock is indicated. If another shock is needed after a defibrillation, it may take several seconds before a pulse is detectable.

• Shocks take priority over CPR. Although CPR delays death, electricity can actually restore the pulse.

• In persistent VF/VT, shocks should be delivered quickly, one after another, in stacked sets of three (200 J, 200 to 300 J, and 360 J). (NOTE: Once the AED gets to the 360-J energy level, all shocks will be 360 J until the device is turned off, at which point it resets to the energy level of 200 J, 200 to 300 J, and 360 J.)

Sherwin Bradley

CASE 1 Continued

The AED delivers a second shock at 200 J, and the police officer presses the analyze button again. After 15 seconds the AED voice prompt states, "Check patient!" The circle of bystanders steps forward as one deep gasp escapes from the man's lips. Another breath follows quickly, and his left hand moves. You check a carotid artery and find that there is a weak pulse. The officer takes the machine out of analyze mode, but leaves it attached with the power on.

An ALS equipped EMS vehicle arrives at the curb. Paramedics quickly walk up with oxygen tanks, drug boxes, and a conventional defibrillator. "We shocked him twice and now he has a pulse of 70!" the police officer shouts.

The paramedics attach their monitor and see an organized narrow-complex rhythm at 70 beats per minute and measure the blood pressure at 90/60 mm Hg. They apply a BVM and assist his spontaneous respirations, which have become more regular and deep. "Congratulations, officer, I think you made a difference here!"

What were the key elements for success in this scenario? What are the major sources of problems in the use of AEDs?

COMMENTS

THE CHAIN OF SURVIVAL

- The survivor's edge for the man in Case 1 came from the strong Chain of Survival in this community: early access, early CPR, early defibrillation, and early ALS. The entire system worked to save him. He had a witnessed arrest, rapid access to EMS, and people who knew what to do.

- Bystanders started effective CPR and activated the EMS system. The EMS system sprang into action. People began CPR; then a police-based early defibrillation program delivered early defibrillation. More and more communities are adopting early defibrillation programs based on public safety personnel.

- At times, however, CPR and defibrillation are not enough to save a person who has sudden cardiac death. To give such persons their best survival edge, ACLS measures are also needed: endotracheal intubation, medications, and further post-resuscitation stabilization.

KNOW YOUR DEFIBRILLATOR

Familiarity with AEDs improves performance (Fig. 3-8). Take every opportunity to examine every device you encounter. Things you want to know include the following:

- How does it analyze VF?

- How does this specific AED operate? Where is its battery?

- How does this one attach to the patient?

- What safety measures are required? How are shocks delivered?

- What messages does the AED give to the rescuers?

MAINTAIN YOUR DEFIBRILLATOR

Get ready for the next cardiac arrest. A regular professional maintenance schedule for defibrillators prevents equipment failures. A dead defibrillator means a dead patient! Operators have the responsibility to check equipment for adequate battery capacity, as well as for a fully charged spare battery, disposable supplies, and any other equipment malfunctions. After each use, restock the machine.

Appendix A provides a recommended AED maintenance checklist of what is required to keep your AED in a state of readiness.

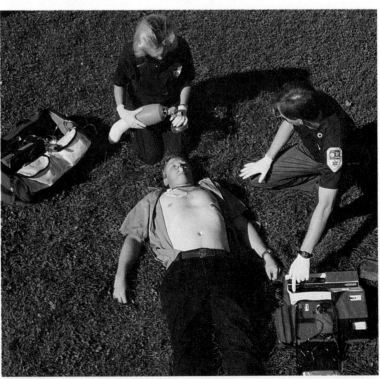

Fig. 3-8: *First responder with AED.*

DISCOVERING DEVICE PROBLEMS: DURING EQUIPMENT CHECKS OR ON THE PATIENT'S CHEST?

Many emergency cardiac care workers fail to recognize the value of routine equipment checks simply to detect device problems. Occasionally equipment problems such as component failures do occur. The purpose of the daily maintenance checks is to detect component problems in a nonclinical setting. Most reported component failures with defibrillators do not occur during clinical use but are instead *discovered* during clinical use. It makes much more sense to discover these problems during daily maintenance checks than during a resuscitation attempt.

DEFIBRILLATOR FAILURES: OPERATOR OR DEVICE?

Defibrillator failures are often attributed to problems with the device. The most common cause of defibrillator failure, however, is operator error. Operator errors include improper device attachment, incorrect operation of the controls, fail-

ure to properly maintain the device, and failure to check out the equipment before the devices are needed. Some suggested remedies follow:

- Remember the basic operation of your AED.
- Is the patient really pulseless and in need of the device?
- Think about what the AED prompts are telling you.
- Is the person correctly attached to the AED?
- Is the defibrillation pad adhering to the chest wall?
- Is the cable snapped to the pad?
- Is the cable attached to the AED?
- Is the person moving or being touched?
- Have you firmly pressed the control buttons?
- Are you following the device's directions?

Thelma Wilson

CASE 2

The Mercy Hospital x-ray room is set up down the hall from the Emergency Department. On weeknights it is staffed with a technician and sometimes an aide or volunteer. Tonight you are a lone x-ray technician working on a quiet Tuesday.

Last year during the annual BLS-CPR update you took a 2-hour class on CPR and AEDs. The well-equipped ACLS hospital code team realized they often arrive too late to help people who collapse outside of critical care areas. AEDs are now strategically located throughout the noncritical care hospital areas and clinics. Mercy Hospital's goal is to follow the AHA recommendation that patients should have a defibrillator available within 1 to 2 minutes of their collapse.

The Emergency Department is busy. You are helping to transport a 60-year-old woman with abdominal pain to the radiology department for radiographs. She leans forward in the wheelchair in obvious discomfort and does not want to talk. She asks to use the bathroom before the procedure. She walks into the restroom and closes the door. In 30 seconds you hear a loud crash. You rush through the door and immediately see that Mrs. Wilson has crumpled to the bathroom floor. She appears unconscious, without movements and with no immediate signs of breathing.

You are alone, with no one immediately available to help. You can perform CPR or go and retrieve the AED that is down the hall.

What would you do at this point?

COMMENTS

THE "LONE RESCUER" WITH AN AUTOMATED EXTERNAL DEFIBRILLATOR

Case 2 presents the challenge of the "lone rescuer." The single rescuer, prepared to start CPR and to operate an AED, faces unique decisions. You must respond to this person, who obviously needs immediate help, and yet you also must summon additional assistance. The recommended action sequence for the lone rescuer trained to do both CPR and automated defibrillation (these recommendations are consistent with the AHA Guidelines) is as follows:

- Assess responsiveness. If unresponsive, do the following:
  - Call out locally for help. (Shout "Help!")
  - **A**—Open the airway. (Don gloves and retrieve pocket mask.)
  - **B**—Give two slow breaths (to confirm open airway).
  - **C**—Confirm pulselessness.
  - **D**—Retrieve and operate the defibrillator.

Many scenarios and variations are possible. For example, what do you do if no one responds to the first local call for help? When do you break away to seek a telephone to activate the in-hospital code team or the 911 system? How much CPR is needed before getting the AED? There is no "best" answer for all possible scenarios. Common sense must come into play.

Experts have debated whether the next step should be a period of CPR or whether the rescuer should leave the patient to retrieve the defibrillator. A minute of CPR, for example, would provide benefit to patients in non-VF rhythms. For patients in VF, however, any delay in defibrillation, even for CPR, is detrimental.

The AHA recommends verification of full cardiac arrest through steps A, B, and C. Once a full arrest is confirmed, the rescuer should place the highest priority on retrieving the AED. An initial period of CPR should not take precedence over the "hunt for VF."

Thelma Wilson

CASE 2 Continued

After verifying full cardiac arrest you position Mrs. Wilson in the hall by gently pulling her a few feet. A few steps down the hall you grab an AED "minicode kit."

The night-shift security guard has responded to your initial cry for help. "Clarence, call a code. Call paging and tell them we have a cardiac arrest in radiology!" You bring the AED to where Mrs. Wilson lies and operate it, using the following steps of AED operation:

Turn power on.

Attach electrodes.

Analyze cardiac rhythm.

Shock up to three shocks if indicated.

You carefully avoid any contact with the patient during the analysis and shock. The AED provides three shocks in a row, at which point you check for a pulse. When no pulse is detected, you return to CPR . After 1 minute of CPR you check for a pulse again, and when none is detected, you press the analyze button again. You deliver three more shocks.

Soon you hear the rumble of the code cart being pushed down the hall. There is still no pulse, as six people crowd into the hallway. "Shock again while we set up," directs Stacey, the code team leader. The woman jerks with the next shock. You begin chest compressions while the respiratory therapist ventilates using the BVM with 100% oxygen.

"Okay, let's see what ECG she has now." Stacey pushes the AED button, which turns the device into a manual defibrillator with an ECG display. "She has a rhythm! Does it produce a pulse?"

COMMENTS

- Automated external defibrillation, like CPR, is now a BLS skill for all first responders. For in-hospital settings the "principle of early defibrillation" means that nonphysician personnel, including floor nursing personnel, should be trained and equipped to perform defibrillation. This guideline is considered the standard of care not only in the community, but also within the hospital.

- Automated external defibrillation technology has developed a wide variety of electronic features such as ECG displays, event data collection methods and the ability to change energy and also to use the device as a manual defibrillator.

- Future additions may include transcutaneous pacing, measurement of physical parameters such oxygen saturation level, estimates of time interval from collapse, and even automatic dialing of 911.

- Automated external defibrillation technology makes possible widespread application of the principle of early defibrillation and should be recognized and understood by all emergency cardiac care providers as core information.

- When ACLS personnel arrive on the scene, patient treatment responsibility shifts from personnel using AEDs to personnel using the advanced resuscitation interventions. The following general rules clarify the interaction:

  - ACLS providers have scene authority over the team and patient.

  - ACLS providers should use the attached AED as the defibrillator of choice for additional shocks and as a manual defibrillator whenever possible.

  - ACLS providers should incorporate the AED operators into the resuscitation efforts, assigning roles such as monitoring, performing CPR, and performing further defibrillations.

  - ACLS providers should count shocks delivered by AEDs as part of the total ACLS treatment of the patient. They should proceed at once to intubation and intravenous access upon arrival if the AED has already been delivering shocks.

  - ACLS providers should remove the AED only when required for patient transfer or ECG monitoring.

• After each use of an AED, responsible personnel should do the following:

  • Restock supplies (defibrillator pads, gauze pads, razors, rhythm paper, cassette tapes, and event documentation modules) in the AED "crash cart."

  • Review AED maintenance checklist (see Appendix A).

  • Complete required code incident reports.

  • Participate in a formal critique with the code team and other AED and BLS-trained personnel.

KEY POINTS

SUMMARY

• Defibrillation with AEDs serves as a critical intervention for people in the first moments of reversible death. AEDs provide a technological breakthrough that allows early defibrillation in settings never before possible and by responders never before permitted.

• The well-trained, competent ACLS provider must know and be familiar with these devices and know how to operate them should an emergency arise.

• Many hospitals are learning that their in-hospital response times and the intervals between patient collapse and shock delivery are embarassingly long. In-hospital early defibrillation programs provide an innovative way to use this new technology to provide earlier defibrillation and to save more lives.

• In addition, AEDs are being adopted by public safety early defibrillation programs. These programs use personnel such as firefighters, police officers, highway patrolmen, and security personnel, as well as emergency medical technicians and emergency first responders. AEDs, however, will only perform successfully if they are incorporated in the ABCD sequence of patient care.

• While managing each patient in cardiac arrest you should:

• Follow the Five Quadrads approach:

  • **Primary ABCD Survey**

  • **Secondary ABCD Survey**

  • **Oxygen/IV/Monitor/Fluids**

  • **Vital signs: Temperature/Heart rate/Bloodpressure/Respirations**

  • **Cardiovascular Quadrad: Tank/Resistance/Pump/Rate**

• During the Secondary Survey you will also accomplish the following:

  • **Intubation**

  • **Obtain brief initial history**

  • **Perform a focused physical examination**

  • **Start oxygen, obtain IV access, identify the rhythm**

  • **Attach pulse oximeter and automatic blood pressure when indicated and available**

  • **Order and review ECG for rhythm diagnosis and exclusion of ischemia/infarction**

• Adult VF cardiac arrest occupies a prominent position in all ACLS training. This prominence reflects a simple statistical reality: most non-traumatic sudden deaths are due to VF; the only way to effectively reverse VF is through early defibrillation.

• This rationale supports the current strong emphasis on automated external defibrillation. Giving this technology to a broad range of responders offers the key to treating adult VF early and definitively.

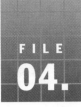

Mega-Ventricular Fibrillation
Refractory Ventricular Fibrillation

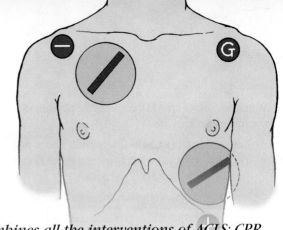

OVERVIEW

"Mega–ventricular fibrillation (mega-VF)" combines all the interventions of ACLS: CPR, defibrillation, endotracheal intubation, and intravenous (IV) medications. "Mega-VF" echoes the ACLS term "megacode," which is used to refer to the "large" (or "mega") resuscitation attempts in which rescuers must provide all ACLS treatments.

The mega-VF cases include patients in ventricular fibrillation or pulseless ventricular tachycardia (VF/pulseless VT), who do not respond to the first round of defibrillatory shocks. They remain in VF/pulseless VT despite CPR and defibrillation. These patients require you to make rapid decisions and perform interventions in an organized manner. CPR, defibrillation, rhythm recognition, advanced ventilation, and drug administration create an intimately entwined resuscitation sequence.

The longer a person remains in VF/VT, the worse the clinical prognosis becomes. When, despite your best initial efforts, you are unable to eliminate VF/VT, you must ask, "Why?". The D of the Secondary Survey reminds you to focus on the "differential diagnosis." Why is this person still in VF? How can we reverse this process of dying? What caused this cardiac arrest? What actions must we take while we consider possible causes?

Mega-VF cases can be thought of as the "putting it all together" cases. This is where all ACLS interventions are brought to bear on the major cause of adult sudden cardiac arrest—VF/VT.

MAJOR CONCEPTS TO MASTER

- Learn the Universal Algorithm.
- Learn the Primary and Secondary ABCD Survey Approach (for patients in full cardiac arrest).
- Apply the Five Quadrads approach for patients in full cardiac arrest and patients in the "peri-cardiac arrest period" and in the post-resuscitation period.
- Learn to perform endotracheal intubation.
- Learn the VF/VT Algorithm sequence (Fig. 4-1).
- Learn an organized team approach to ACLS care.
- Learn to perform defibrillation safely and effectively.
- Learn to obtain IV access for the cardiac arrest patient.
- Learn the "Why?" "When?" "How?" and "Watch out!" for the medications used in refractory VF: (epinephrine, lidocaine, bretylium, procainamide, magnesium sulfate, and sodium bicarbonate).
- Learn the sequence of IV/drug bolus/flush/elevate.
- Learn to consider the major causes of refractory VF/VT.
- Learn immediate post-resuscitation care of patients who regain a spontaneous pulse.

Critical actions

Every case of persistent VF/VT requires that you do the following:

- Perform the Primary and Secondary ABCD Surveys.

- Rapidly defibrillate VF and VT, using either a manual defibrillator or an automated external defibrillator (AED).

- Provide effective CPR, interrupting only for intubation, defibrillation, and essential patient or personnel movements.

- Maintain the airway (A) and ventilations (B) with non-invasive airway adjuncts until able to perform endotracheal intubation.

- Perform endotracheal intubation both to stabilize the airway and to provide a route for drug delivery.

- Obtain IV access.

- Administer appropriate resuscitation medications when indicated, in the proper dose and manner.

- Defibrillate rapidly after each drug if VF or VT remains.

- Systematically consider the possible reversible causes of the arrest and major reasons why the VF is unresponsive to defibrillation.

- Participate skillfully, effectively, and professionally in all resuscitation attempts.

- Master each role in the mega-VF cases: team leader, CPR provider, airway maintenance, defibrillator and monitor, IV access, and drug administration.

Skills and procedures to learn

- The Primary and Secondary ABCD Surveys

- Recognition of VF/VT in its many variations (near-asystole, fine, medium, coarse, and extra coarse) (Figs. 4-2 and 4-3)

- How to operate a defibrillator and monitor to obtain rapid rhythm assessment (by means of three-lead ECG monitor and "quick-look" paddles)

- How to operate standard manual defibrillators to deliver countershocks

- How to maintain operator safety during defibrillation

- How to maintain your defibrillator in a state of readiness

- How to troubleshoot the most common defibrillator problems

- Advanced airway maintenance (endotracheal intubation, suctioning, tube confirmation, and tube fixation)

- Intravenous access techniques

- How to prepare and administer the six (Class II) pharmacologic agents used for persistent VF/VT

Rhythms to learn

The following "arrhythmias" may occur with many variations, often in the same patient:

- Ventricular fibrillation (fine, medium, coarse, and extra coarse) (Fig. 4-2)

- Ventricular tachycardia

- Artifactual ECG signals that may be mistaken for VF (loose leads, CPR artifact, radio transmissions, and 60-cycle electrical interference)

Medications to learn

Bretylium	Magnesium sulfate
Epinephrine	Procainamide
Lidocaine	Sodium bicarbonate

Nelson Gore

CASE 1

The emergency medical dispatcher sends your ALS mobile intensive care unit to an emergency reported as a "man down." You and your partner hear that it was a witnessed arrest of a man who is 50 years old. His wife, a nurse, is performing CPR. As you move through the open front door, she yells, "What took you so long?" She continues to compress and ventilate, tears streaming down her face. He is not breathing, although she manages to get his chest to rise with each mouth-to-mouth ventilation. You feel a femoral pulse with each of the wife's chest compressions. You place your equipment on the living room carpet: a drug box, an ACLS ventilation kit, and a defibrillator and monitor.

What are your priorities here? What are the first things you are going to do?

The Five Quadrads approach

- You should begin every resuscitation attempt in a systematic manner. We recommend the *Five Quadrads approach* and follow that approach throughout this book.

- The Five Quadrads approach is the most comprehensive approach to cardiopulmonary emergencies because it incorporates the following systematic techniques:

  - Primary ABCD Survey

  - Secondary ABCD Survey

  - Universal Algorithm

- The power of the Five Quadrads approach is that it applies to every cardiopulmonary emergency and is not limited just to people in full cardiac arrest. In addition, the Five Quadrads approach, with only slight modifications, can cover a large variety of special resuscitation situations. These modifications are presented in Chapters 10 to16 in this book.

- The first quadrad is the Primary ABCD Survey. Notice that this survey incorporates much of the Universal Algorithm.

PRIMARY ABCD SURVEY

A—Airway. Open the airway.

B—Breathing. Provide positive-pressure ventilations.

C—Circulation. Give chest compressions.

D—Defibrillation. Shock VF/VT.

- Defibrillation (D) moves you to the VF/VT Algorithm (Fig. 4-1). After the first three shocks, you branch into either persistent VF/VT (Figs. 4-2 and 4-3), return of spontaneous circulation, pulseless electrical activity (PEA), or asystole.

- Even though the wife appears to be providing effective CPR, you cannot assume that the Primary ABCs are acceptable. You should ask her to briefly stop CPR so that you can verify breathlessness, pulselessness, and the need to continue CPR. You then should move immediately to determine whether Mr. Gore is in VF/VT.

- The AHA emphasis on early defibrillation does not mean that you can neglect the basics of airway, breathing, and circulation. A responsible team leader always makes sure that other team members are providing good basic care. In the scenario in Case 1, you have only two helpers—the wife, who is doing CPR, and your paramedic partner. Direct the wife to continue chest compressions, and direct your partner to take over airway management.

- Your partner should insert an oropharyngeal airway and begin bag-valve-mask (BVM) ventilations (or pocket face mask) with 100% oxygen attached.

  You can make other combinations of job assignments. (For example, your partner could assume all CPR efforts and let the wife stop and rest.)

- You should maintain the "hunt for VF" constantly in your mind.

- Any resuscitation team has the responsibility to properly attach the defibrillator monitor or the quick-look paddles within 30 to 60 seconds of arriving on the scene, whether out of hospital or in hospital.

Nelson Gore

CASE 1 Continued

You place the defibrillator and monitor on the floor, by the left ear of the patient. Your partner inserts an oropharyngeal airway and places a BVM over the patient's mouth and nose. He attaches the oxygen tube from the tank to the oxygen inlet on the bag. He begins ventilations in a 5-to-1 ratio with the wife's chest compressions.
What are the steps to follow in operating all currently available, conventional defibrillators?

- Perhaps the most important question in emergency cardiac care is the following: *Do you know how to operate your defibrillator?*

- The *number 1 cause of defibrillation errors* is lack of operator familiarity with the equipment. You cannot respond correctly if you have not learned to operate your defibrillator. Both you and the defibrillator must be ready for action.

- Go over any defibrillator you expect to operate, referring to the recommended daily maintenance checklist (Appendix B). Know all the following major operation controls on your device:

  - Power button (labeled "1" on most defibrillators)

- Energy selection dial (labeled "2" on most defibrillators)

- Charge switch (labeled "3" on most defibrillators)

- Discharge controls (both on device face and on paddles)

- Lead select switch

- Size of the ECG

- Synchronization controls

- Patient-monitor cable

- Note that these controls are standard on all available conventional defibrillators. This does not mean that once you have learned to use one product you therefore know every product. This just means that with review, you can locate each of these controls on any device.

FIGURE 4-1

Ventricular Fibrillation and Pulseless Ventricular Tachycardia Algorithm

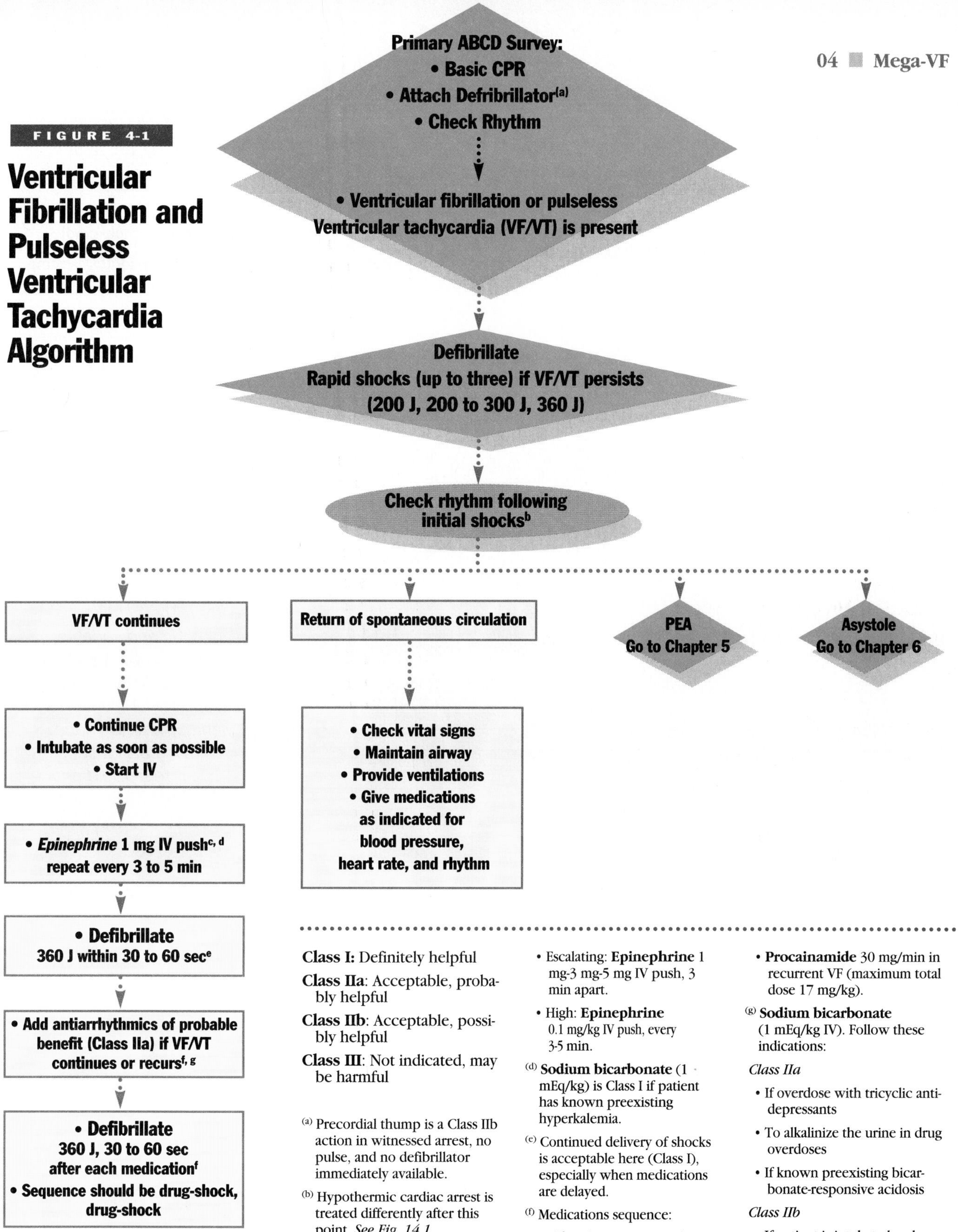

Primary ABCD Survey:
- Basic CPR
- Attach Defribrillator[a]
- Check Rhythm

↓

- Ventricular fibrillation or pulseless Ventricular tachycardia (VF/VT) is present

↓

Defibrillate
Rapid shocks (up to three) if VF/VT persists
(200 J, 200 to 300 J, 360 J)

↓

Check rhythm following initial shocks[b]

VF/VT continues	**Return of spontaneous circulation**	**PEA** Go to Chapter 5	**Asystole** Go to Chapter 6

VF/VT continues path:

- Continue CPR
- Intubate as soon as possible
- Start IV

↓

- *Epinephrine* 1 mg IV push[c, d] repeat every 3 to 5 min

↓

- **Defibrillate** 360 J within 30 to 60 sec[e]

↓

- Add antiarrhythmics of probable benefit (Class IIa) if VF/VT continues or recurs[f, g]

↓

- **Defibrillate** 360 J, 30 to 60 sec after each medication[f]
- Sequence should be drug-shock, drug-shock

Return of spontaneous circulation path:

- Check vital signs
- Maintain airway
- Provide ventilations
- Give medications as indicated for blood pressure, heart rate, and rhythm

---

Class I: Definitely helpful

Class IIa: Acceptable, probably helpful

Class IIb: Acceptable, possibly helpful

Class III: Not indicated, may be harmful

[a] Precordial thump is a Class IIb action in witnessed arrest, no pulse, and no defibrillator immediately available.

[b] Hypothermic cardiac arrest is treated differently after this point. *See Fig. 14.1.*

[c] The recommended dose of **epinephrine** is 1 mg IV push every 3-5 min. If spontaneous circulation does not return consider several Class IIb dosing regimens:

- Intermediate: **Epinephrine** 2-5 mg IV push, every 3-5 min.

- Escalating: **Epinephrine** 1 mg-3 mg-5 mg IV push, 3 min apart.

- High: **Epinephrine** 0.1 mg/kg IV push, every 3-5 min.

[d] **Sodium bicarbonate** (1 mEq/kg) is Class I if patient has known preexisting hyperkalemia.

[e] Continued delivery of shocks is acceptable here (Class I), especially when medications are delayed.

[f] Medications sequence:

- **Lidocaine** 1.0-1.5 mg/kg IV push. Repeat in 3-5 min to maximum dose of 3 mg/kg. A single 1.5 mg/kg dose in cardiac arrest is also acceptable.

- **Bretylium** 5 mg/kg IV push. Repeat in 5 min at 10 mg/kg.

- **Magnesium sulfate** 1-2 g IV in torsades de pointes, suspected hypomagnesemic state, or refractory VF.

- **Procainamide** 30 mg/min in recurrent VF (maximum total dose 17 mg/kg).

[g] **Sodium bicarbonate** (1 mEq/kg IV). Follow these indications:

Class IIa

- If overdose with tricyclic antidepressants

- To alkalinize the urine in drug overdoses

- If known preexisting bicarbonate-responsive acidosis

Class IIb

- If patient is intubated and arrest continues for long intervals

- If circulation restored after prolonged arrest

Class III

- Hypoxic lactic acidosis

- Whether you can locate each control quickly and easily depends on practice that you *must* perform prior to an actual cardiac arrest. A critical rule in emergency cardiac care is the following:

  Do not meet your defibrillator for the first time at the side of a patient who needs you to know what you are doing.

- Since the controls are standard (Fig. 4-4), the steps of operation, as follows, are standard:
  - Turn power on (switch 1).
  - Remove the quick-look paddles from their cradle.
  - Place the lead select switch on the "paddles" setting.

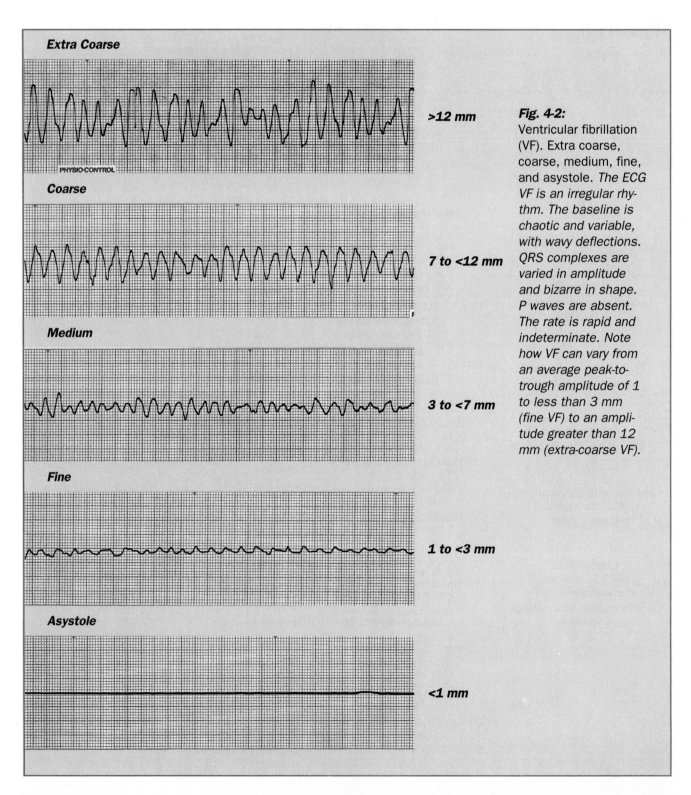

Extra Coarse — >12 mm

Coarse — 7 to <12 mm

Medium — 3 to <7 mm

Fine — 1 to <3 mm

Asystole — <1 mm

Fig. 4-2: Ventricular fibrillation (VF). Extra coarse, coarse, medium, fine, and asystole. *The ECG VF is an irregular rhythm. The baseline is chaotic and variable, with wavy deflections. QRS complexes are varied in amplitude and bizarre in shape. P waves are absent. The rate is rapid and indeterminate. Note how VF can vary from an average peak-to-trough amplitude of 1 to less than 3 mm (fine VF) to an amplitude greater than 12 mm (extra-coarse VF).*

- Apply defibrillator gel to the paddles (or apply adhesive chest pads).

- Place the paddles in a "sternal-lateral" position on the patient's chest (Fig. 4-5).

- Direct other personnel to stop all contact with the patient while you assess the rhythm on the monitor screen (Fig. 4-6).

- If VF/VT: Select energy level by pressing energy select switch (switch 2).

- Charge the defibrillator to selected energy level by pressing charge switch (switch 3).

- Deliver shock by pressing shock control buttons.

- Details on the use of a defibrillator with quick-look paddles or with attached monitor leads are presented in the box on p. 64.

What about the precordial thump? Should that be performed early in all resuscitation attempts? The ACLS Guidelines indicate the precordial thump as an acceptable, possibly helpful action in witnessed arrest with no pulse, and if you lack a defibrillator. The issue, for which we lack a clear answer, is simple: *Is the precordial thump just as likely to make a bad rhythm good as it is to make a good rhythm bad?* We do not know the answer. The AHA recommendation is "Why not do a precordial thump?" when you lack a defibrillator, and "Why do one?" when you do have a defibrillator.

THE OVERALL TREATMENT SEQUENCE FOR VF/VT IS SIMPLE

- **Cardiopulmonary resuscitation:** Perform CPR at all times when indicated unless performing other resuscitation interventions.

- **Defibrillation:** Defibrillate VF/VT if present.

- **Endotracheal Intubation:** Perform endotracheal intubation as follows:

    To protect the airway

    To ventilate the patient's lungs

- **Medications:** Administer drugs (which act only as adjuncts to defibrillation).

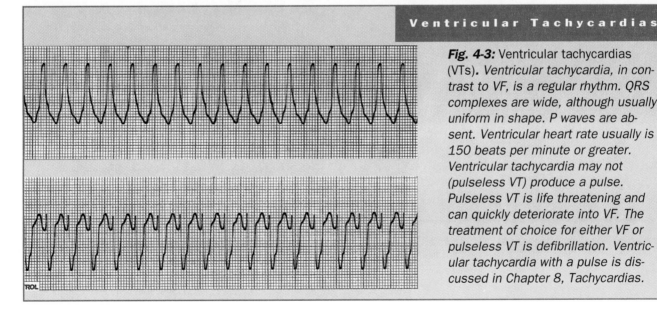

Ventricular Tachycardias

Fig. 4-3: Ventricular tachycardias (VTs). *Ventricular tachycardia, in contrast to VF, is a regular rhythm. QRS complexes are wide, although usually uniform in shape. P waves are absent. Ventricular heart rate usually is 150 beats per minute or greater. Ventricular tachycardia may not (pulseless VT) produce a pulse. Pulseless VT is life threatening and can quickly deteriorate into VF. The treatment of choice for either VF or pulseless VT is defibrillation. Ventricular tachycardia with a pulse is discussed in Chapter 8, Tachycardias.*

BOX 4-1

Steps To Follow for Conventional Defibrillators

CONTROLS

Before you ever get close to a real patient with a defibrillator take a look at the controls. During a crisis you can make many little (and some big) mistakes because you do not know how to operate your device (Fig. 4-4).

SEQUENCE OF ACTIONS FOR MANUAL DEFIBRILLATION

- *Attach the ECG monitor to the patient if assessing the rhythm through monitor leads:* **white** *to right shoulder,* **red** *over lower left ribs, and* **black** *or* **green** *lead to left shoulder.*

- *Turn the power on.*

- *Select lead I, II, or III on the lead selector switch (or select "paddles" if using quick-look paddles to assess the rhythm).*

- *Select the energy level (200 J, 300 J, or 360 J).*

- *Apply a conductive material to the paddles or chest.*

- *(If using quick-look paddles, you would now place the paddles firmly against the chest to assess the rhythm. Lead selector switch must be on "paddles" and not on "lead I, II, or III").*

- *Press the charge button. (NOTE: Charging is recommended* **before** *assessing the rhythm. This is to save time. Some protocols suggest delaying the charging until after the rhythm assessment. This ensures greater safety. Both approaches are acceptable.)*

- *Stop CPR and patient contact. ("Clear" the patient.)*

- *Assess the ECG rhythm.*

- *Place paddles firmly on the chest in the sternal-apex position (Fig. 4-5); use 25 pounds of pressure.*

- *Safety: Clear all persons including yourself from patient contact.*

- *Press both discharge buttons at once.*

SAFETY

- *Use a clearing chant for defibrillation. Announce loudly*

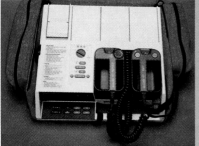

Fig. 4-4: *A conventional portable defibrillator.*

something similar to the following chant before each shock:

- *"I'll shock on three. One, I am clear."*

- *"Two, you're clear."*

- *"Three, everybody's clear." Look around to be sure no one is touching the patient or stretcher.*

Defibrillate up to three times (200 J, 200 to 300 J, and 360 J). Recharge with the paddles on the chest. Multiple-sequenced shocks (200 J, 200 to 300 J, and 360 J) are acceptable (Class I), especially when ACLS drugs are delayed.

No pulse checks are required between shocks for persistent ventricular fibrillation. Do not take the time to check for a pulse if the monitor continues to display VF/VT, as this will delay rhythm assessment. Push the charge control as soon as a shock is delivered. Do not stop for a pulse check; it will delay rhythm assessment if the monitor is still hooked up and displays persistent VF/VT. This does not mean a pulse check is prohibited between shocks, just that pauses for pulse checks are not required if the patient is properly connected and continues to display VF/VT.

Leave paddles on chest while recharging. While recharging the defibrillators, check for persistent VF/VT. Take the paddles from the chest (leave adhesive pads in place) and disarm the defibrillator. Then, check for a pulse.

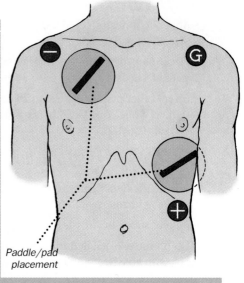

Paddle/pad placement

Fig. 4-5: *Correct lead placement and correct manual paddle placement.*

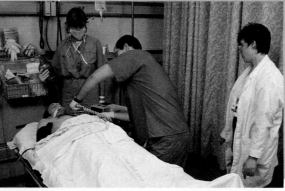

Fig. 4-6: *Person performing defibrillation with conventional defibrillator paddles.*

PADDLE OR PADS AND PLACEMENT ISSUES

- Nitroglycerin patches: If the patient has a nitroglycerin patch on his or her chest, remove it or make sure the defibrillation electrode does not touch the patch. The patches do not conduct electrical current effectively and have been known to cause electrical arcing.

- Nitroglycerin paste: EMS providers should have on gloves to prevent contact with nitroglycerin paste; otherwise, they may experience a nitroglycerin-induced headache or hypotension.

- Implanted pacemakers or cardioverter-defibrillators (AICDs): Avoid putting defibrillator pads or paddles over the generator unit of implanted pacemakers or AICDs. When possible, place pads or paddles more than 5 inches away from these sites.

AUTOMATED IMPLANTABLE
CARDIOVERTER-DEFIBRILLATORS (SEE BOX 4-2)

- These implantable devices are becoming more common, and most EMS and emergency care providers will encounter patients with AICDs.

- Always apply standard care protocols to these patients, even if they appear to be receiving a series of shocks from their devices.

- If you are touching someone, you can sometimes feel small discharges from their AICD during a shock, but there is little chance of harm to you.

- The patient or bystanders may tell you that the implantable defibrillator has discharged or is in the midst of a charge-discharge cycle. If so, wait 30 to 60 seconds following the last discharge before proceeding with VF/VT protocols. This wait allows the device to complete any assessment-treatment cycle that it may be conducting and prevents personnel from interfering.

DEFIBRILLATION ENERGY LEVELS

For VF/VT, defibrillation energy levels are as follows:

- 200 J: First shock
- 200 to 300 J: Second shock
- 360 J: Third shock

(If the person refibrillates, defibrillate at the same energy level that was used for the last successful shock.)

THE PURPOSE OF DEFIBRILLATION

- The purpose of a defibrillation is to stop all electrical activity in the heart—to place the heart in complete electrical silence—that is, to produce asystole. This electrical "stunning" of the heart eliminates the chaotic activity of the VF. During this postshock asystolic pause the natural pacemaker centers of the heart should recover and take over spontaneous, coordinated contractile activity.

- The recovery is difficult, however, if the fibrillating myocardium has exhausted the energy stores. If all stored energy is depleted during the period of prolonged fibrillation, the natural pacemaker centers will be incapable of recovery and taking over spontaneous beating.

- The emphasis on rapid defibrillation is really a "fuel conservation" message.

- The heart must be defibrillated before all the energy stores are gone. Since the fibrillating myocardium uses up energy stores at an alarming rate, there simply is not much time. Eliminating VF early saves myocardial energy and leaves something to drive the normal heartbeat.

Nelson Gore

CASE 1 Continued

Two firefighters arrive to help. As they don gloves, you direct one to take over chest compressions and the other to continue with the BVM ventilations. Mr. Gore does not respond to three rapid countershocks, oxygenation, and CPR. His ECG rhythm is still VF.

Defibrillation and CPR have not worked. Where are you now in the Five Quadrads? How would you proceed from this point?

COMMENTS

You have now completed the Primary Survey in ACLS. You have assessed for VF/VT in a pulseless patient and delivered three defibrillatory shocks. He now requires multiple interventions. His chances for survival are dwindling as the minutes pass.

At this point in the VF/VT Algorithm you must think in terms of the Secondary Survey. The intervention sequence is as follows.

SECONDARY ABCD SURVEY

- Airway: Establish advanced airway control; perform endotracheal intubation.

- Breathing: Assess adequacy of ventilations via endotracheal tube.

- Circulation: Continue CPR and defibrillation; obtain IV access for fluids and medications; provide rhythm-appropriate cardiovascular drugs.

- Differential diagnosis: Consider and identify possible reversible causes for the arrest.

Advanced Cardiac Life Support and Automated Implantable Cardioverter-Defibrillators

WHY?

People at risk for recurrent malignant ventricular tachyarrhythmias may get a surgically implanted automated cardioverter-defibrillator (AICD). Some ICDs have a pacemaker function as well. Patients usually carry a card defining the specifics of the device and giving contact numbers for their physician.

WHEN?

- The AICDs constantly monitor for lethal rhythms such as VF, VT, and profound bradycardia. If VF/VT is detected by the device, it will verify the lethal arrhythmia by several additional analytic steps. During this analysis time the patient usually becomes unconscious and collapses.

- The device will analyze and deliver shocks as long as VF/VT is present. (Some AICDs may be programmed to deliver a set number of shocks.)

HOW?

- The AICD pulse generator is usually located in the left or right upper abdominal quadrant. The two electrodes provide multiple functions: sensing, defibrillation (for VF), cardioversion (for VT), and pacing (for bradycardia or overdrive pacing for tachycardia).

- One electrode is threaded transvenously into the base of the right ventricle. The other electrode is sewn directly onto the pericardial surface of the heart. (Newer models have the treating electrode tunneled under the skin and placed subcutaneously over the heart, but outside the chest wall.)

- Shocks from an AICD are at low energy (2 to 5 J). While these low-energy shocks may be painful to a conscious patient, they will not harm people who touch the patient while providing CPR or other care. In fact, most of these shocks cannot even be felt by the person in contact with the patient. Automated implantable cardioverter-defibrillators will not harm monitoring devices or external defibrillation equipment.

RECOMMENDED TREATMENT GUIDELINES FOR UNCONSCIOUS PATIENTS WITH AN AICD

- Apply the Primary ABCD Survey, assessing airway, breathing, and circulation and performing CPR as follows:

- Apply the external monitor-defibrillator.

- Assess the ECG rhythm.

- Deliver defibrillatory shocks per standard guidelines, unless a discharge from the AICD is observed. (This will be displayed as a modest, sudden thoracic movement, if at all; the monitor screen will also reveal a sharp, upward deflection indicating the shock delivery.) Conventional defibrillatory shocks will not harm the AICD.

- If an AICD discharge is observed, wait 30 seconds after the last AICD shock. This waiting period allows the AICD to repeat its rhythm assessment and deliver further shocks per the AICD treatment algorithm. Allow these AICD shocks to continue until the rhythm is no longer VF or the device does not appear to be responding anymore. (The patient's rhythm status and response of the AICD are easily observed if the patient is attached to a monitor.)

- If VF/VT persists, change the placement of the external paddles or pads. (Sometimes, internal electrodes will shield the myocardium from the full force of the external shock.) If you are using an anterior sternal-apex pathway, switch to an anterior-posterior pathway unless you have an AED. An AED's defibrillator pads must remain anterior but can be repositioned.

- Continue the code following the VF/VT Algorithm.

WATCH OUT!

- The biggest precaution for patients with AICDs is the following: Always provide them with standard, aggressive ACLS.

- Do not be afraid of harmful AICD shocks to the resuscitation team. These will not occur.

- Allow some time for the AICD to "do its thing." Often the AICD is the most effective intervention. The balance to achieve is to allow the AICD time for assessment and treatment, but to not delay standard airway management, ventilation, CPR, and IV medications.

Nelson Gore

CASE 1 Continued

Your partner proceeds with endotracheal intubation. He sprawls prone on the floor, stretched out on his abdomen, supporting his upper body with his elbows. He successfully intubates the man's trachea, which is confirmed by distinct bilateral breath sounds at the midaxillary line on each side, plus a silent epigastrium. Your partner secures the endotracheal tube and continues ventilations. Your partner states, "Let's try starting an IV; he still looks like he has good veins."

Technically speaking, you should be in charge of this code, but your partner appears to anticipate all your orders and keeps moving forward with the protocols. Who is in charge here? Should he be anticipating all the interventions without waiting for orders from the team leader?

CODE ORGANIZATION

- In such scenarios as in Case 1 the prehospital team of two responders has usually made advanced agreements regarding who will be in charge. Prearrival understandings are standard procedures in EMS systems. The team leader should be designated or understood in advance for in-hospital resuscitations as well.

The team leader has the following major responsibilities:

- To assign tasks
- To ensure that each rescuer performs his or her tasks safely and effectively
- To order interventions according to protocols
- To think about why the person arrested and possible reversible causes

- Sometimes the designated team leader arrives after other rescuers have initiated the resuscitation attempt, most often, CPR and defibrillation. The team leader should still perform the Primary and Secondary Surveys, reviewing who is doing what and how effectively. This can be done verbally, by asking about the status of each part of the ABCD Surveys.

- The leader of the resuscitation team also must assign the four critical tasks of resuscitation (Fig. 4-7) as more and more personnel become available. These tasks are as follows:

- Airway and intubation
- Chest compressions
- Defibrillation and monitoring
- Intravenous access

- The preceding list reflects the priority of the tasks. If less than four team members are present, follow the order of priorities listed next:

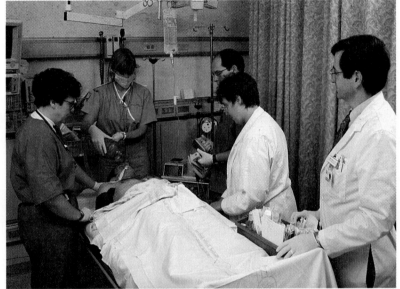

Fig. 4-7: *Leader always assigns four jobs: (1) airway and ventilation; (2) chest compressions; (3) IV access; and (4) defibrillations.*

- *One person*: Person A does basic CPR (airway, breathing, and chest compressions).
- *Two people:* Person A does basic CPR; person B does monitoring and defibrillation.
- *Three people:* Person A does CPR; person B does defibrillation; person C does airway management, including endotracheal intubation. (Person B moves to IV access when able.)
- *Four people:* Person A does basic CPR; person B, defibrillation; person C, airway management, including endotracheal intubation; person D, IV access and medications.
- *Five people:* Same as four people, with the fifth person assuming role of leader.

Nelson Gore

CASE 1 Continued

After CPR and defibrillation, you moved immediately to endotracheal intubation and ventilation. In the past it seemed that the ACLS provider had a choice between endotracheal intubation and starting an IV line. Here, however, the sequence clearly puts intubation before IV medications. Why?

- After CPR and three defibrillation attempts, the team leader assigns a qualified rescuer to perform endotracheal intubation.

- Endotracheal intubation has many benefits and should have the second highest priority after CPR and defibrillation. Intubation has the following advantages:

  - It provides a patent airway.

  - It decreases the chance of aspiration.

  - It allows direct administration of oxygen.

- It allows efficient ventilation to remove carbon dioxide (CO_2) and correct acidosis.

- It allows direct tracheal suctioning.

- It provides a route for drug administration of the following VF/VT cardiac arrest drugs: atropine, lidocaine, and epinephrine, or ALE.

- Once the trachea is intubated, ventilations do not have to be synchronized with chest compressions. The person's lungs can be ventilated at a rate of 12 to 15 ventilations per minute.

Nelson Gore

CASE 1 Continued

You observe that ventilations are producing good chest excursions with bilateral breath sounds and there are palpable pulses with each chest compression. One medic has attached the three-lead monitor cable, which reveals persistent VF. The medic attempting to insert a 16-gauge over-the-needle catheter in the right antecubital space is having problems. He has made one attempt and gives a quick expression of frustration as he fails on the second attempt. He pulls the needle from the arm, exclaiming, "This guy has nothing for veins here. I'll try on the other arm."

How would you proceed at this point?

- Administer epinephrine at this point: the patient has persistent VF, despite three defibrillation shocks. Intravenous access, however, is not yet available after two IV attempts and will still be unavailable for at least 1 to 2 minutes.

- At this point, endotracheal administration of epinephrine is indicated. This is consistent with the AHA recommendations to provide endotracheal drug administration whenever IV medications are not readily available.

- Why this emphasis on epinephrine? Why does this agent have such high priority in cardiac arrest?

- Remember all ACLS drugs should be considered in the context of the four questions that follow:

  Why do you give the drug? (mechanism)

  When do you give the drug? (indications)

  How do you give the drug? (dose)

  Watch out! (precautions)

Epinephrine

WHY?

- Epinephrine is the drug of choice for patients in cardiac arrest. No medication does a better job of increasing blood flow to the brain and heart.

- Epinephrine is a catecholamine (sympathomimetic) with α-adrenergic and ß-adrenergic action.

- The vasoconstrictive actions improve coronary and cerebral blood flow and increase the chance for survival.

- Epinephrine also increases coronary perfusion pressure, systemic vascular resistance, systemic blood pressure, heart rate, and myocardial contractility.

- This medication also increases myocardial oxygen consumption and automaticity.

WHEN?

- Give epinephrine early in any cardiac arrest, and every 3 to 5 minutes thereafter if the person remains in VF.

HOW?

- The recommended dose of epinephrine is 1 mg IV push every 3 to 5 minutes. If this dose and at least one subsequent shock do not convert the VF/VT, use one of the following acceptable and possibly helpful (Class IIb) dosing regimens:

  - Intermediate: Epinephrine 2 to 5 mg IV push, every 3 to 5 minutes

  - Escalating: Epinephrine 1 to 3 to 5 mg IV push, 3 minutes apart

  - High: Epinephrine 0.1 mg/kg IV push, every 3 to 5 minutes

WATCH OUT!

- Delays are probably the biggest error in epinephrine administration.

- Sodium bicarbonate and epinephrine must not be mixed in the same IV line.

- Watch out for an increase in myocardial oxygen demand.

- Higher doses of epinephrine are considered acceptable but can be neither recommended nor discouraged.

ENDOTRACHEAL EPINEPHRINE ADMINISTRATION

- Draw up 2 to 2.5 mg of epinephrine (1:1000 concentration) from either 1-mL glass ampules (1 mg/mL) or a multidose 30 mL vial (1 mg/mL). Use a 10-mL or larger syringe.

- Add normal saline to a total volume of 10 mL.

- Ventilate the lungs, using the resuscitation bag several times.

- Cease chest compressions.

- Remove the bag from the end of the endotracheal tube.

- Insert a long central-line catheter deep into the endotracheal tube. A variety of catheters are available and acceptable for endotracheal drug administration. The point is to select a catheter long enough for the tip to extend beyond the end of the endotracheal tube. Inject the drug forcefully. Follow with 5 to 10 mL of air from the syringe to flush out the drug in the catheter.

- You may follow with an additional 10 mL of normal saline to flush the drug deeper into the lungs.

- The patient may now have a reflex cough. Put a gloved finger over the end of the endotracheal tube to prevent the drug from being blown out of the tube.

- Rapidly attach the ventilation bag and ventilate the lungs three, four, or even five times, in quick succession.

- As an alternative, insert a 20-gauge needle through the wall of the endotracheal tube. Administer the medication with ventilations to help aerosolize the drug further into the lungs for better absorption.

- Other endotracheal medications for cardiac arrest that you can administer down the endotracheal tube are abbreviated ALE, as noted earlier. The endotracheal doses are as follows:

  Atropine : 2 to 3 mg diluted in 10 mL normal saline

  Lidocaine: 2 to 3 mg/kg

  Epinephrine: 2.0 to 2.5 mg diluted in 10 mL normal saline

Nelson Gore

CASE 1 Continued

After administration of the endotracheal epinephrine, you continue chest compressions and ventilations for 30 seconds, and reassess the rhythm by stopping CPR. The monitor continues to display medium coarse VF but of less amplitude than before. You resume CPR and observe that the medic attempting to insert an IV line into the left arm has still not succeeded. What would be your response and your next intervention?

COMMENTS

- At this point in the code you have successfully intubated the patient's trachea, delivered three shocks, and administered an endotracheal dose of epinephrine. You are still faced, however, with persistent VF and no IV access.

- KEEP SHOCKING!! Defibrillation is the only intervention known to convert VF to a spontaneously perfusing rhythm.

- The AHA protocols for refractory VF recommend the addition of two drugs here: an adrenergic agent (epinephrine) to provide vasoconstriction and an antifibrillatory antiarrhythmic drug to decrease the chances of postshock refibrillation.

- The AHA Guidelines do not require additional medications before further countershocks. Do not get distracted by the lack of IV access and think that further shocks should be delayed until medications have been administered. If VF persists, then shock it.

- NOTE: You can always administer epinephrine and lidocaine through the endotracheal tube.

Nelson Gore

CASE 1 Continued

You direct the person handling the airway to rapidly "bag" the patient, and you glance to make sure the oxygen tube is connected and flowing at 15 L per minute.

"Let's shock some more at 360 joules. Give him three stacked shocks at 360 joules if he needs them and give them quickly. I want Helen [one of the firefighters] to tell me when it has been 3 minutes since the last dose of epinephrine."

Your medic partner charges the defibrillator to 360 and places the paddles on the chest, being careful to avoid the monitor leads running between the patient and the defibrillator. He firmly states, "I'm going to shock on 3. One, I'm clear; two, you're clear; three, everybody's clear."

CONTINUED

| Nelson Gore | *The fourth shock is delivered safely. The paramedic immediately pushes the charge button on the fourth shock is delivered safely. The paramedic immediately pushes the charge button on the defibrillator* |
| CASE 1 Continued | |

paddles without lifting the paddles from the chest. Every eye stares at the monitor, which continues to show exactly the same pattern of VF. There is no loose-lead artifact. A firefighter puts his fingers on the carotid artery and states, "There is no pulse."

The high-pitched tone of the defibrillator charging stops. The charging light glows a steady yellow. The rhythm remains in VF. Your partner says, "I'm going with a fifth shock. Everybody clear," and he delivers an additional shock. The medic never removed the paddles from the chest. He charges and shocks using only the controls on the defibrillator paddles.

After this shock you state, "Replace the paddles in their cradles. Restart CPR immediately, resume bagging, and please hyperventilate."

After 15 seconds, you direct the team to stop bagging and stop compressing the chest, adding, "Let's check the rhythm." This time, the monitor displays a slow junctional escape complex at a heart rate of 30 beats per minute. "Check a pulse," someone states, and three hands reach out to palpate the nearest artery.

"Hey, I think there is a pulse with this! Someone check a blood pressure. We may have gotten this person back."

COMMENTS

The preceding section of Case 1 illustrates several critical details on how to manage persistent VF. The AHA Guidelines make specific recommendations here, even though the recommendations are "best guesses" in some areas. Many ACLS providers have focused on certain details (such as stacked shocks, energy levels, pulse checks between shocks, and leaving paddles on the chest), as if there were a true "right way" and a "wrong way." The answer, like so many areas in emergency cardiac care, revolves around what seems reasonable and what makes common sense in determining the following:

Stacked shocks versus single shocks?

Shocks with and without interposed CPR?

Pulse checks between shocks?

STACKED SHOCKS VERSUS SINGLE SHOCKS?

"Stacked shocks" refers to charging, shocking, recharging, and reshocking as fast as possible. You do not take the paddles or pads off the chest; you operate the device controls as quickly as possible. Animal data provide support for this approach through the "critical mass" theory of VF. Each shock eliminates VF from a certain portion of the myocardium. If a "critical mass" remains in VF, that portion will restart fibrillatory waves in the other, nonfibrillating portions of the heart. By putting the shocks close together, you increase the probability that you will defibrillate successfully and reduce the amount of fibrillating myocardium to an amount below the critical mass.

SHOCKS WITH AND WITHOUT INTERPOSED CPR?

If one shock does not succeed, you could argue that before giving the next shock you should provide some intervention that would increase the probability of successful defibrillation. This is the rationale behind the antiarrhythmic agents given during cardiac arrest. Returning to CPR and providing ventilation, oxygenation of the blood, and circulation, in theory, should make persistent VF easier to defibrillate on the next shock. Laboratory data, however, suggest that the fibrillating myocardium continues to deteriorate during the interposed CPR attempts. Therefore, if you perform CPR for 1 minute on a fibrillating heart, that heart will be "worse" than it was before you started the 1 minute of CPR.

PULSE CHECKS BETWEEN SHOCKS?

The AHA ACLS Guidelines had a long-standing recommendation to always check pulses between defibrillation shocks. Experts feared that the monitor leads may be dislodged during the resuscitation, especially during the sudden muscular contractions that occur with each shock. Artifactual signals produced by loose leads could be misinterpreted as VF, and further shocks could be delivered, even though the true underlying rhythm had reverted to an organized rhythm. Shocks to organized rhythms, of course, have the potential to harm the patient by putting them into VF, although the chances of this are extremely low (estimated at less than one chance in a thousand).

The new technology of AEDs forced a reexamination of the pulse check question in the late 1980s when the AHA developed national guidelines for the use of AEDs. The analysis phase of AEDs requires that the operator *not* touch the patient during the analysis phase and allow the device to continue analysis undisturbed following the first shock. A pulse check would require delays in using the device between shocks. This pause between further shocks would be detrimental to the patient. Pulse checks without turning off the AED would, first, interfere with the analysis of the cardiac activity by the AED and, second, expose the operators to the possibility of shocks, since they might be touching the patient during subsequent shocks. All protocols using AEDs mandate *no pulse checks* between stacked shocks.

Experience with AED use in thousands of patients has validated the no-pulse-check concept. Rarely people have reported incorrect AED shocks that could have been prevented by a pulse check. In all cases reported to date, however, the operators have incorrectly placed the AED in analysis mode on patients who were not in full cardiac arrest.

In addition, the ECG circuitry on modern defibrillators has been improved, so "false VF" produced by a loose electrode would be very unlikely. Defibrillator engineers have broadened the "band width" of the signals picked up by the monitor leads and enhanced the display capabilities of defibrillator monitor. The chance of detecting a change in clinical state with a pulse check that would not be detected by a properly connected defibrillator is remote. Besides, loose electrodes now produce a sharp display on monitors that is easily recognized as artifact and not confused with VF.

Nevertheless, in our scenario in Case 1, one of the rescuers did perform a pulse check during the recharging of the defibrillator. This is perfectly acceptable, since it did not delay the sequence of rapid shocks to persistent VF. Rescuers should not think that pulse checks are prohibited during shock sequencing (especially if they do not delay care). The guideline is as follows: Pulse checks are not required after every shock *if* you have all of the following conditions:

- Patient was originally confirmed to be in full cardiac arrest, without a pulse.
- Postshock rhythm appears to be VF that is consistent with the preshock VF signal.
- Defibrillator continues to be properly connected to the patient.
- Emergency personnel are operating an AED.

The following summarize the treatment sequence followed in Case 1 (this sequence is Class I, that is, acceptable and definitely helpful according to 1992 to 1994 AHA Guidelines):

- Shock, shock, shock
- Intubate, IV attempts, epinephrine-down-the-tube
- Shock, shock, shock

Bart Johnson

CASE 2

The root canal is almost complete. Bart Johnson, a 55-year-old hospital administrator, suddenly becomes briefly agitated and stops breathing. His dental hygienist pulls free the dental dam. He is not breathing at all. In the drawer is a pocket face mask, which the hygienist places over Mr. Johnson's nose and mouth, and she gives two slow, deep breaths. She feels no carotid pulse. "Help! Call 911. Let's move him to the floor." The dentist takes the feet; the hygienist removes the chair arm. They pull him to the office floor. A receptionist is calling EMS from the front desk. "Get the AED from the closet!" says the dentist. The hygienist continues to ventilate the lungs, using her pocket mask, while the dentist, Dr. Schmidt, begins compressions. The AED model has no monitor. Dr. Schmidt turns the power on, attaches the electrodes, "clears" the patient, and delivers three shocks as directed by the device. After the third shock they resume CPR.

What are the best features of this code so far?

COMMENTS

The Primary ABCD Survey is performed by the dental clinic personnel. They also activated the EMS system. They are equipped with an AED and treat the person with three shocks within the first 2 minutes of his cardiac arrest.

The nonemergency team in Case 2 performs all the tasks that this man requires in the first few minutes of arrest. Regular practice in this specific environment makes this rare event a smooth, coordinated performance. Each person knows the tasks he or she must complete and reacts with minimum discussion during a crisis. Planning and forethought contribute to saving this man's life.

Bart Johnson

CASE 2 Continued

"They're in the back exam room!" says the receptionist as you and your ALS-trained partner arrive. A quick assessment reveals that the man remains breathless and pulseless. "Stop CPR!" you call out. "Press analyze on your defibrillator." The AED delivers three more shocks at 360 J. A quick pulse check reveals no pulse. Your partner quickly intubates the man's trachea, confirms tube placement, and hooks up oxygen to the ventilation bag. You start an IV line in the left antecubital space. You give "Epi" 1 mg IV, elevate the arm, and run a 20-mL bolus of normal saline.

Since the AED lacks a monitor screen, you remove the AED patches and attach the monitor leads of your portable monitor and defibrillator. The patient remains in VF. Your partner states, "He is still in VF after six shocks from the AED. Should we shock with our defibrillator, or just go ahead with the ACLS drugs?" How would you respond? What would be your next treatment steps?

COMMENTS

- Delivering additional shocks with the conventional defibrillator is acceptable.

- Note that the ALS unit arrived on the scene and simply continued with the AED as a method to assess for the presence of VF and treat with three more shocks.

- Common sense demands that all physicians, nurses, and ALS personnel learn to use AEDs. Scenarios like that in Case 2 are going to occur with more frequency.

- The question is how do you "count the shocks" that were delivered by the AED in the dentist's office? The AED had delivered three shocks prior to ALS arrival. Should the ALS unit simply have "counted" those three shocks and moved directly to endotracheal intubation and IV drug administration before delivering additional shocks?

The delivery of additional shocks (using the "stacked shocks" method). This minor protocol point does not merit the amount of discussion it has generated. In the scenario in Case 2 you decided to continue to deliver shocks, first with the AED and then with your conventional defibrillator. The patient thus received six shocks before receiving epinephrine and nine shocks before receiving any additional medications. The AHA considers this approach of continued shocks for persistent VF, especially when there are medication delays, to be acceptable (Class I: acceptable, definitely helpful). All EMS systems that allow first-responder defibrillation have adopted this AHA protocol. These systems have experienced considerable success in saving lives, thus proving the acceptability of additional shocks without intervening medications.

Bart Johnson

CASE 2 Continued

After three more stacked shocks the rhythm is still VF. Your partner comments, "Hey, it is now 3 minutes since I gave the first dose of Epi. Do you want some more Epi, and if so how much?"

COMMENTS

- The recommended first dose of epinephrine is always 1 mg IV push (2.0 to 2.5 mg per endotracheal tube).

- The second (and subsequent) doses of epinephrine should come 3 to 5 minutes later.

- The big question: What should be the second dose of epinephrine in persistent cardiac arrest? Resuscitation researchers and clinicians have debated this question intensely over the past decade. Results from animal research strongly suggested that the 1-mg dose of epinephrine was ineffective and should be increased to 0.1 to 0.2 mg/kg (7 mg for a 70-kg person). However, three prospective, randomized, well-designed clinical trials in

humans produced disappointing results. These studies observed no differences in outcomes for patients receiving standard-dose epinephrine (1 mg) and those receiving a high dose (generally 0.1 to 0.2 mg/kg).

- The preceding studies did, however, observe the following interesting results that account for the AHA accepting a variety of doses of epinephrine for the second dose:

  - First, high-dose epinephrine did no harm. The high-dose epinephrine patients fared no worse than the standard-dose patients among the survivors.

  - Second, high-dose epinephrine seemed to offer some benefit for those patients who were younger, who were in non-VF rhythms, and who were receiving epinephrine sooner rather than later. These benefits were not statistically significant; therefore the authors could not present strong recommendations. Nevertheless, the trends were positive and promising.

- The AHA-ACLS recommendations therefore accept a variety of dosing regimens for the second dose of epinephrine. The following are considered acceptable and possibly helpful (Class IIb):

  - Intermediate dose: *Epinephrine* 2 to 5 mg IV push, every 3 to 5 minutes

  - Escalating dose: *Epinephrine* 1 to 3 to 5 mg IV push, 3 minutes apart

  - High dose: *Epinephrine* 0.1 mg/kg IV push, every 3 to 5 minutes

- *Different clinical interpretations:* Since the 1992 AHA Guidelines were published, it has become apparent that clinicians have interpreted these recommendations in a variety of ways. Some ACLS providers have considered a Class IIb recommendation to be a prohibition of the use of high-dose epinephrine—since the clinical trials showed no benefit, high-dose epinephrine should not be used. Other experts have focused on the observation that high-dose epinephrine does no harm and therefore should be given selectively to the promising subgroups of cardiac arrest.

- *What seems reasonable?* (See Box 4-3.) A frequent practice now in ACLS is to use escalating doses of epinephrine for persistent cardiac arrest. The elderly patient in VF stands as a commonly accepted exception. In our opinion the ACLS provider should move quickly to higher doses of epinephrine (2 to 5 mg IV push, every 3 minutes) in the following situations:

  - Non-VF cardiac arrest (asystole, PEA, tachycardias, and bradycardias)

  - Younger patients (maybe <60 years of age; definitely <50 years of age)

  - Patients with a brief interval between the collapse and the availability of epinephrine (less than 10 minutes)

- NOTE: the preceding guideline of the authors of this book, while not a specific recommendation of the AHA, is consistent with the Class IIb status of alternative dosing regimens for epinephrine.

BOX 4-3

The Second Dose of Epinephrine in Cardiac Arrest: What Should It Be?

- *The recommended first dose of epinephrine is always epinephrine 1 mg IV push (2.0 to 2.5 mg per endotracheal tube).*

- *The second (and subsequent) doses of epinephrine should come 3 to 5 minutes later.*

- *The AHA ACLS recommendations accept a variety of dosing regimens for the second dose of epinephrine. The following are considered acceptable and possibly helpful (Class IIb):*

  - *Intermediate dose: Epinephrine 2 to 5 mg IV push, every 3 to 5 minutes*

  - *Escalating dose: Epinephrine 1 mg - 3 mg - 5 mg, IV push, 3 minutes apart*

  - *High dose: Epinephrine 0.1 mg/kg IV push, every 3 to 5 minutes*

- *The authors suggest that the ACLS provider should move quickly to higher doses of epinephrine (2 to 5 mg IV push, every 3 minutes) in the following situations:*

  - *Non-VF cardiac arrest (asystole, PEA, tachycardias, and bradycardias)*

  - *Younger patients (maybe all people <60 years of age; definitely those patients <50 years of age)*

  - *Patients with a brief interval between the collapse and the availability of epinephrine (less than 10 minutes)*

- *The more of the preceding factors that are present, the more aggressive should be the second dose of epinephrine. (For example, for pediatric resuscitation the standard PALS recommendation is the high dose of 0.1 mg/kg for the second IV/IO dose.)*

The preceding guidelines are those of the authors of this book and are not a specific recommendation of the AHA. These guidelines, however, are consistent with the Class IIb status of alternative dosing regimens for epinephrine.

Bart Johnson

CASE 2 Continued

You decide that this patient may do better with a somewhat higher dose of epinephrine, so you direct your partner to administer 2 mg epinephrine and to continue to do so every 3 minutes as long as Mr. Johnson remains in cardiac arrest. After your partner pushes in the 2 mg of "Epi," he gives a 20-mL bolus of normal saline and elevates the arm to enhance drug delivery.

You direct another shock to be delivered 30 seconds after the epinephrine bolus and flush. This shock does not defibrillate the heart, and the patient remains in VF.

Your partner mutters, "Okay, we need to pull out the antiarrhythmic stuff. What should it be? Lidocaine or bretylium?" What would your directions be?

COMMENTS

- **Vasoconstriction versus antiarrhythmics.** Many ACLS providers fail to appreciate that they give epinephrine and lidocaine (or bretylium) for two different reasons, as follows:

  - Epinephrine provides strong vasoconstriction. During CPR, this leads to greater blood flow to the brain and the coronary arteries.

  - Lidocaine, bretylium, and procainamide (and to some extent magnesium) are antiarrhythmic agents. In the setting of VF/VT, their role is to *decrease* the chances of refibrillation after defibrillation.

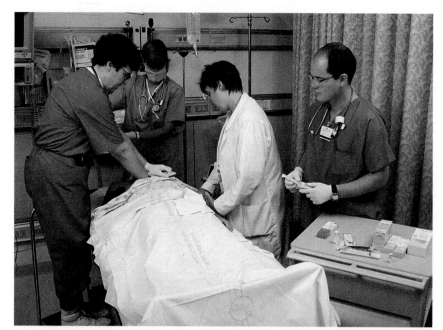

Fig. 4-8: *A patient surrounded with items of the mega-VF (items of Secondary Survey): IV line and fluid bottles, IV setup, defibrillator and monitor, endotracheal intubation equipment, and array of the drugs of mega-VF (epinephrine, lidocaine, sodium bicarbonate, bretylium, magnesium, and procainamide).*

- **Defibrillation versus antiarrhythmic medications.** In a patient with refractory VF/VT, defibrillation is the best intervention to eliminate the profoundly disturbed rhythm. This concept is so important to understand that it will be restated: It is electricity—not medications—that eliminates the chaotic cardiac activity we call VF. The antiarrhythmic agents given during cardiac arrest resulting from VF/VT must be combined with rapid shocks. The antiarrhythmic drugs possess two important mechanisms of actions, as follows:

- *They lower the defibrillation threshold.* The agents increase the chances that a single electrical shock will stun the heart out of VF and into asystole. NOTE: You must still provide electrical current. Drugs do not defibrillate.

- *They raise the refibrillation threshold.* The agents increase the chance that once the heart has been stunned by the electrical shock into electrical silence (asystole), the chaotic activity of VF will not return.

- The approach here must be to combine one (or several) antiarrhythmic agents with defibrillation. The high-energy shocks get rid of the VF activity; the antiarrhythmic agents keep that activity from returning.

- These observations account for the two ACLS recommendations that follow:

  - Start epinephrine early, and keep giving it at regular intervals (persistent vasoconstrictive effect).

  - Provide defibrillation and medications in an alternating drug-shock–drug-shock pattern.

- The AHA recommends several antiarrhythmic agents to be selected and given at this point in a resuscitation attempt. In practice, this flexibility allows for several treatment patterns, but the vast majority of care providers "max out" on each drug before moving to the next one, usually in the following sequence: lidocaine (×2); bretylium 5 to 10 mg/kg (×2); and procainamide 30 mg/min to a maximum dose of 17 mg/kg.

- The next section provides the "Why?" "When?" "How?" and "Watch out!" for the two most widely used antifibrillatory agents, lidocaine and bretylium.

Lidocaine

WHY?

- Key: Antifibrillatory properties.
- Raises the fibrillation threshold (the amount of current needed to cause fibrillation). This decreases the probability that a heart will refibrillate after a shock has eliminated fibrillation.
- Lowers the defibrillation threshold (lowers the amount of current needed to defibrillate the heart). This means it increases the probability that a shock will defibrillate the heart.
- Decreases excitability in ischemic tissue.
- Suppresses ventricular irritability.

WHEN?

- Cardiac arrest due to VF/VT.
- Administer after initial defibrillation shocks, intubation, and epinephrine.
- First antiarrhythmic to use for refractory VF/VT.

HOW?

- First dose: 1.0 to 1.5 mg/kg IV push (or 2 to 4 mg/kg endotracheal).
- Repeat bolus in 3 to 5 minutes to a maximum combined dose of 3 mg/kg.
- An additional countershock should be administered between these doses.
- A single dose of 1.5 mg/kg in cardiac arrest is acceptable. NOTE: Some experts consider 3 mg/kg to be potentially toxic in the cardiac arrest patient, since there is no spontaneous blood flow. Consequently, some clinicians prefer to use 1.5 mg/kg as the maximum dose for lidocaine. A definitive answer on this question is lacking. Toxic effects of lidocaine become irrelevant if the patient cannot be resuscitated from VF. Most ACLS providers use two doses of lidocaine at 1.5 mg/kg.
- If you get return of circulation, start a continuous infusion at 2 to 4 mg/min.

WATCH OUT!

- Watch out for the following signs of lidocaine intoxication: seizures and respiratory compromise in patients who do regain circulation after the use of higher doses of lidocaine.
- Use lower loading doses of lidocaine for older persons or those with decreased liver function. These people can have a single dose of 1 mg/kg.

Bretylium

WHY?

- Bretylium possesses antifibrillatory actions, primarily by increasing the fibrillation threshold.
- Bretylium also produces adrenergic blockade, which can produce severe hypotension. This effect places bretylium in a second-line position behind lidocaine in the VF/VT Algorithm.

WHEN?

- Refractory malignant ventricular arrhythmias.
- Use bretylium for patients as follows:
  - When VF/VT persists despite epinephrine, countershock, and lidocaine
  - When VT continues to occur after maximum doses of lidocaine
  - When recurrent VT occurs despite lidocaine and procainamide
- First antiarrhythmic agent for VF in hypothermic patients.

HOW?

- Five mg/kg rapid IV push. Follow in 30 to 60 seconds with defibrillation. (Some protocols simplify dosing by recommending one 500-mg ampule in adults and avoiding the weight calculation. This is acceptable, since the margin of error with bretylium is wide.)
- Repeat in 5 minutes at 10 mg/kg (or simplify by giving two 500 mg ampules for the second dose).
- May continue to repeat at 5- to 30-minute intervals to a maximum total dose of 30 to 35 mg/kg. (Some clinicians administer the second dose of bretylium at 2 to 3 minutes rather than waiting a full 5 minutes.)
- If you get return of circulation, start a continuous infusion at 1 to 2 mg/min.
- Bretylium may require several minutes for the antifibrillatory properties to take effect.
- Do not delay shocks after administering the medication more than 30 to 60 seconds.

WATCH OUT!

- Watch out for nausea, vomiting, and postural hypotension.

> **Bart Johnson**
>
> **CASE 2 Continued**
>
> *For Mr. Johnson, you now follow the sequence of interventions listed here:*
>
> - *Lidocaine 100 mg IV push followed by 20 mL saline flush*
> - *Shock at 360 J in 30 to 60 seconds*
> - *Epinephrine 2 mg IV push followed by 20 mL saline flush*
> - *Lidocaine 100 mg IV push followed by 20 mL saline flush*
> - *Shock at 360 J*
> - *Shock at 360 J*
>
> *This last shock finally converts Mr. Johnson's heart to an organized junctional escape rhythm that slowly increases to 50 beats per minute. The blood pressure is 90 mm Hg systolic. You start a maintenance lidocaine infusion at 2 mg/min and prepare him for transport to the base hospital. What were the major reasons for the success of this resuscitation?*

COMMENTS

Well-trained lay responders (the dental office team) provided the first strong links in the Chain of Survival for the man in Case 2: early access, early CPR, and early defibrillation.

- The Primary ABCD Survey was completed by those who witnessed the event.

- An AED's shocks were used as part of the ACLS treatment sequence.

- Professionals who seldom work together acted as a team to deliver a rapid sequence of care.

- Advanced airway and IV access were established almost at the same time.

- Two ACLS drugs (epinephrine and lidocaine) were administered in a drug-shock–drug-shock sequence.

- The second and subsequent doses of epinephrine were higher doses (Class IIb choices).

> **Wolfgang Block**
>
> **CASE 3**
>
> *IN-HOSPITAL MONITORED CARDIAC ARREST*
>
> *You are working as a critical care nurse in the coronary care unit. You are caring for Mr. Wolfgang Block, a 49-year-old supervisor at a local construction company. Mr. Block is a large man, weighing 240 pounds. He was admitted several hours ago as a "rule-out AMI" with a history and pain consistent with AMI and an ECG that showed 2 mm ST-segment elevation in leads V_1 to V_4.*
>
> *Unfortunately, Mr. Block suffered a 30-second episode of monomorphic VT that responded to synchronized cardioversion at 200 J. He also received lidocaine 100 mg (approximately 1 mg/kg), followed by a maintenance infusion of 2 mg/min. His heart returned to sinus rhythm with a blood pressure of 110/70 mm Hg for approximately 10 minutes when it suddenly went back into the regular, monomorphic VT. You deliver a synchronized shock of 200 J, and the postshock rhythm has deteriorated to VF. A "local code" is called, and you quickly reach for the defibrillator controls to deliver three shocks: 200 J, 300 J, and 360 J. Despite these shocks, VF persists, and you order epinephrine 1 mg, which is given quickly through an existing IV line. The anesthesiologist arrives and successfully intubates Mr. Block's trachea.*
>
> *How would you direct the care of Mr. Block at this point?*

COMMENTS

As the critical care nurse, you have followed Mr. Block's case since he was admitted. The first step here is to review the Primary and Secondary Surveys, as follows:

- *Airway:* His trachea has been intubated successfully.

- *Breathing:* His lungs are being ventilated well through the endotracheal tube, and bilateral breath sounds are present with each BVM ventilation. You have ordered portable chest x-ray and initial arterial blood gas levels.

- *Circulation:* The unit assistant is performing vigorous chest compressions with good, palpable carotid pulses.

A 14-gauge short catheter is in place in each antecubital vein, and the normal saline infuses well. The first dose of epinephrine was given. Rhythm remains coarse VF.

- *Defibrillation and differential diagnoses.* Since he remains in VF, you must continue to deliver defibrillation shocks at 360 J. You review the sequence of events and consider that, given his large body mass, he may have received an inadequate dose of lidocaine following the first episode of VT.

After the Primary and Secondary Surveys, continue with the VF/VT protocols, making sure to give full doses of lidocaine.

Wolfgang Block

CASE 3 Continued

You direct the following interventions: shock at 360 J; lidocaine bolus of 150 mg (roughly 1.5 mg/kg); shock at 360 J, 30 seconds later; second dose of epinephrine of 3 mg; shock at 360 J.

Following the last shock, the rhythm converts to an organized rhythm, with a narrow-complex QRS at 110 beats per minute. This lasts about 45 seconds, when he breaks again into a run of VT for 10 seconds and then VF.

You immediately charge the defibrillator to 360 J and deliver a shock that converts him to the previous perfusing rhythm. Because of the clinical instability and the repeated episodes of refibrillation, you decide to fully load with lidocaine by ordering another bolus of 150 mg (roughly 1.5 mg/kg).

Despite the full (3 mg/kg) loading dose of lidocaine, Mr. Block continues this pattern of instability. You add bretylium 500 mg (about 5 mg/kg) IV bolus; shock at 360 J again, and get conversion back to the perfusing rhythm. Several minutes later, he has another run of VT and refibrillates again, requiring another shock at 360 J. This shock converts the heart to the perfusing rhythm again, and you now follow with bretylium 1000 mg (10 mg/kg). How would you manage this pattern of fibrillation-conversion-refibrillation?

COMMENTS

- Mr. Block does not clearly fit the definition of "refractory VF/VT" because he does not stay continuously in VF/VT.

- Instead, Mr. Block displays the rather common problem of a "stuttering code"—he is in and out of VF/VT with periods of adequate perfusion interspersed with a full cardiac arrest.

- Mr. Block has "maxed out" with both lidocaine and bretylium, having received the recommended loading dose of both agents: 3 mg/kg for lidocaine and 15 mg/kg for bretylium. Repeat doses of each drug can be given but only if the initial two doses appear to succeed.

- This type of "stuttering-refractory" VF presents a model indication for the use of procainamide. However, the requirement to administer procainamide slowly (to prevent its hypotensive effects) poses a problem.

Procainamide

WHY?

- Procainamide is an antiarrhythmic agent that suppresses cardiac automaticity and ventricular ectopy.

- It slows intraventricular conduction, which can lead to bidirectional block.

- Bidirectional block may terminate reentrant arrhythmias.

WHEN?

- Procainamide is a third-line agent to use for persistent VF/VT (after lidocaine and bretylium).

- Use for "stuttering" codes when patient's condition is severely unstable and patient is in and out of cardiac arrest. These interposed periods of perfusion allow for the longer time it takes for procainamide to be administered.

- Procainamide is also useful for tachycardias in patients who are not in full cardiac arrest, both ventricular and supraventricular tachycardias. Again, it is a third-line agent in these situations and a second-line agent in stable VT.

HOW?

- The loading dose of procainamide is 17 mg/kg given at a rate of 30 mg/min. This requirement to give procainamide slowly, over time, decreases its usefulness in full cardiac arrest patients. Certainly, the outcome in the vast majority of cardiac arrests would have been determined by the time procainamide had reached therapeutic levels.

- Some clinicians administer procainamide much more aggressively in patients in full cardiac arrest, giving the loading dose over 15 to 30 minutes and following with a pressor agent such as norepinephrine or dopamine. This cannot be recommended because the known hypotensive effects of procainamide might render a person in full cardiac arrest unable to be resuscitated, even with elimination of the VF/VT.

- In patients not in full cardiac arrest give procainamide at 20 to 30 mg/min to one or more the following endpoints:
  - The arrhythmia is suppressed.
  - Hypotension becomes excessive.
  - QRS complex becomes widened by 50% of its original width.
  - Loading dose has been administered (17 mg/kg).
- Follow the loading dose with a maintenance infusion of 1 to 4 mg/min.

WATCH OUT!

- Observe the ECG monitor closely, and measure the blood pressure when administering procainamide, especially when using rapid infusion rates.
- Procainamide can produce strong vasodilator effects and negative inotropic effects.
- It can widen the QRS complex and lengthen baseline PR and QT intervals.
- The preceding effects lead to AV conduction problems such as heart blocks and proarrhythmia effects like cardiac arrest.
- Be particularly cautious when patients have low potassium or magnesium levels.

Wolfgang Block

CASE 3 Continued

You start an infusion of procainamide at 30 mg/min during a period when Mr. Block has his spontaneous rhythm. At a weight of 108 kg and a loading dose of 17 mg/kg, Mr. Block will require about 1800 mg. Given at 30 mg/min this will take just over 1 hour. However, Mr. Block appears to stabilize and, after 15 minutes, you notice a more regular rhythm. The blood pressure is 90/60 mm Hg at a heart rate of 75 beats per minute. The blood pressure does not drop any further. You order a maintenance procainamide infusion of 2 mg/min to follow the loading dose. After routine post-resuscitation review, Mr. Block's condition remains stable.

COMMENTS

- Mr. Block is representative of scenarios that are promising but also challenging. The "stuttering" nature of his arrest with intermittent periods of spontaneous circulation clearly delayed the onset of irreversible damage and gave the resuscitation team optimism that "this is one person we're going to get back."

- The challenge is to try to figure out why his heart kept refibrillating and going back into cardiac arrest, despite appropriate therapy. Sometimes, ischemic damage in the myocardium produces markedly irritable areas of myocardium. These damaged areas can produce electrical instability no matter what agents are used.

- In addition, however, the conscientious clinician always returns to the basics of resuscitation when faced with a patient who does not seem to be responding. Ask whether there is adequate CPR, effective ventilation through an adequate airway, associated electrolyte abnormalities, or even side effects from medications that you have administered.

- One additional clue can come from analysis of the spontaneous rhythm that occurs between episodes of VF/VT. For example, you get some clues simply by looking at whether the interposed non-VF rhythms during a VF/VT resuscitation are fast or slow, as follows:

  - *Rapid tachycardia precedes refibrillation.* This event may be caused by the epinephrine that has been administered or by excessive natural catecholamines. Treatment is to withhold further doses of epinephrine (especially if using doses greater than 1 mg); consider beta blockers (such as *metoprolol* 5 mg IV).

  - *Sinus or nodal bradycardia precedes the refibrillation.* Excessive parasympathetic system activity may be present, or nodal dysfunction on ischemic basis. Treatment is to add *atropine* or to *pace* with transcutaneous pacing during the non-VF rhythms.

BOX 4-4

Refractory Ventricular Fibrillation or Ventricular Tachycardia Arrest

Using the ABCD part of the Secondary Survey to identify reversible causes

STEP ONE

Troubleshoot the ABC of the Secondary Survey: Check the Following

AIRWAY

- *Airway is open and air is moving easily.*
- *Endotracheal tube is patent and unobstructed.*

BREATHING

- *Bilateral, symmetric chest expansions are present.*
- *Airway manager is "bagging" at correct rate and force.*

CIRCULATION

- *Chest compressions in CPR are adequate in rate, force, depth, and location.*
- *Intravenous access is established correctly.*
- *Medications are administered properly.*
- *Monitor is used correctly (leads all connected, correct control settings).*

STEP TWO:

Review D of the Secondary Survey (Differential Diagnoses): Ask "What else could be causing this lack of response?"

AIRWAY

- *Tube in the wrong place, in the esophagus or right mainstem bronchus*
- *Tube obstructed or kinked*
- *Foreign body aspiration*
- *Anaphylaxis (angioedema)*
- *Inflammatory conditions of the hypopharynx (epiglottitis or retropharyngeal abscess)*
- *Craniofacial trauma, laryngeal or tracheal disruption*

BREATHING

- *Preexisting chest wall mechanical abnormalities (scoliosis, emphysema, congenital)*
- *Tension pneumothorax from resuscitation efforts*
- *Subcutaneous emphysema*

CIRCULATION

- *Pericardial tamponade from resuscitation efforts*
- *Pulmonary embolus*
- *Prolonged hypoxia*
- *Massive acute myocardial infarction*
- *Electrolyte disturbances (potassium, calcium, magnesium)*
- *Drug overdoses of many types: tricyclic antidepressants, aspirin, beta blocker, or calcium channel blocker*
- *Illicit drugs: cocaine, heroin, cyanide poisoning (following fires with synthetic materials)*
- *Anesthetic agent toxicity*
- *Carbon monoxide poisoning*
- *Occult trauma: cardiac tamponade, hypovolemia, exsanguination*

Melvin Wayne	ALCOHOLIC, MALNOURISHED; VENTRICULAR FIBRILLATION REQUIRES MAGNESIUM
CASE 4	

Melvin Wayne is a 50-year-old "character," well-known to your Emergency Department. He lives under the 520 bridge overpass and supports himself by panhandling on University Avenue. Fortified wine supplies the majority of his daily caloric intake. The medics bring him to the Emergency Department where you are on duty. He had collapsed on the street in front of Jack-in-the-Box, in apparent cardiac arrest. Despite the lack of bystander CPR, Melvin was successfully resuscitated by the emergency medical technicians using an AED to deliver five shocks. The medics arrived, intubated his lungs, started an IV line, and gave a bolus of lidocaine, followed by a lidocaine infusion at 2 mg/min.

Under your care in the Emergency Department, Melvin's condition remains unstable; he has had two more episodes of VF cardiac arrest, despite lidocaine, bretylium, and epinephrine.

How would you approach this problem of instability and recurrent episodes of VF?

COMMENTS

- As with all unstable patients who remain in cardiac arrest, or who seem to go in and out of arrest, you should troubleshoot and review the differential diagnosis.

- The Primary and Secondary Surveys (ABCD) provide a good framework around which to perform this troubleshooting, and the box on p. 79 provides details on the major points to consider.

- A clinical theme with Mr. Wayne is the chronic alcoholism and associated chronic malnutrition. In the setting of a persistent cardiac arrest with instability, you should think that electrolyte abnormalities may be playing a role, in particular, magnesium, potassium, and calcium.

- With this history it would be empirically acceptable to administer magnesium, even though you have no laboratory documentation that he is hypomagnesemic.

Magnesium

WHY?

- Known association between magnesium deficiency, arrhythmias, and sudden death

- Provides antiarrhythmic effects

- Leads to vasodilation

- Improves electrical stability in the heart

- Reduces spasm

WHEN?

- In cardiac arrest, give magnesium to patients with known or clinically suspected low levels of magnesium (hypomagnesemia). This is a Class IIa (acceptable, probably helpful) recommendation.

- Suspect magnesium deficiency in patients with poor dietary intake and habits and chronic diseases (alcoholics, renal failure, and chronic gastrointestinal problems associated with malabsorption).

- Torsades de pointes: Magnesium is a treatment of choice in this form of VF/VT.

HOW?

- Refractory VF/VT cardiac arrest with known or suspected hypomagnesemia is treated as follows:

  - One to 2 g IV push (2 to 4 mL 50% MgSO$_4$).

  - NOTE: The usual "recommended" approach is to give magnesium over 1 to 2 minutes. However, 1 to 2 minutes is an inordinate amount of time to delay giving this drug in refractory VF, and many experienced clinicians always administer magnesium IV push.

  - Mix (2 to 4 mL of a 50% solution diluted in 10 mL normal saline).

  - Some experts recommend IV push administration in cardiac arrest.

- Torsades de pointes pattern of VF/VT: 1 to 2 g IV over 5 to 60 minutes. (Even higher doses, up to 5 to 10 g, may be needed to control torsades de pointes.)

- Continue infusion for 24 hours at 0.5 to 1.0 g/hour if magnesium deficiency is documented after resuscitation.

- How supplied: 10-mL glass ampule of 50% MgSO$_4$ = 5 g.

WATCH OUT!

- Toxic effects are rare.

- Side effects include flushing, sweating, mild bradycardia, and hypotension.

- Signs of excessive serum magnesium levels include diarrhea, vomiting, depressed reflexes, paralysis, circulatory collapse, and respiratory depression.

Suhail Idris

CASE 5

VENTRICULAR FIBRILLATION ASSOCIATED WITH PREEXISTING HYPERKALEMIA

You are a resident covering the cardiology service. Mr. Idris is a 38-year-old graduate student admitted to the coronary care unit from the Emergency Department. He is a kidney dialysis patient who missed his last treatment. He has been depressed about his condition and has been occasionally noncompliant with treatment. He came to the hospital because of extreme weakness and a fainting spell. He has not been hungry and has eaten only a couple of bananas today. Lab results return with a potassium level of 8.5 mEg/L. His ECG shows peaked T waves, wide QRS complex, and small P waves.

Approximately 30 minutes after transfer from the Emergency Department to the coronary care unit, you hear an overhead page that there has been a cardiac arrest in Room 354, Mr. Idris's room. You arrive and take on the role of team leader. The monitor shows coarse VF.

As you direct the initial steps of the Primary and Secondary Surveys, what unique aspect of Mr. Idris's care should you consider?

COMMENTS

- Mr. Idris has suffered a cardiac arrest with known, preexisting hyperkalemia. This is a Class I indication for the use of sodium bicarbonate and introduces the complex topic of the use of bicarbonate in adult cardiac arrest.

- Bicarbonate therapy has provoked a great deal of debate in cardiac resuscitation. Although some of this debate has actually been useful, most has been waged in an unproductive "black and white" fashion. Participants in this debate contend that bicarbonate either damages people or stands as the only key to restoring a spontaneous circulation.

- The 1992 AHA Guidelines brought some sense to this debate by presenting bicarbonate like any other medication. Bicarbonate has both indications and contraindications. Use bicarbonate when those indications are present and avoid it when the indications are absent.

- Mr. Idris clearly should be given sodium bicarbonate, 1 mEq/kg IV bolus, with half that dose repeated every 10 minutes. As arterial blood gas levels become available, they can be used to guide the dosing by calculating base deficits and bicarbonate concentrations.

- The following section summarizes the use of sodium bicarbonate in cardiac resuscitation. The following comments apply to all cardiac arrests, regardless of the type of rhythm.

Sodium Bicarbonate

WHY?

- Bicarbonate is a buffer agent administered to neutralize hydrogen ions.

- Hydrogen ions accumulate during the "no-flow" state of cardiac arrest and create severe acidosis. This acidosis adversely affects the myocardium, disrupting cardiac activity.

- In theory, bicarbonate combines with the hydrogen ions, producing carbonic acid and then water (H_2O) and carbon dioxide (CO_2). This CO_2 must then be excreted through the lungs.

- In the nonventilated lungs of a cardiac arrest patient, however, the CO_2 cannot be excreted efficiently. The excess CO_2 crosses from the bloodstream into the cells of the myocardium and nervous system, where it converts back to hydrogen ions. These hydrogen ions produce a paradoxic intracellular acidosis—you gave bicarbonate to neutralize the extracellular acidosis and wind up producing an intracellular acidosis.

- This leads to the following critical principle in cardiac resuscitation: the treatment of the acidosis of cardiac arrest is ventilation and restoration of normal circulation. The best "buffer therapy" we possess is good CPR and ventilations.

- There are specific clinical situations, however, in which bicarbonate is clearly indicated. These are discussed next.

WHEN?

- Ventilation with endotracheal intubation provides the major treatment of acidosis associated with cardiac emergencies.
- There is no definite basis for routine use. Consider routine use only after known beneficial therapy; hyperventilate the lungs instead.

Class I intervention (definitely helpful)

- Known, preexisting hyperkalemia: Sodium bicarbonate is a Class I intervention.

Class IIa (acceptable, probably helpful)

- Cardiac arrest associated with overdose of tricyclic antidepressants

- Cardiac arrest associated with preexisting bicarbonate-responsive acidosis

Class IIb (acceptable, possibly helpful)

- Patient's trachea has been intubated successfully; effective ventilations and chest compressions have been administered; the patient remains in cardiac arrest.

  NOTE: Whereas in the past, everyone received bicarbonate during cardiac arrest, emergency care providers now give routine bicarbonate only in the following situation: you have intubated the trachea and ventilated the lungs and continue good chest compressions, yet the patient is not responding. A long arrest interval presents an acceptable clinical indication for bicarbonate.

- Patient finally gets return of spontaneous circulation after a long arrest interval.

  - Animal research demonstrates an "acid washout" phenomenon, which occurs when circulation returns to tissue that has been severely deprived of blood flow during cardiac arrest. This presents an acceptable clinical situation to give bicarbonate.

Class III (not acceptable, harmful)

- Patient is in cardiac arrest, and lungs are not effectively ventilated.

  - While you can sometimes provide effective ventilations for a nonintubated person, the majority of patients require endotracheal intubation. Unless there is some other indication, bicarbonate should not be administered to a nonintubated person. In nonventilated lungs it is the accumulation of metabolic byproducts rather than bicarbonate deficit that produces the acidosis. Administration of bicarbonate to the nonintubated patient has been characterized as equivalent to intracellular injection of acid.

HOW?

- 1 mEq/kg IV bolus.
- Repeat half of dose every 10 minutes or per arterial blood gas levels.

WATCH OUT!

- Sodium bicarbonate can produce a variety of side effects, including the following:
  - Mixed venous intracellular acidosis
  - Hyperosmolarity
  - Hypernatremia
  - Metabolic alkalosis
  - Acute hypokalemia
- Do not mix with other emergency medications.

SUMMARY

You will face your most frequent and most difficult resuscitation challenges in patients with persistent VF. Most survivors come from the group of patients who had their lives temporarily interrupted by this chaotic arrhythmia. You will achieve most of these possible survivals by rapid, effective defibrillation. Learning your defibrillator stands as the single most important skill in cardiac resuscitation.

Advanced cardiac life support providers make one of their most critical errors with refractory VF: they learn the algorithm without learning to think about the arrest. The Primary and Secondary Surveys provide a powerful conceptual tool. Consider the effectiveness of each component of the arrest—airway, breathing, CPR, defibrillation, and medications. Most of all, however, think about why the person went into cardiac arrest and why they are staying in arrest. Only through this process will you discover and save those "hearts too good to die."

Pulseless Electrical Activity
The Hunt for Reversible Causes

OVERVIEW

• *This chapter presents patients with pulseless electrical activity (PEA). The person lacks a detectable pulse, yet the heart still possesses electrical activity. In each of these cases you are challenged with a person either in or "on their way to" a full cardiac arrest. The monitor displays "some sort of electrical activity," and on checking the pulse you cannot feel one.*

• *Before 1992, people referred to "electrical activity without an associated pulse" as "electromechanical dissociation" or "EMD." For the 1992 AHA Guidelines, the ACLS subcommittee decided that ACLS providers needed a broader term. To many experts and clinicians, "EMD" was a specific clinical state characterized by narrow, organized-appearing QRS complexes and the absence of mechanical cardiac contractions during that QRS activity. Organized electrical depolarization occurs throughout the myocardium but without synchronous shortening of the myocardial fiber.*

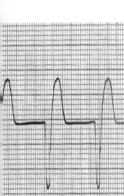

• *Emergency cardiac care providers, however, have had to deal with a much greater variety of "electrical activity during cardiac arrest," yet ACLS treatment algorithms were missing for these other rhythms. Many clinicians thought that the 1986 algorithm for EMD did not apply to the large variety of pulseless patients with some electrical activity on the ECG monitor screen.*

• *Recent research with cardiac ultrasonography and indwelling pressure catheters has led to a reconsideration of "electromechanical dissociation." These data demonstrate that often the electrical activity is associated with mechanical contractions, but these contractions do not produce a blood pressure detectable by the usual methods of palpation or sphygmomanometer.*

• *Therefore the 1992 ACLS Guidelines adopted a new, more encompassing term. "Pulseless electrical activity" includes not only the more specific "EMD" but also a broad range of non–ventricular fibrillation/non–ventricular tachycardia (non-VF/non-VT) electrical activity that has variously been labeled as "pseudo-EMD," "idioventricular rhythms," "ventricular or junctional escape rhythms," "bradyasystolic" or "agonal" rhythms, and a plethora of "post-defibrillation idioventricular rhythms."*

• *This new term provides an opportunity to present guidelines for arrest rhythms that have baffled ACLS providers in the past. Furthermore, the therapeutic approach to all of the electrical activity included under this term is the same: CPR, intubation, epinephrine, atropine (if the activity is slow), and then **hunt for reversible causes.***

• *The core concept behind managing patients with PEA is that the patient may well have a reversible cause of his or her cardiac arrest. If the team leaders (with contributions from the team members) cannot identify a reversible cause, the prospects for successful resuscitation are dismal.*

• *This is the major clinical point to remember about these arrhythmias—they are often associated with specific clinical states that can be reversed when identified early and treated appropriately.*

• *In the cases in this chapter you will learn how to apply the Primary and Secondary Survey Approach to help evaluate patients and provide treatment during the initial resuscitation efforts. In addition, we will describe how to use the Five Quadrads to guide ACLS providers in their hunt for reversible causes of PEA cardiac arrest.*

MAJOR CONCEPTS TO MASTER

- Learn to use the Primary and Secondary Survey Approach in the hunt for reversible causes of PEA arrest (see Box 5-1 on p. 87).
- Learn to apply the Five Quadrads to the initial management of PEA cardiac arrest.
- Always search for reversible causes of PEA cardiac arrest.
- Initiate appropriate treatment on discovery of any reversible cause of PEA cardiac arrest.

Critical actions

The critical actions for patients with PEA are as follows:

- Apply the Five Quadrads approach; in particular, perform the steps of the Primary and Secondary ABCD Surveys and the Universal Algorithm, as follows:
- Perform CPR when indicated.
- Properly attach and operate defibrillator and monitor.
- Recognize PEA rhythms.
- Recognize the need for and successful performance of endotracheal intubation.
- Establish intravenous (IV) access.
- Provide indicated medications.
- Hunt for reversible causes.
- Treat any identified reversible causes.

Skills to learn

- Recognize signs of the following:
  - Hypovolemia
  - Pericardial tamponade
  - Tension pneumothorax
  - Problems with tank/resistance/pump/rate
- Perform the following:
  - Intravenous fluid infusion
  - Pericardiocentesis
  - Needle decompression of pneumothorax

Rhythms to learn

- Pulseless electrical activity includes electromechanical dissociation and other rhythms associated with absent pulse, including the following:
  - Idioventricular rhythms
  - Pulseless asystolic rhythms
  - Bradyasystolic rhythms
  - Ventricular junctional escape rhythms
  - "Pseudo-EMD"
- NOTE: Each electrical complex can be fast or slow and narrow or wide. Treatment approaches and prognoses sometimes vary based on fast-versus-slow and narrow-versus-wide complexes.

Medications to learn

- *Epinephrine* and *atropine* are the two medications recommended in the PEA Algorithm (Fig. 5-1).
- Other medications may be needed, depending on the specific cause of the PEA arrest.

Deborah Luten	PULSELESS ELECTRICAL ACTIVITY RESULTING FROM VENTILATION MISADVENTURES
CASE 1	You are called to a 27-year-old woman in the intensive care unit (ICU) whose condition has deteriorated abruptly. During nasotracheal suctioning she suddenly became agitated and distressed and then lost consciousness. She has had nasotracheal intubation for the past 5 days for severe varicella (chickenpox) pneumonitis. She had been placed on continuous positive airway pressure (CPAP) to improve her oxygenation. The cardiac monitor shows a sinus bradycardia of 40 beats per minute; a blood pressure cannot be obtained, and the nurse cannot feel a pulse.

As the team leader in the ICU, how would you begin your evaluation of Ms. Luten?

COMMENTS

- By definition, Ms. Luten has PEA: she has no detectable pulse by palpation, and yet she displays a narrow-complex, regular sinus bradycardia of 40 beats per minute. You are going to use the AHA PEA Algorithm (Fig. 5-1) to help guide your evaluation and treatment.

FIGURE 5-1

Pulseless Electrical Activity Algorithm

The term pulseless electrical activity (PEA) includes the following:
- Electromechanical dissociation (EMD)
- Pseudo-EMD
- Idioventricular rhythms
- Ventricular escape rhythms
- Bradyasystolic rhythms
- Post-defibrillation idioventricular rhythms

Continue Basic Life Support
Perform Secondary ABCD Survey:
- Intubate if needed
- Access ventilations
- Obtain IV access

Check for occult blood flow using Doppler ultrasound, echocardiograph, end tidal CO_2 device

Consider the differential diagnoses:
(Possible treatments shown in parentheses)

Five H's:
- Hypovolemia, includes anyaphylaxis (volume infusion)
- Hypoxia (oxygen and ventilation)
- Hypothermia (see hypothermia algorithm in Chapter 14)
- Hyper-/hypokalemia (and other electrolyte abnormalities)
- Hydrogen ion (acidosis)

Five T's:
- Tension pneumothorax (needle decompression)
- Tamponade, cardiac (pericardiocentesis)
- Thrombosis, pulmonary (surgery, thrombolytics)
- Thrombosis, acute myocardial (thrombolytics, see Chapter 9)
- Tablets, drug overdoses (drug-specific interventions)

- *Epinephrine* 1 mg IV push[a,c]
- Repeat every 3 to 5 min

- If rate of electrical activity is slow (< 60 beats/min), give *atropine* 1 mg IV
- Repeat every 3 to 5 min to a total of 0.03 to 0.04 mg/kg[d]

Class I: Definitely helpful
Class IIa: Acceptable, probably helpful
Class IIb: Acceptable, possibly helpful
Class III: Not indicated, may be harmful

(a) **Sodium bicarbonate** 1 mEq/ kg is Class I if patient has known preexisting hyperkalemia.

(b) **Sodium bicarbonate** (1 mEq/ kg) is given as follows:

Class IIa
- If known preexisting bicarbonate-responsive acidosis

- If overdose with tricyclic antidepressants
- To alkalinize the urine in drug overdoses

Class IIb
- If patient is intubated and arrest continues for long intervals
- If circulation is restored after prolonged arrest

Class III
- Hypoxic lactic acidosis (unventilated patient)

(c) The recommended dose of **epinephrine** is 1 mg IV push every 3 to 5 min. If spontaneous circulation does not return, consider several Class IIb dosing regimens:

- Intermediate: **Epinephrine** 2-5 mg IV push, every 3 to 5 min.
- Escalating: **Epinephrine** 1 mg-3 mg-5 mg IV push, 3 min apart.
- High: **Epinephrine** 0.1 mg/kg IV push, every 3 to 5 min.

(d) The shorter atropine dosing interval (3 minutes) is possibly helpful in cardiac arrest (Class IIb).

Adapted with permission, Journal of the American Medical Association, 1992, Volume 268, *Guidelines for Cardiopulmonary Resuscitation and Emergency Cardiac Care*, p. 2219, copyright© 1992, Amercian Medical Assocation.

• Throughout this book we recommend the Primary and Secondary Surveys as the best unifying approach to evaluate cardiopulmonary emergencies, in particular, the patient in cardiac arrest. Start there. The Five Quadrads incorporate the Primary and Secondary Surveys, and offer an easy-to-remember, efficient method to review 20 clinical items.

PRIMARY ABCD SURVEY

• The ICU patient in Case 1 already has a nasotracheal tube in place and has been placed on the ventilator for 5 days; you quickly check that **Airway** and **Breathing** appear satisfactory because the nasotracheal tube extends from the nose and is attached to the ventilator.

The chest appears to rise with the ventilations. *(This is an incomplete evaluation, and will be discussed later.)*

• You then go to **C**irculation and check the pulse. You confirm again the absence of a pulse and direct the clinical assistant to start chest compressions.

SECONDARY ABCD SURVEY

• **Airway:** Patient has been placed on nasotracheal intubation already.

• **Breathing:** Patient has been placed on a ventilator with CPAP, and you see that the nurse who had been performing the suctioning reattached the endotracheal

---

BOX 5-1

The Primary and Secondary ABCD Surveys Applied to Pulseless Electrical Activity

The Five Quadrads

Apply the Five Quadrads to the initial evaluation and management of PEA arrest, as follows:

• *Primary ABCD Survey*
• *Secondary ABCD Survey*
• *Oxygen/IV/Monitor/Fluids*
• *Temperature/Blood Pressure/Heart Rate/ Respirations*
• *Tank (Volume)/Resistance/Pump/Rate*

Primary ABCD Survey

AIRWAY
• *Open the airway.*

BREATHING
• *Provide two breaths with positive-pressure ventilation.*

CIRCULATION
• *Give chest compressions.*

DEFIBRILLATION
• *Shock VF/pulseless VT.*

Secondary ABCD Survey

AIRWAY
• *Assess adequacy of the primary ventilation and airway techniques.*
• *Perform endotracheal intubation if indicated.*

BREATHING
• *Provide positive-pressure ventilations through the endotracheal tube.*
• *Establish that placement of the endotracheal tube is correct as follows:*
  • *Check end-tidal CO_2 volume; use esophageal detection device.*
  • *Assess that the chest wall moves with each ventilation.*
  • *Listen for bilateral breath sounds.*

CIRCULATION
• *Perform chest compressions.*
• *Attach monitor leads.*
• *Identify heart rhythm and rate.*
• *Obtain IV access.*
• *Administer medications appropriate for the rhythm and vital signs.*
• *Measure blood pressure if pulse is detected.*

DIFFERENTIAL DIAGNOSES
• *Consider the following possible causes of the cardiac emergency, including "five Hs and five Ts" (Table 5-1) of possible causes of PEA arrest:*
  • *Hypovolemia*
  • *Hypoxia*
  • *Hypothermia*
  • *Hyperkalemia, hypokalemia*
  • *Hydrogen ion (acidosis)*
  • *Tamponade: cardiac tamponade*
  • *Tension pneumothorax*
  • *Thrombosis: lungs (massive pulmonary embolism)*
  • *Thrombosis: heart (acute, massive myocardial infarction [AMI])*
  • *Tablets: drug overdose*

tube to the ventilator, which appears to be operating properly. You listen to each side of the chest in the midaxillary line and hear the sounds of each ventilation from the ventilator.

- **Circulation:** Chest compressions are in progress; IV already in place. You know, however, that in PEA arrests you should verify the absence of blood flow by some technique in addition to hand palpation of a peripheral artery. You ask for a quick Doppler confirmation that there is indeed no blood flow during the QRS complexes.

- **Differential Diagnoses:** Already you are beginning to consider what could have caused such an acute deterioration in an intubated patient who is receiving ventilation with CPAP. You think the most likely problem would relate to airway and ventilation, but you are not sure how that would immediately affect the pulse and cause the patient to go into cardiac arrest. You remember that familiar ICU axiom: Acute deterioration in a patient on CPAP is an acute pneumothorax until proven otherwise.

- **Oxygen/IV/Monitor/Fluids**: All have been initiated.

- **Temperature/Blood Pressure/Heart Rate/ Respirations:** 36.8° C, not detectable, 40 beats per minute, and 15 breaths per minute, respectively.

- **Tank (Volume)/Resistance/Pump/Rate:** Analyze the cardiovascular quadrad: What is the nature of the problem? (The "cardiovascular quadrad" is less useful in full cardiac arrest patients, but it is mentioned here because the ACLS providers will be using it routinely for all cardiopulmonary emergencies. (See Chapters 1 and 10 for additional examples.)

    Tank: Is there a *tank* problem? None, apparently. There are no immediate data to suggest that Ms. Luten is hypo-volemic or hypervolemic, either from an absolute or a relative volume perspective.

    Resistance: Is there a *resistance* problem? None, apparently. You note no clinical signs of vasoconstriction, and there was no reason for profound vasodilation that would have led to the pulseless state.

    Pump: Is there a *pump* problem? Probably, although it is not clear at this point. The heart does not appear to be pumping blood, despite the monitor display of 40 beats per minute.

    Rate: Is there a *rate* problem? Yes. The rate of 40 beats per minute on the cardiac monitor is *not* appropriate for a hypotensive or arrested patient and should be much higher. This is a "too slow" rhythm, and you mentally direct your attention to the Bradycardia Algorithm.

- To evaluate the D—Differential Diagnoses of the Secondary Survey—you order a "stat" chest x-ray, 12-lead ECG, and arterial blood gas levels.

- The PEA Algorithm (Fig. 5-1) provides us with two review boxes, the first stating the following:

    - Continue CPR.

    - Intubate at once.

    - Obtain IV access.

    - Assess blood flow using Doppler ultrasound, end-tidal CO_2 volume, echocardiography, or arterial line.

    NOTE: *All of these points and more have been covered by the Five Quadrads.*

- The PEA Algorithm lists two medications to administer for PEA: epinephrine 1 mg IV push, followed by a second dose (at several acceptable levels) 3 to 5 minutes later; and atropine 1 mg IV (up to a total dose of 0.03 to 0.04 mg/kg IV).

Deborah Luten

CASE 1 Continued

To better time the chest compressions and ventilations, you direct the respiratory therapist to disconnect the ventilator and to ventilate the lungs using a resuscitation bag attached to the nasotracheal tube. Chest expansion is small with these ventilations. The respiratory therapist uses 100% oxygen at 15 L/min.

You order epinephrine 1 mg IV push, followed at once by atropine 1 mg IV. This produces a slight increase in the heart rate to 45 beats per minute, but then the rate drops back and continues to slowly decline.

A single thought keeps returning to you: The abrupt deterioration must be related to the continuous positive-pressure ventilations being delivered to this ill woman with severe pneumonitis. You think that a tension pneumothorax could have occurred. By shifting the mediastinum dramatically, this may be compromising return of blood flow to the heart. Without venous return you have an "empty pump" syndrome. Mechanical contractions occur that the cardiac monitor displays as normal-looking electrical activity, but no blood flow occurs and the patient is therefore "pulseless."

You state, "I'm going to check for a tension pneumothorax. Please hand me a 14-gauge Intracath, some size 7 sterile gloves, and two Betadine swabs." You ask for a pause in chest compressions long enough to prep the skin and insert the 14-gauge needle through the right second

CONTINUED

D e b o r a h   L u t e n

C A S E   1   C o n t i n u e d

intercostal space in the midclavicular line just above the top of the third rib (Fig. 5-2). You listen closely as you insert the open needle, but you hear no hiss of escaping air.

With mounting concern, you ask for chest compressions to resume while you prepare to repeat the procedure on the left side. You move to the left side, and again you hear no sounds of air escaping when you puncture the chest wall with the needle.

It is now only 3 minutes since you arrived at the bedside of Ms. Luten, although it seems much longer. You appropriately considered possible causes for her PEA, but your initial diagnosis of a tension pneumothorax related to positive-pressure ventilation appears incorrect. The bilateral needle decompression attempts did not confirm air under pressure in the thorax and did not seem to help. Her heart rate is now 20 beats per minute, and the QRS complexes are beginning to widen out.

What would you now do in this code that is not going well?

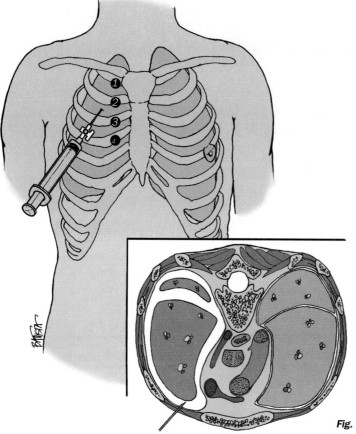

COMMENTS

- In addition to the basics of the Primary and Secondary Surveys, the most important principle to follow in PEA and asystolic arrest is to repeatedly pursue *the hunt for reversible causes!* Even if your first diagnosis of a tension pneumothorax proved incorrect, you must continue the hunt.

- The ACLS Guidelines provide a list of possible causes of PEA in the PEA Algorithm (Fig. 5-1 and Table 5-1).

- While the ACLS Guidelines provide Table 5-1 as a list of *some* possible causes that have immediate therapies, many ACLS providers have interpreted this list as the *only* possible causes. This interpretation is far removed from the true intent of providing a partial list to stimulate thought, but not to limit thought.

- Advanced cardiac life support providers and instructors enjoy memory aids to help remember aspects of emergency care. The following are two memory techniques that people have used to remember some of the possible causes of PEA:

  - The first technique simply notes that the possible causes can be listed as the "five Hs and five Ts" (See the box on p. 91 and Table 5-1).

Fig. 5-2: *Landmarks for needle decompression of pneumothorax.*

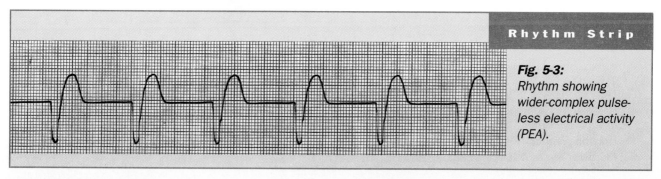

R h y t h m   S t r i p

Fig. 5-3: *Rhythm showing wider-complex pulseless electrical activity (PEA).*

TABLE 5-1

Conditions That Cause Pulseless Electrical Activity: "Five Hs and Five Ts"

CONDITION	FEATURES OF THE ELECTRICAL ACTIVITY	HISTORICAL/PHYSICAL CLUES	MANAGEMENT
HYPOVOLEMIA	Narrow complex Rapid rate	History, flat neck veins	Volume infusion
HYPOXIA	Slow rate (hypoxia)	Cyanosis, blood gas levels, airway problems	Oxygenation, ventilation
HYPOTHERMIA	J or Osborne waves	History of exposure to cold, core body temperature	See Hypothermia Algorithm, Chapter 14, p. 247.
HYPERKALEMIA OR **H**YPOKALEMIA	Both states cause wide-complex QRS **High-potassium ECG** • T waves taller and peaked • P waves get smaller • QRS widens • Sine-wave PEA **Low potassium ECG** • T waves flatten • Prominent U waves • QRS widens • QT prolongs • Wide-complex tachy	History of renal failure, diabetes, recent dialysis, dialysis fistulas, medications Abnormal loss of potassium; diuretic use	**Hyperkalemia** sodium bicarbonate, glucose plus insulin, calcium chloride Kayexalate/sorbitol, dialysis (long-term) **Hypokalemia** Rapid but controlled infusion of potassium; add magnesium if cardiac arrest
HYDROGEN ION Acidosis	Smaller amplitude QRS complexes	History of bicarbonate-responsive preexisting acidosis, renal failure	Sodium bicarbonate, hyperventilation
TAMPONADE Cardiac tamponade	Narrow complex Rapid rate	History, no pulse with CPR, vein distention	Pericardiocentesis
TENSION **P**NEUMOTHORAX	Narrow complex	History, no pulse with CPR, slow rate (hypoxia), neck vein distention, tracheal deviation, unequal breath sounds; difficulty in ventilating the patient	Needle decompression
THROMBOSIS Lungs: Massive pulmonary embolism	Narrow complex Rapid rate	History, no pulse felt with CPR, distended neck veins	Pulmonary arteriogram, surgical embolectomy, thrombolytics
THROMBOSIS Heart: Acute, massive myocardial infarction	Abnormal 12-lead ECG: Q waves, ST-segment changes, T waves, inversions	History, ECG, enzyme levels	Thrombolytic agents; See AMI cases Chapter 9.
TABLETS Drug overdose (tricyclic, digoxin, beta blockers and calcium channel blockers)	Various effects on the ECG, predominately prolongation of the QT interval	Bradycardia, history of ingestion, empty bottles at the scene, pupils, neurologic examination	Drug screens, intubation, lavage, activated charcoal, lactulose per local protocols; specific antidotes and agents per toxidrome

FIVE CAUSES THAT START WITH "H"
Hypovolemia
Hypoxia
Hypothermia
Hyper/hypokalemia
Hydrogen ion (acidosis)

FIVE CAUSES THAT START WITH "T"
Tamponade (cardiac)
Tension pneumothorax
Thrombosis-lungs (pulmonary embolus)
Thrombosis (AMI)
Tablets (drug overdoses)

- The second technique uses the 10-letter acrostic "PEA ITTT VOD!" where by some stretch of pronunciation you can pretend that "VOD" reminds one of "BAD." The sentence "PEA it bad" has a clinical context as follows, which should make the phrase easier to remember:
  - **P**otassium
  - **E**mbolus
  - **A**cidosis

  - **I**schemia (AMI)
  - **T**emperature
  - **T**amponade
  - **T**ension (pneumothorax)

  - **V**olume
  - **O**xygen (hypoxia)
  - **D**rugs
- A third technique involves learning a table that provides clues from the ECG, the history, and the physical examination, and combines these clues with management tips. In Table 5-1 we have arranged the possible causes of PEA in the "five Hs" followed by the "five Ts", and combined this list with ECG, historical, and physical examination clues.
- We recommend that everyone devise a system to review the possible causes. To maintain ease of memory and to provide some uniformity, we recommend referring, once again, to the Primary and Secondary Surveys. Within each component of these two surveys you can mentally list a number of causes that may be playing a role either in the original arrest or in persistence of cardiac arrest.
- Table 5-2 provides a detailed list to review possible causes of PEA cardiac arrest, using the ABCD mnemonic of the two surveys. This technique can also be used during arrests of any origin or cause. For example, we adapted this table from a similar table in Chapter 4.

TABLE 5-2

Pulseless Electrical Activity Cardiac Arrest: Hunting for Reversible Causes Using ABCD of the Secondary Survey

STEP ONE

Troubleshoot: Check to see that ABCs are working correctly.

AIRWAY
- *Airway is open, and air is moving easily through airway adjuncts.*
- *Endotracheal tube, if in place, is open and unobstructed.*

BREATHING
- *Bilateral, symmetric chest expansions with ventilations are present.*
- *Person is "bagging" at correct rate and force.*

CIRCULATION
- *CPR chest compressions are adequate in rate, force, depth, and location.*
- *Intravenous access is established correctly.*
- *Medications are administered properly.*
- *Monitor is used correctly (leads connected, correct control settings).*

STEP TWO

Differential Diagnoses:
Review D, asking "What else could be causing this PEA?"

AIRWAY (Problems lead to hypoxia.)
- *Tube in the wrong place; in the esophagus or right mainstem bronchus*
- *Tube obstructed or kinked*
- *Foreign body aspiration*
- *Anaphylaxis (angioedema)*
- *Inflammatory conditions of the hypopharynx (epiglottis or retropharyngeal abcess)*
- *Craniofacial trauma, laryngeal or tracheal disruption*

BREATHING (Problems lead to hypoxia.)
- *Preexisting mechanical abnormalities of the chest wall (scoliosis, emphysema, congenital)*
- *Tension pneumothorax from resuscitation efforts*
- *Subcutaneous emphysema*

CIRCULATION
- ***Hypovolemia***
- ***Pericardial tamponade*** *from resuscitation efforts*
- ***Pulmonary embolus***
- ***Prolonged hypoxia*** *causing cardiac failure*
- ***Massive acute myocardial infarction***
- ***Electrolyte disturbances (potassium, calcium, and magnesium)***
- ***Drug overdoses*** *of many types: Cyclic antidepressants, aspirin, beta blocker or calcium channel blocker overdoses*
- ***Occult trauma:*** *Cardiac tamponade, hypovolemia, exsanguination*
- *Illicit drugs: cocaine, heroin, cyanide poisoning (from fires or synthetics)*
- *Carbon monoxide poisoning*
- *Anesthetic agent toxicity*

Items in bold italics are the 10 causes (five Hs and five Ts) listed in Table 5-1.

Deborah Luten

CASE 1 Continued

With a growing sense of despair, you take a slow, deep breath and again return to the ABCDs. "Okay, let's take it from the top. Chuck [the respiratory therapist], would you please take your laryngoscope and check the tube placement? Double-check that we're not down in the right mainstem bronchus. Make sure we are still getting good, bilateral breath sounds. Where is the portable chest x-ray, by the way? Please call them again."

"How are the chest compressions? It seems like we might need a stiffer board under her back. What about 'lytes and ABGs? Let's find those reports. Has she been having trouble with her 'crit' or other bad numbers? Also, it's time for more epinephrine and make it 3 mg IV this time. Also I want the next dose of atropine to be 2 mg."

"Get her attending physician on the phone so I can talk to her. Did she get any new medications today that she might be allergic to? By the way, if any of you have any suggestions or ideas please share them—we need to figure out what went wrong here. I didn't think her pneumonitis was so bad."

As the team members move about with their responsibilities you hear a quiet, "Oh my God!" from Chuck, who is peering into the mouth with a laryngoscope. He glances up and meets your eyes. "The tube is in the esophagus."

Now, 5 minutes into the code, the picture becomes clear: somehow, during the suctioning and coughing the end of the nasotracheal tube must have become dislodged. Since she was sedated to comply with the ventilator, she did not display signs of respiratory distress. The ventilator sounds were transmitted bilaterally, leading to the initial false finding of equal breath sounds.

Quickly the nasotracheal tube is untaped and removed. Bagging is performed through a face mask while an orotracheal tube is prepared. The reintubation proceeds without difficulty, and her lungs are immediately hyperventilated with 100% oxygen. Within 60 seconds you notice her heart rate beginning to increase. Two minutes later a palpable pulse causes you to order CPR compressions to stop. At 3 minutes after reintubation the blood pressure is 90/60 mm Hg, and the heart rate is 75 beats per minute.

In retrospect, were there any clues that this was a pure airway and breathing problem? What should you have done differently?

COMMENTS

- Ms. Luten made a full recovery from this episode of respiratory compromise and 6 minutes of CPR. Some oxygenation and ventilation must have been occurring through the dislodged nasotracheal tube, which was located a few centimeters from the glottic opening.

- The biggest clue here was the sinus bradycardia with a narrow QRS complex. Steadily slowing bradycardia is a classic finding with respiratory compromise and hypoxic failure. The narrow cardiac complexes indicated a normal-functioning myocardium. Lack of oxygen and the progressive acidosis caused deterioration, but there was no intrinsic problem with the heart.

- A better approach would have been to perform more aggressive Primary and Secondary ABCD Surveys on first arriving on the scene. The assumption that the endotracheal tube is correctly placed in a person already placed on a ventilator seemed reasonable. Nevertheless, do not manage codes based on assumptions that can be checked easily. This was an acute, sudden deterioration. Such situations require a return to the basics and a reconfirmation that all interventions have been and are continuing to be performed correctly.

Raymond Jackson CASE 2	You are on duty in the Emergency Department when the medics enter with a 55-year-old man who is unconscious but withdrawing to painful stimuli. Medics report they picked him up as "a man down" call in the University District. In the field his initial blood pressure was 80 mm

Hg, and pulse rate was 120 beats per minute, but the medics report his pulse has gotten progressively weaker. He became unresponsive just as they drove up to the Emergency Department ambulance bay. When you place your fingers on his femoral artery during the transfer, you cannot feel a pulse. His extremities are cool, his fingertips are cyanotic, and his skin is clammy with sweat. How would you approach this patient?

COMMENTS

The Five Quadrads approach provides your starting point.

PRIMARY ABCD SURVEY

Patient is unconscious, unresponsive and looks cyanotic. Perform Primary Survey as follows:

- **Airway:** Open the airway.
- **Breathing:** There are no breaths; ask for the pocket face mask from where it is "Velcro-ed" to the Emergency Department wall; assign airway management to one of the team members; give two quick breaths through the one-way valve; observe for obstruction and bilateral symmetric chest expansion.
- **Circulation:** Check a carotid pulse; if there is no pulse, assign chest compressions to a team member and begin chest compressions.
- **Defibrillation:** Turn on the defibrillator and monitor. Switch lead selector switch to "paddles," apply electrode-defibrillation paste to paddles, and apply paddles to the chest for a "quick-look." Narrow QRS complex and sinus tachycardia at 120 beats/min are evident. Assign monitor management and defibrillation to other team members.

SECONDARY ABCD SURVEY

- **Airway:** Start ventilations with bag valve mask and 100% oxygen; instruct airway manager to proceed with endotracheal intubation.
- **Breathing:** Assure proper tube placement; ask airway manager to report any problems; order stat portable chest x-ray.
- **Circulation:** Assign starting of an IV to two team members; first person who starts IV informs the group. Check to see what rhythm is displayed (sinus tachycardia). Chest compressions are in progress; verify the absence of blood flow by Doppler ultrasound. Stop CPR briefly and time Doppler with QRS complexes on monitor.

- **Differential Diagnoses:** The team members have conducted a smooth transfer from the medics to the Emergency Department, and you have continued the resuscitation efforts. As the team leader, you have not touched any equipment or done any procedure. (You did hand the nurse starting the IV a bag of normal saline from the cabinet.) *Your role is to think.* Your thoughts are moving quickly to gather clues about why this man is in cardiac arrest.

OXYGEN/IV/MONITOR/FLUIDS

All of these tasks have been assigned and are in progress. Note how "assign four tasks" was done smoothly: chest compressor, airway manager, rhythm manager (monitor and defibrillator), and IV access and medications.

VITAL SIGNS

Temperature is 35.8° C, heart rate is 120 beats per minute, blood pressure cannot be obtained; there are no spontaneous respirations.

TANK (VOLUME)/RESISTANCE/PUMP/RATE

Analyze the cardiovascular quadrad: What is the nature of the problem?

- *Is there a tank problem?* Unclear at this point. Tank problems are among the reversible causes of PEA. You must consider whether the tank is absolutely empty from loss of volume or relatively empty because of a resistance problem.
- *Is there a resistance problem?* Probably. There are signs of increased peripheral vascular resistance, which suggest shock from hypovolemia.
- *Is there a pump problem?* Unclear at this point. This is PEA—electrical activity is normal but no pulse is being produced. Pump problems are among the reversible causes of PEA.
- *Is there a rate problem?* No. The sinus tachycardia at 120 beats per minute is a clue to a normal cardiac electrical system. Sinus tachycardia is always a response to some other process and never necessitates defibrillation or cardioversion.

Raymond Jackson

CASE 2 Continued

The actions and interventions of the Five Quadrads are in progress. One of the nurses remarks that Mr. Jackson is a heavy-drinking street person, well known to the Emergency Department staff. He had been in the Emergency Department 3 days ago looking for "a place to stay and dry out and get the booze out of my system." You notice dark, tarry stains on Mr. Jackson's ragged underwear as his clothing is removed.

You ask the resident helping in the room to slip on a glove and perform a quick stool guaiac test. The stool sample is tarry black and markedly positive. You notice that the endotracheal tube is in place, and you ask one of the nurses to "please place an NG tube." She responds that she is too busy starting the IV and asks whether you can do it instead. You do not reply but ask the resident who just performed the stool examination to "please place an NG tube as soon as you get a moment." Once placed, the tube is aspirated for dark, almost black liquid that tests positive for blood.

What are your thoughts about Mr. Jackson now, and how would you proceed with evaluation and treatment?

COMMENTS

- Mr. Jackson has suffered an acute gastrointestinal hemorrhage that may or may not fully account for this PEA. Certainly profound hypovolemia can cause PEA. As it is one of the reversible causes of cardiac arrest, it would be a tragedy to overlook hypovolemia.

- *Order rapid fluid replacement.* An empirical fluid bolus is always appropriate in PEA. Many experts have argued that the treatment of PEA should always include an *empirical fluid bolus.* Such an action would be immediately and strongly indicated on any clinical clue that hypovolemia was playing a role in the pulseless state.

- The other important clue you have with Mr. Jackson is the rhythm (Fig. 5-4) a narrow QRS complex. Not all PEAs are alike. As noted earlier, PEA is a heterogeneous grouping of electrical activity ranging from perfectly viable normal sinus rhythm to broad, agonal "slurring" that represents "the last dying gasp" of the myocardium.

- The AHA PEA Algorithm already makes a distinction between fast and slow PEA, recommending an additional medication—atropine—for bradycardic PEA.

- In addition to the electrical activity rate as a criterion by which you can subclassify PEAs, you can also use the width of the QRS complex. This approach is conveyed in Fig. 5-5.

- Although no study has clearly demonstrated differences in survival among PEAs classified by QRS width and by electrical activity rate, these features can have useful empirical treatment and prognostic implications.

- Mr. Jackson has a mild tachycardia with a narrow QRS complex. This is exactly what you would expect in a person who is exsanguinating from severe gastrointestinal hemorrhage.

- Do not neglect to use the width and rate of the PEA to provide clues for treatment.

Rhythm Strip

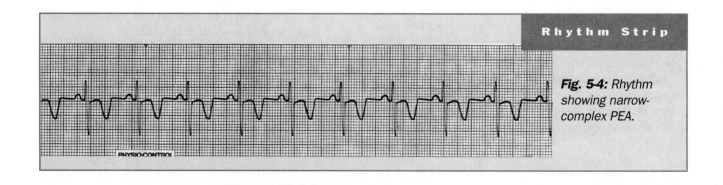

Fig. 5-4: Rhythm showing narrow-complex PEA.

PHYSIO-CONTROL

FIG. 5-5

Classification of Pulseless Electrical Activity by Electrical Activity Rate and QRS Width

RATE OF COMPLEXES (PER MINUTE)	WIDTH OF COMPLEXES	
	Narrow	Wide
Fast (>60)	Sinus EMD Pseudo-EMD Paroxysmal supraventricular tachycardia	VT VF
Slow (<60)	EMD Pseudo-EMD Post-defibrillation	Bradyasystolic Idioventricular Vent escape

Pulseless Electrical Activity (PEA) is a term used to encompass the broad range of rhythms that display electrical activity but without a clinically detectable pulse. There are several subsets of PEA. One is "electromechanical dissociation" (EMD), which is now reserved for rhythms with a narrow and more organized QRS complex. Pulseless electrical activity can be more precisely described in terms of the *width* of the QRS complexes and the *rate* of the associated electrical activity.

Although "PEA" may appear to be an imprecise term, it has great clinical utility because most PEAs are treated the same, according to the PEA Algorithm. By this definition, ventricular tachycardia (VT) and ventricular fibrillation (VF) are PEA rhythms. However, by following the Universal Algorithm and the Primary and Secondary Survey Approach, ACLS providers will not get confused. They will have already identified and treated VT/VF before getting to the PEA decision point.

Raymond Jackson

CASE 2 Continued

You instruct the team to push high volumes of normal saline (NS) as rapidly as possible. They begin infusions through two 14-gauge needles and have administered 750 cc over about 8 minutes. CPR has been performed continuously. You administer epinephrine, 1 mg at first, and then 5 mg IV 3 minutes afterward. The first Doppler reading shows that Mr. Jackson does have effective mechanical contractions as the Doppler detects pulsatile blood flow when CPR is stopped. The Doppler beats coincide with the QRS complexes on the monitor. After the 750 mL of NS and the second dose of epinephrine the nurse reports she can feel a weak femoral pulse. Mr. Jackson begins to demonstrate some spontaneous movements and withdrawal in response to painful stimuli.

The hematocrit is reported back as a "critical lab value" of 13%. You order four units of O-negative blood brought to the Emergency Department immediately. Within 5 minutes the O-negative blood is infusing at "wide-open" rate.

Should not Mr. Jackson's condition be classified as profound hypotension or shock rather than as PEA?

COMMENTS

- Case 2 represents a good example of the "overlap" syndromes that exist in emergency cardiopulmonary care. (See Chapter 7 for a more in-depth discussion of this topic. Also see the box on p. 123.) Mr. Jackson had, indeed, profound hypotension—so profound you could not feel a pulse. He also had a "too fast" heart rate: a tachycardia that was profoundly symptomatic: he was without a pulse.

- A powerful adrenergic agent, *epinephrine*, stands as the common agent of treatment for all these conditions— hypotension, PEA, and symptomatic tachycardia. Epinephrine provides a therapeutic unity to the treatment of all these conditions. You aggressively administered epinephrine (two doses of 1 and 5 mg) in this case because epinephrine is an appropriate agent for profound hypotension. Remember, however, that vasopressors are only an adjunct in persons with hypotension and shock. Rapid, aggressive fluid replacement will always be the first-line therapy.

- Remember to refer to the *Hypotension/Shock/Acute Pulmonary Edema Algorithm* (Chapter 10) for additional guidelines in patients like Mr. Jackson. As an "overlap" syndrome, his condition includes not only PEA, but also shock and severe hypotension. As such you must consider the following:

  - **Massive fluid replacement** (initial treatment of choice here)

  - **Blood** and **blood products transfusions** (as soon as possible)

  - **Vasopressors** (for example, **dopamine, norepinephrine,** and **epinephrine**)

- The critical action in Case 2 was the identification of a reversible cause of PEA. Mr. Jackson had, in effect, quietly, and without complaints to his friends, bled to death. Only by quick focus on the Five Quadrads were you able to identify the cause and institute appropriate, lifesaving interventions.

Rachel Pomeranz	One of your colleagues in the Emergency Department has started treatment in a woman with acute renal colic resulting from a kidney stone.
CASE 3	Because the nurses could not obtain peripheral venous access, your colleague had started a right subclavian central IV line. You suddenly

hear an overhead page, "We need a doctor in Room 7 immediately." You enter the rather confused scene in the room and learn that the lady abruptly became distressed, short of breath, and then confused and incoherent. She is not attached to a monitor, and you cannot feel a pulse.

With this history, what would you think is the most likely cause of this sudden collapse? How would you approach this patient?

COMMENTS

- Once again, Case 3 will reveal PEA when a monitor is attached. You arrive on the scene and take charge of the resuscitation activities. You quickly run through the Primary and Secondary ABCD Surveys. You make sure you assign the four basic tasks of all resuscitation attempts, as follows:

  - Someone for the airway: Proceed with intubation.

  - Someone for chest compressions: Start chest compressions.

  - Someone for monitor and defibrillator: Patient is not in VF.

  - Someone for IV access and medications: Person is in process of trying to start another IV line; you order a dose of 3 mg epinephrine injected down the endotracheal tube.

- Your ABCD surveys revealed the following information:

  - She was perfectly normal except for severe renal colic until moments before her collapse.

- The central line had been started in her right subclavian vein and she was doing well until several minutes after the IV infusion of NS and 50 mg IV meperidine.

- Blood pressure is unobtainable; heart rate is 120 beats per minute on monitor, which showed low QRS voltage and sinus tachycardia; respirations are 22 breaths per minute: shallow, labored, and insufficient.

- Jugular venous distention is present and easily observed.

- Cardiac sounds to auscultation were faint and difficult to hear.

- The challenge here is to focus on the D (Differential Diagnosis) of the Secondary Survey and try to identify a reversible cause for this woman's sudden collapse. The circumstances strongly suggest that some event occurred related to the insertion of the right subclavian line. Your main thoughts are right-sided pneumothorax or right-sided hemothorax as complications of the subclavian line insertion. You think you may need to perform a needle decompression followed by insertion of a chest tube.

Rachel Pomeranz	The IV bag shows that about 400 mL NS has been infused through the right subclavian line, and you order the nurse to stop infusing flu-
CASE 3 Continued	ids through that line. You order a "stat" portable chest x-ray. You con-

sider what else could be going on, and you review the long list of possible problems according to ABCD: Airway problems, Breathing or ventilation, and Circulation (Table 5-2). You decide to place a chest tube for either pneumothorax or hemothorax on the right side and ask the nurse to get a chest tube set up.

The radiology technician returns at once with the portable chest x-rays, stating, "It's in way too far!" However, on close inspection you see that the endotracheal tube is located 2 cm above the carina, exactly where it should be. "Well, the tube looks okay to me," you state, "and I don't see a pneumo- or hemothorax." The x-ray technician glances at you with a look of infinite patience practiced over many years, saying, "Doc, I was referring to the IV catheter." He points carefully to the lateral chest x-ray, where you note that the course of the radiopaque catheter extends to the lowest part of the ventricle, exactly at the level of the diaphragm.

What emergency procedure would you consider now? Describe how you would perform it.

Rachel Pomeranz

CASE 3 Continued

You take a 60 mL syringe and ask for an 18-gauge, long spinal needle. With sterile techniques you insert the needle in the space just between the xiphoid process and the left costal margin. You maintain a slight pull on the syringe plunger and feel a slight "pop" as you penetrate the pericardial sac. Several mL of bloody fluid enter the syringe. You quickly aspirate 60 mL of the pericardial fluid. Almost immediately the nurse reports return of a pulse.

You are not sure whether the perforation in the right atrial appendage has sealed over and whether there will be continued bleeding from the presumed small hole. Since you think the pulseless state occurred because fluid was infused into the pericardial sac, you hope the problem is solved. Nevertheless, you almost wish you had prepared to place a small flexible catheter in the pericardial sac. "Too late now," you mumble as you pull the needle and syringe from the chest. "Please contact the cardiothoracic surgeon on call for me. She may need to do this stick again in a short while. Let's get a bed in the ICU for the patient."

Is this a common scenario for cardiac tamponade and the need for pericardiocentesis?

COMMENTS

- The PEA arrest described in Case 3 now seems to have been caused by acute pericardial tamponade. Clearly the right subclavian central line was inserted too far, as demonstrated on the lateral chest x-ray. The most likely sequence of events was perforation of the right atrial appendage by the catheter tip. When the IV fluids were infused, the normal, nondistensible pericardium quickly filled to capacity and tamponade ensued. This compromised the ventricular filling during diastole, producing the clinical emergency of an "empty pump." A normally beating heart was not being refilled with blood after each beat.

- The immediate step is to stop the infusion of fluids through the central line. Next, perform an emergency pericardiocentesis.

- The preferred pericardiocentesis technique is drainage directed by fluoroscopy in the catheterization laboratory. Echocardiography, used to guide flexible catheters inserted by the Seldinger technique, can also be used. Most pericardiocenteses are performed for subacute pericardial effusions in which symptoms are more gradual and the need for drainage less emergent.

- In the case of Ms. Pomeranz, however, you are faced with the life-threatening challenge of arrest resulting from PEA. A cardiac arrest does not permit time for arrangements for a catheterization laboratory and consultant cardiologist.

- *Pericardiocentesis.* The simplest and most direct technique is to do the following:
  - Attach a 16- to 18-gauge long (9 cm) needle to a 60 mL syringe.
  - Insert the needle gradually into the fifth intercostal space (Fig. 5-6), immediately to the left of the sternum.

- With constant aspiration pressure you can tell when you enter the pericardial sac by a distinct "give" sensation and aspiration of grossly bloody pericardial fluid.

- Remove as much of the pericardial fluid as possible. This may require changing the syringes, but usually aspiration of 60 mL is sufficient to produce a dramatic change in symptoms.

- Spin the bloody fluid for a hematocrit; observe whether the fluid clots. (Pericardial fluid does not clot and has a different hematocrit from venous blood.)

- An alternative method is the subxiphoid approach in which the needle is inserted at a 30- to 45-degree angle to the skin and pointed toward the left shoulder.

- Many textbooks have recommended an elaborate technique in which a sterile "alligator" connector on one of the ECG lead V is attached to the metal shaft of the pericardiocentesis needle.
  - In theory, when the needle passes through the pericardial sac and makes contact with the epicardium, the ECG signal will change with PR- or ST-segment elevations displayed on the ECG.
  - Many clinicians have found the preceding technique to be unsatisfactory, often because of the immediate lack of the required alligator clip.
  - Currently it is more effective to use the same amount of time to arrange for the procedure to be performed in the catheterization laboratory.

- If needed emergently, as with Ms. Pomeranz, the simple, direct needle insertion to check for the fluid (diagnosis) and remove as much as possible (therapy) is the technique of choice.

COMMENTS

- Case 3 was an unusual scenario for several reasons:
  - Trauma, usually of the chest wall, is the most common cause of acute pericardial tamponade.
  - Acute tamponade is a more likely cause of PEA than the chronic form is, since the pericardial sac is tighter and less distensible.
  - Chronic pericardial tamponade is more gradual in onset and occurs because of infection, neoplastic disease, renal failure (uremia), and collagen-vascular disease syndromes, and following surgery, CPR, radiation therapy, or drug reactions (most commonly hydralazine or procainamide).
- The scenario in Case 3 illustrates how, by being thoughtful and systematic, you can figure out the underlying causes of PEA in even the most difficult and obscure situations.

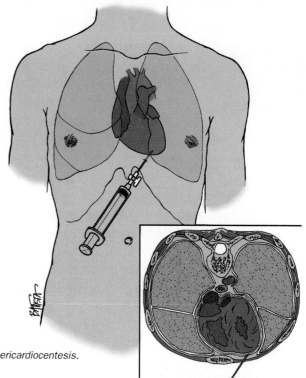

Fig. 5-6: *Landmarks for pericardiocentesis.*

Rachel Pomeranz

CASE 3 Continued

Ms. Pomeranz recovered quickly with a blood pressure of 110/70 mm Hg and a heart rate of 105 beats per minute, and she regained consciousness about 10 minutes later. Once in the ICU, the cardiologist repeated the pericardiocentesis one more time; when the patient's blood pressure began to drop and a narrow systolic-diastolic gradient developed. She had some memory problems for several days but recovered completely. She never complained of renal stones again.

COMMENTS

- The key action in Case 3 is to have the "hunt for reversible causes" at the forefront of your approach at all times.

- Once a reversible cause is identified, move quickly and decisively to correct it.

Nawanda Harris

CASE 4

You are working in your family medicine group practice, trying to keep up with a full schedule. You are about to see Nawanda Harris, your next patient, for follow-up of her long-standing diabetes, hypertension, and peripheral vascular disease. Mrs. Harris is 72 years old and recently was in the hospital for prosthetic knee replacement for degenerative arthritis. She was discharged only 3 days ago. You hear some commotion down the hall by the bathroom and note that Mrs. Harris is lying supine on the floor, gasping for breath, and complaining of chest pain. As more and more people crowd into the room, you realize that you cannot feel a carotid pulse, and Mrs. Harris appears to have lost consciousness.

How would you approach Mrs. Harris? What do you think could have caused her collapse?

COMMENTS

- Your approach to Mrs. Harris should be systematic and methodical. This scenario requires that you assume leadership of a confused and distressing situation. You will have to use all your skills and experience as an ACLS provider and team leader.

- The Primary and Secondary Surveys with the Five Quadrads guide you in the approach you should take.

- The scenario in Case 4 presents a "classic" background and story for massive acute pulmonary embolus. A large saddle embolus, producing acute cardiovascular collapse with PEA, is almost invariably fatal.

• In some settings emergency thoracotomy with embolectomy might be possible. Furthermore, clinicians in some centers are performing pilot studies of thrombolytic therapy that is used for acute pulmonary emboli. These approaches are mentioned to encourage you to find out just what is available and what is being done in your institution.

• The scenario in Case 4, fatal pulmonary embolus, is probably one of the most common scenarios involving PEA. Most of these patients will not be resuscitated. A failed resuscitation necessitates use of your other critical ACLS skills: telling the living, dealing with survivors, and conducting critical incident stress debriefing for your colleagues. Do not neglect these skills, for they are as important to the ACLS provider as any others.

KEY POINTS

SUMMARY

• **Always begin by performing the Primary and Secondary Surveys.**

• **Continue with the rest of the Five Quadrads.**

• **Check for the possibility of positive blood flow with a negative pulse by using a Doppler ultrasound.**

• **If you detect blood flow with Doppler ultrasound, treat aggressively for shock with the following:**

  • *Rapid, aggressive fluid resuscitation* (much more important than the other steps)

  • *Epinephrine*

  • *Dopamine*

  • *Norepinephrine*

• **Consider trial of *transcutaneous pacing*.**

• ***Hypovolemia* is the most common cause of electrical activity without measurable blood pressure. Through prompt recognition you often can identify and correct the many causes of hypovolemia. These causes include hypovolemia from hemorrhage and other fluid losses, cardiac tamponade, tension pneumothorax, and massive pulmonary embolism.**

• **If there is no blood flow per Doppler, do the following:**

  • Provide a fluid challenge (at least 250 to 500 mL rapid IV infusion).

  • Start *epinephrine* therapy.

  • Give atropine if the rhythm is bradycardic.

• **Send arterial blood gas samples to check for acidosis, and serum samples to check for hyperkalemia, hypokalemia, hypercalcemia, and hypocalcemia.**

• **Ask about the patient's drug, alcohol, and medication history.**

• **Consider overdose of tricyclics, digitalis, beta blockers, and calcium channel blockers.**

• **Consider anaphylaxis or profound cardiovascular collapse from some atypical agent (vitamin K, x-ray contrast material, or *any* injectable agent such as ketorolac tromethamine).**

• **Review the 12-lead ECG and monitor strips. The QRS width and the QRS rate can supply important clues to what has caused the PEA (Fig. 5-5).**

• **Fast, narrow complexes often indicate hypovolemia.**

• **Slow, narrow complexes often indicate hypoxia.**

• **Slow, wider complexes often indicate specific critical rhythm disturbances such as the following:**

  • Severe hyperkalemia, hypothermia, hypoxia, preexisting acidosis, and a large variety of drug overdoses can present as a broad-complex PEA.

  • Overdoses of tricyclic antidepressants, beta blockers, calcium channel blockers, and digitalis, as well as many other agents, produce PEA—that is their mechanism of death.

• **Provide proper airway management and aggressive hyperventilation because hypoventilation and hypoxemia are frequent causes of PEA.**

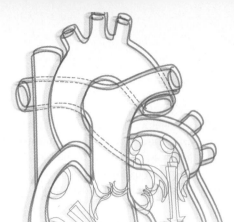

Asystole
When To Start? When To Stop?

O V E R V I E W

- *This chapter presents cardiac arrest patients in **asystole**—flatline, no cardiac electrical activity, the rhythm of death.*

- *The major theme in efforts to resuscitate patients in asystole is to find a reversible cause. The best—perhaps the only—way to treat asystole is to find and treat a reversible cause of the arrest. Unless you are able to find such a cause, your patient will remain in what some have called the eternal rhythm.*

- *What is the treatment sequence for asystole? The **Asystole Treatment Algorithm** lists the appropriate therapy to use for this group of treatments, as follows:*

  - *Continue CPR.*
  - *Intubate at once.*
  - *Obtain intravenous access.*
  - *Consider possible causes of the arrest.*

  - *Consider transcutaneous pacing (TCP). If you are going to use pacing, do it early.*
  - *Administer epinephrine.*
  - *Administer atropine.*
  - *Administer bicarbonate.*

- *Your guiding approach, however, will again be the **Five Quadrads**. As noted in Chapter 1, we focus on cardiac arrest patients with the first two of the Five Quadrads: the Primary-Secondary ABCD Survey. You should always apply the Five Quadrads to every cardiopulmonary emergency to provide a systematic, uniform approach. Such an approach prevents mistakes and omissions and provides the patient with the best chances of survival.*

- *Patients with asystole however, also introduce another critical ACLS topic—termination of resuscitation efforts. If you are unable to successfully resuscitate your patient within a reasonable period of time (see below for a discussion of what a "reasonable period of time" is), you must begin to consider when to stop the resuscitation. Whenever you encounter asystole, even at the start of a resuscitation attempt, you should ask the following questions:*

  - *Why are we doing this?*
  - *Should we even begin?*
  - *When should we stop?*

PHYSIO-CONTROL

MAJOR CONCEPTS TO MASTER

- **Understand the priorities of the Asystole Algorithm (Fig. 6-1).**
- **Hunt for and recognize potentially reversible causes of asystole, such as the following:**
  - **Hypoxia**
  - **Hyperkalemia**

- **Preexisting acidosis**
- **Drug overdose**
- **Hypothermia**
- **Understand that ventilation is the best method to manage acid-base problems.**
- **Recognize indications for terminating resuscitation efforts.**

Critical actions

- Apply the Five Quadrads within the first minutes of cardiac arrest, as follows:
  - Primary ABCD Survey (and initiation of CPR)
  - Secondary ABCD Survey (search for reversible causes of asystole)
  - Oxygen/IV/Monitor/Fluids

    Temperature/Blood Pressure/Heart Rate/Respirations

    Tank (Volume)/Pump/Rate
- Continue effective CPR.
- Recognize asystole and confirm it in more than one lead.
- Use ventilatory support as the main management for acid-base balance.
- Initiate IV access.
- Administer the following medications when the appropriate conditions (Why? When? How? and Watch Out!) exist:
  - Epinephrine
  - Atropine
  - Sodium bicarbonate
- Palpate for a pulse whenever the ECG changes; if there is a pulse, measure the blood pressure.
- Know the indications for terminating resuscitation efforts.

Skills to learn

- Know the indications for and operation of a transcutaneous external pacemaker (TCP).
- In particular, you must know how to operate any TCPs available for you to use in your clinical work.
- We do not cover the insertion and operation of emergency transvenous pacemakers here. (These pacemakers require skill that is specialized and beyond the scope of the typical ACLS provider. In addition, the true value of transvenous pacing in asystolic arrest remains unproved.)

Rhythm to learn: Asystole

Medications to learn:
(Why? When? How? and Watch out!)

- Epinephrine
- Atropine
- Sodium bicarbonate

Milton Barclay

CASE 1

HYPOXIA

You are a second-year emergency medicine resident acting as medical control for the EMS for 1 month. A call comes in from the dispatcher for an ALS unit to respond to "CPR in progress."

"Come with us, Doc!" says Harold, one of the paramedics. You hop in the rig and roll toward a nearby housing subdivision. Traffic is light, since it's 3 AM.

Several minutes earlier, Julie Barclay had awakened, feeling something was wrong. Her husband Milt, aged 60, was not on his side of the bed. She wandered out into the hallway and found him slumped over on the floor. She called 911 and received dispatcher-assisted CPR instructions. Seven minutes later the ALS team arrives at their house. You begin CPR while your partner hooks up an ECG monitor. The rhythm is asystole (Fig. 6-2). The other paramedic inserts an oral airway and begins ventilations using a bag-valve-mask hooked to oxygen at 15 L/min.

What are the prospects for resuscitating Mr. Barclay?

COMMENTS

- Mr. Barclay had an unwitnessed arrest. The sound of his fall may have been what woke his wife. He may also have been in cardiac arrest for a long time.

- Mr. Barclay has an initial rhythm of asystole, defined as a complete absence of ventricular electrical activity. At times P waves may be present. During the slowing of bradycardia into asystole, rare ventricular escape beats may be present. Most often asystole presents only as a slightly wavering "flatline."

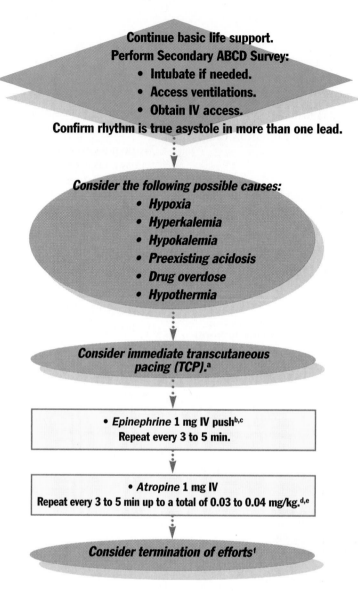

FIGURE. 6-1

Asystole Treatment Algorithm

Continue basic life support.
Perform Secondary ABCD Survey:
- **Intubate if needed.**
- **Access ventilations.**
- **Obtain IV access.**

Confirm rhythm is true asystole in more than one lead.

Consider the following possible causes:
- *Hypoxia*
- *Hyperkalemia*
- *Hypokalemia*
- *Preexisting acidosis*
- *Drug overdose*
- *Hypothermia*

Consider immediate transcutaneous pacing (TCP).[a]

- *Epinephrine* 1 mg IV push[b,c]
  Repeat every 3 to 5 min.

- *Atropine* 1 mg IV
  Repeat every 3 to 5 min up to a total of 0.03 to 0.04 mg/kg.[d,e]

Consider termination of efforts[f]

Class I : Definitely helpful

Class IIa: Acceptable, probably helpful

Class IIb: Acceptable, possibly helpful

Class III: Not indicated, may be harmful

[a] Pacing is an acceptable intervention (Class IIb). Perform TCP as early as possible, without waiting for the effects of medications. Not recommended as routine treatment for asystole.

[b] The recommended dose of **epinephrine** is 1 mg IV push every 3 to 5 min. If spontaneous circulation does not return, consider several Class IIb dosing regimens:
- Intermediate: **Epinephrine** 2 to 5 mg IV push, every 3 to 5 min

- Escalating: **Epinephrine** 1 to 3 mg to 5 mg IV push, 3 min apart
- High: **Epinephrine** 0.1 mg/kg IV push, every 3 to 5 min

[c] **Sodium bicarbonate** 1 mEq/kg is definitely indicated (Class I) if patient has known preexisting hyperkalemia.

[d] The shorter **atropine** dosing interval (3 min) is Class IIb in asystolic arrest.

[e] **Sodium bicarbonate** (1 mEq/kg) follow these indications:

Class IIa

- If known preexisting bicarbonate responsive acidosis
- If overdose with tricyclic antidepressants
- To alkalinize the urine in drug overdoses

Class IIb

- If patient intubated and arrest continues for long intervals
- If circulation restored after prolonged arrest

Class III

- Hypoxic acidosis (unventilited patient)

[f] Consider stopping resuscitative efforts when patient remains in documented asystole or other agonal rhythms for more than 10 minutes <u>after</u>:

- Patient successfully intubated
- Initial IV medications given
- No reversible causes identified
- Physician concurs

Adapted with permission, Journal of the American Medical Association, 1992, Volume 268, *Guidelines for Cardiopulmonary Resuscitation and Emergency Cardiac Care*, p. 2220, copyright © 1992, American Medical Association.

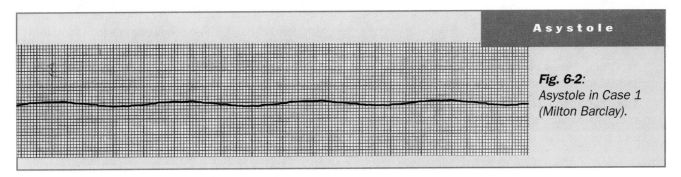

Fig. 6-2: Asystole in Case 1 (Milton Barclay).

- Do not make the mistake of diagnosing asystole in only one lead. When you see a flatline on the monitor, confirm that asystole is actually the rhythm by changing to other leads on the lead-select switch. (Another way is to switch each defibrillation paddle to the opposite side of the sternum.)
- "False asystole" is most frequently produced by a defibrillator operator who has made an error. Errors that produce "false asystole" include the following:
  - Failure to properly connect the monitor cable to the patient
  - Failure to properly connect the monitor cable to the defibrillator
  - Failure to turn the power switch on
  - Failure to ensure adequate ECG size
- Defibrillating true asystole is not recommended. It can lower the already remote chances of survival even more. Shocks to asystole can end any chance for spontaneous

return of electrical activity. Sometimes high levels of parasympathetic tone cause both ventricular and supraventricular pacemaker activity to stop. Shocks stun the heart and cause a large parasympathetic discharge. Some EMS systems evaluated the effect of empirical countershocks to asystole; they found no change in the rate of survival.

- With asystole the team leader must rapidly and aggressively consider the differential diagnosis.
- A possible differential diagnosis for this man is hypoxia. Since his arrest was unwitnessed, he may have had ventricular fibrillation (VF) that then deteriorated into asystole.
- Adequate ventilation is required to treat or prevent a severe acid-base problem.
- Administer 100% oxygen during resuscitation efforts, as quickly as it can be hooked up.
- Hypoxemia leads to anaerobic metabolism and metabolic acidosis, which can interfere with the effects of medication and defibrillation.

Milton Barclay

CASE 1 Continued

Over the next 10 minutes, you and your team treat Milton Barclay aggressively. You continue CPR, and you prepare to perform endotracheal intubation and start an IV line. Ray has difficulty with the intubation. He makes two attempts and moves over to let you have a try. You manage to intubate Mr. Barclay; at about the same time Harold has started an IV infusion of normal saline.

Once IV or endotracheal access is established, you can administer medications. What are the two drugs listed in the ACLS Guidelines for asystole? Which do you use first?

COMMENTS

- **Epinephrine** is the first drug of choice for all patients in cardiac arrest.
- **Atropine** is recommended to reverse a possible hyper-parasympathetic state.

Epinephrine hydrochloride

WHY? (Actions)

- Epinephrine is the first drug to choose for patients in cardiac arrest.
- No medication has displayed better results in increasing blood flow to the brain and heart.
- As a catecholamine (sympathomimetic) with alpha-

adrenergic and beta-adrenergic action, epinephrine produces vasoconstriction, improving coronary and cerebral blood flow.
- Epinephrine increases coronary perfusion pressure, systemic vascular resistance, blood pressure, heart rate, and myocardial contractility. Epinephrine also increases myocardial oxygen consumption and automaticity.

WHEN? (Indications)

- Any pulseless cardiac arrest

HOW? (Dosing)

- 1.0 mg IV push, repeated every 3 to 5 minutes.
- If the preceding approach fails, the following Class IIb dosing regimens can be considered:

- Intermediate: Epinephrine 2 to 5 mg IV push, every 3 to 5 minutes

- Escalating: Epinephrine 1 mg to 3 mg to 5 mg IV push, 3 minutes apart

- High: Epinephrine 0.1 mg/kg IV push, every 3 to 5 minutes

WATCH OUT!

- Give epinephrine as soon as possible during an arrest.

- Delays in giving epinephrine increase hypoxia. Hypoxia may delay or prevent any possible response.

- Do not mix epinephrine with sodium bicarbonate.

- Watch out for the increase in myocardial oxygen demand if spontaneous electrical activity returns.

- High doses of epinephrine are considered Class IIb, that is, "acceptable, considered not harmful, and possibly helpful."

Atropine sulfate

WHY?

- Atropine is a parasympatholytic drug, a vagolytic drug, and an anticholinergic drug.

- Atropine helps only those conditions in which there is excess vagal activity. Atropine may not be effective for asystolic conditions that lack a vagal component.

- Atropine increases sinus node automaticity and atrioventricular (AV) conduction when they have been suppressed by abnormal parasympathetic or vagal discharges.

WHEN?

- Give atropine routinely to all asystolic cardiac arrest patients.

HOW?

- For asystole or pulseless electrical activity (PEA) give 1.0 mg as the first dose. Repeat every 3 to 5 minutes.

- For persistent asystole give up to 0.03 to 0.04 mg/kg as a full vagolytic dose.

WATCH OUT!

- Avoid atropine in hypothermia.

- Use with caution in patients with ischemic heart disease resulting from coronary artery disease.

Milton Barclay

CASE 1 Continued

You administer epinephrine 1 mg IV push followed by atropine 1 mg IV push and continue vigorous CPR and hyperventilations. You switch the monitor lead switch, first, to lead I and then to lead III. The rhythm, however, remains flatline. Three minutes later, you administer a much higher dose of epinephrine (3 mg) IV and add a second dose of atropine 1 mg IV. The rhythm does not change. You have now been treating Mr. Barclay for 12 minutes.

Why is Mr. Barclay not responding to therapy? Should the resuscitation efforts be terminated at this point?

COMMENTS

- Asystole represents the complete absence of electrical activity in the myocardium. Prolonged asystole usually means the myocardium has suffered an irreversible ischemic insult (unless hypothermia is a factor; see Chapter 14).

- You can stop resuscitation attempts when a patient does not respond after a "reasonable" trial of ACLS interventions. A reasonable trial includes the following:

  - Countershocks for VF have been given.

  - Endotracheal intubation has been successfully accomplished, and aggressive ventilation performed.

  - Intravenous access has been achieved.

  - Rhythm-appropriate medications have been administered according to ACLS protocols.

  - Reversible causes have been thoroughly considered and ruled out.

- Persistent asystole or other agonal ECG patterns are present for *at least 10 minutes*, uninterrupted by periods of perfusing or organized complexes.

- Temperature (core) has been documented to be greater than 34° C.

- NOTE: There is no specific time limit beyond which successful resuscitation is impossible. However, any decision to prolong resuscitation efforts because "there is always a chance" requires common sense and sound clinical judgment. The lead physician must assume the role to officially "cease efforts." First, however, consult with the entire code team, and ask them to contribute their thoughts to the particular clinical situation.

- Among experts on emergency cardiac care, as of 1994, there is a prevailing opinion that ACLS providers have erred on the side of prolonging codes inappropriately. The 1992 Emergency Cardiac Care Guidelines have taken a major step to correct this pattern of resuscitation errors. The guidelines section on "Ethical Considerations in

Resuscitation" acknowledges this problem of resuscitations that are started when they should not have been started and continued when they should have been stopped.*

- Asystole most often represents a confirmation of death rather than a "rhythm" to be treated.

- Prehospital resuscitation protocols that require transport of *all* patients with ongoing CPR in ambulances are ethically inappropriate and a misuse of resources.

Irla Sharp

CASE 2

ARREST IN ASSOCIATION WITH DIALYSIS

You are a respiratory therapist working on the code team next to the coronary care unit (CCU) when you hear "Code Blue" called out in the CCU. You respond to find a 68-year-old woman who was admitted to the CCU this afternoon following an out-of-hospital cardiac arrest and resuscitation. She is unresponsive, and the monitor shows asystole (Fig. 6-3).

Earlier that day, she had "arrested" while in the dialysis clinic. She had not, however, completed her dialysis "run." She has been on a regimen of renal dialysis for 4 years and has adjusted well to the treatments. She responded well to that resuscitation and had regained consciousness in the unit.

The code team arrives, begins CPR, intubates the patient's trachea, and administers epinephrine and atropine. Since this was a witnessed cardiac arrest in a fully staffed CCU with rapid response times, you decide to try TCP.

Why are you starting TCP for asystole?

Asystole

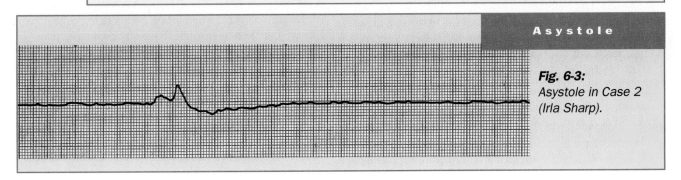

Fig. 6-3:
Asystole in Case 2 (Irla Sharp).

WHY?

- TCP provides direct stimulation to the heart that may cause a mechanical cardiac contraction. It acts as a stand-in for the heart's stimulating conduction system and can maintain cardiac output if it successfully stimulates the ventricles to contract.

- Because of ease of implementation and attachment, TCP is the fastest method of emergency pacing. Many defibrillators have a TCP mode integrated into the defibrillator.

- TCP can be used to treat severe conduction system problems because pacing bypasses the conduction system and directly stimulates the myocardium.

- Unlike transvenous pacing, TCP requires no special equipment insertion or monitoring (such as portable fluoroscopy equipment) and does not require transfer to the fluoroscopy suite.

- TCP is not an invasive procedure. The device is attached to the patient's skin through two large skin-adhesive pacing electrodes. Monitoring electrodes are also used to provide a display of the rhythm.

WHEN?

- Asystolic or bradyasystolic cardiac arrest: Patients most likely to benefit are those with witnessed asystole or the more promising "P-wave asystole" (Fig. 6-4).

- It is not appropriate to use TCP for "last ditch efforts in a code," simply because you have exhausted all other measures.

HOW?

- Apply two adhesive pacing electrodes to the patient's chest.

- One is applied directly on the skin, just to the left of the sternum, right over the apex (point of maximal impact).

- The second electrode is applied posteriorly, directly behind the front electrode. Place it to the left of the spinal column and medial to the left scapula.

---

* Emergency Cardiac Care Committee and Subcommittees, American Heart Association: Guidelines for cardiopulmonary resuscitation and emergency cardiac care. VIII. Ethical considerations in resuscitation, *JAMA* 268:2282, 1992.

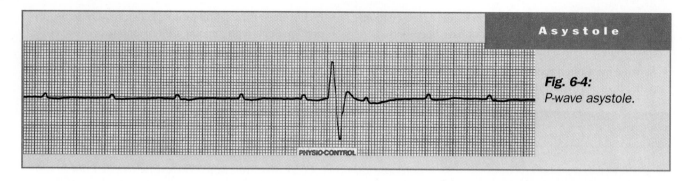

Asystole

Fig. 6-4:
P-wave asystole.

PHYSIO-CONTROL

- Attach the pacer's ECG cardiac monitor leads (three) to the chest wall in a lead II configuration.

- Select a pacing rate, usually 80 to 100 beats per minute. (Chest compressions can be delivered; compressions can push directly on the anterior pad.)

- Select a pacing energy output, usually expressed in milliamperes. During treatment of cardiac arrest patients start at maximum energy output.

- Turn on the power. Observe for pacer spikes. These spikes indicate that the device is discharging.

- Observe for electrical and mechanical capture.

- *Electrical capture* occurs when the TCP produces a broad QRS complex with a T wave of opposite polarity appearing consistently after each pacer strike. TCP of asystole is shown in Fig. 6-5.

- *Mechanical capture* occurs when the pacing produces a measurable hemodynamic response such as a palpable carotid or femoral pulse or a measurable blood pressure.

- Once mechanical capture has been identified, note the milliampere setting. Turn the current milliampere setting about 10% above the noted capture setting.

- NOTE: TCP produces jerking muscle contractions of the chest and shoulder girdle muscles. These movements can be confused with a palpable pulse; thus check for hemodynamic response at the femoral or brachial arteries.

WATCH OUT!

- TCP can be painful for conscious people. If your patient regains consciousness, an analgesic may be required.

- The pacing artifact may actually prevent your recognition of an underlying ECG of VF. Turn off the pacer periodically, and check the underlying nonpaced ECG.

COMMENTS

- Many scientific studies have confirmed that an asystolic heart rarely responds to pacing. To have any chance of effectiveness, TCP must be performed early, at the same time drugs are given. The 1992 AHA recommendations use the term "consider" when listing pacing in the guidelines for asystole. Very few studies have observed more than anecdotal success.

- Scientists have conducted multiple studies of TCP since 1986. These studies showed that in the setting of prehospital cardiac arrest, TCP is only rarely effective. Note, however, that if pacing is to work, it must be applied early, simultaneous with drug administration.

- REMEMBER: Pacing is a Class IIb recommendation (acceptable, possibly helpful).

Irla Sharp

CASE 2 Continued

Within a few minutes of the resuscitation attempt, CPR is initiated, endotracheal intubation performed, and an IV started. Epinephrine and atropine are administered through the IV.

In addition, you have started early TCP. The pacing stimulus appears to produce a definite broad-QRS complex on the monitor screen with a large T wave opposite in polarity to the QRS complexes. You direct the chest compressor to continue chest compressions but make sure the chest compressions are timed to coincide with the pacing signal. You reassure him that he will not feel any pacing stimulus. You stop CPR briefly and check whether the pacing beats are producing a pulse. You check a femoral pulse with the paced beats and you can actually feel a pulse.

What additional interventions should you give at this time?

COMMENTS

- Always return to the Primary-Secondary Survey. In particular, you should review the D (differential diagnoses) of the Secondary Survey, for that directs you to consider the causes of the cardiac arrest.

- The preceding approach coincides with the Asystole Treatment Algorithm, which also directs the team leader to consider the possible causes of the cardiac arrest (Fig. 6-1).

- Upon review of the circumstances of this arrest, you believe that some metabolic abnormality related to the patient's known renal failure, such as hyperkalemia, hypovolemia, or possible acidosis, could be playing a role in this arrest.

- Certainly, you have sufficient empirical information to administer sodium bicarbonate, which is appropriate both for possible acidosis and for hyperkalemia.

- The initial electrolyte levels from 2 hours earlier in the day show that Mrs. Sharp was hyperkalemic at 6.0 mEq/L, and her pH was 7.1. Mrs. Sharp has a known, preexisting hyperkalemia for which sodium bicarbonate is a Class I (definitely helpful) intervention.

Sodium bicarbonate used in asystolic cardiac arrest

WHY?

- Bicarbonate is a Class I agent only when a patient has known, preexisting hyperkalemia or known acidosis.

- Bicarbonate is a buffering agent that is thought to neutralize acid accumulated during ineffective ventilations.

- Ventilation with endotracheal intubation is the major treatment of acidosis associated with cardiac emergencies.

- Sodium bicarbonate is also beneficial in patients with preexisting metabolic acidosis, hyperkalemia, or aspirin overdose.

WHEN?

- No definitive evidence supports the routine use of bicarbonate in cardiac arrest.

- Consider bicarbonate only *after* the established beneficial intervention—hyperventilation via endotracheal tube—has been initiated.

- Bicarbonate is a Class IIa agent for known or suspected preexisting bicarbonate-responsive acidosis and metabolic acidosis that is due to bicarbonate losses (gastrointestinal or renal).

HOW?

- Give 1 mEq/kg initially, and repeat half the dose every 10 minutes or per arterial blood gas levels. Keep in mind, however, that arterial blood gas levels are notoriously unreliable during cardiac arrest even with continuing CPR.

WATCH OUT!

- Do not give sodium bicarbonate to patients with inadequate ventilations and the hypoxic lactic acidosis that occurs in extended cardiac arrests.

Irla Sharp

CASE 2 Continued

Remarkably, Mrs. Sharp shows a definite response to the sodium bicarbonate and the TCP. She establishes a palpable pulse in response to the pacing. Her pupils become responsive as the atropine is metabolized. Following the first dose of 60 mEq of bicarbonate you give an additional 30 mEq 10 minutes later.

You also administer calcium chloride 5 mL IV of a 10% (100 mg/mL) solution, 50 mL of a 50% glucose solution, and 10 units of regular insulin, all in an attempt to further reduce the serum potassium level and the toxic effects of the hyperkalemia.

Now, 20 minutes after the arrest was announced, you find that Mrs. Sharp has a spontaneous pulse and circulation. You turn off the TCP and stop chest compressions.

What was it that made a difference in resuscitating this patient with asystole?

COMMENTS

- The exact role of TCP in asystolic cardiac arrest has not been defined. In Case 2 pacing was performed as an "augmentation" to the chest compressions of CPR. Certainly TCP cannot replace chest compressions in a person with cardiac arrest unless the pacing alone produces satisfactory, measurable blood pressure. This rarely happens.

- However, TCP may indeed stimulate mechanical ventricular contractions of the myocardium sufficient to produce

some coronary and carotid blood flow. Certainly in a scenario like this one, in which the myocardium is relatively good but the cardiac conduction has been rendered ineffective (the effect of the elevated potassium level and the acidosis), TCP may help.

- The other major difference in the arrest in Case 2 was the early focus on the "Why?" (the D [differential diagnosis] of the Secondary Survey). Only by carefully evaluating the circumstances of the arrest could you identify the acidosis and hyperkalemia that were the major causes of this arrest.

Vickie Wildebor

CASE 3

BETA BLOCKER OVERDOSE
A 38-year-old woman is admitted to the Emergency Department after taking an overdose of propranolol, a beta blocker. After taking the tablets, her resolve to die faded, and she immediately called 911. Bradycardia with third-degree heart block developed en route to the Emergency Department, but then deteriorated into asystole a few minutes later. Her initial ECG was asystole. Respirations, heart rate, and blood pressure are all absent.
How would you approach Mrs. Wildebor?

Asystole

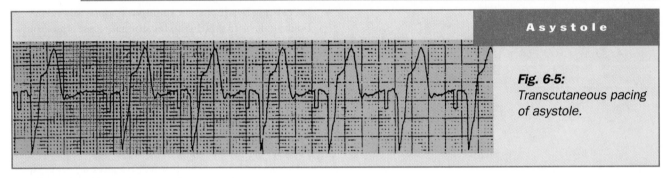

Fig. 6-5:
Transcutaneous pacing of asystole.

COMMENTS

- As with all cardiopulmonary emergencies, start with the Five Quadrads, featuring the Primary-Secondary Survey ABCDs.

- **Primary ABCD Survey** reveals that the patient in Case 3 is in full cardiac arrest and needs CPR; defibrillation is not indicated.

- **Secondary ABCD Survey** reveals that she needs intubation, IV access, and the medications appropriate for asystole (epinephrine and atropine).

- **D (differential diagnoses) of Secondary Survey:** Clearly this case is a bradyasystolic arrest in association with the overdose of a beta blocker. This scenario leads to an immediate therapeutic approach as follows:
  - Normal saline bolus (500 mL)
  - TCP (because the myocardium is only temporarily affected by the beta blockade and should respond to the pacing stimulus)
  - Glucagon 1 to 5 mg IV
  - Epinephrine 1 mg IV bolus repeated every 3 minutes
  - Calcium chloride 10 mL of a 10% solution

- Chapter 11 presents details on the management of toxicologic emergencies like Case 3.

- **Oxygen/IV/Monitor/Fluids:** Begin these as soon as possible, as noted earlier. The rhythm strip reveals an interesting phenomenon of "P-wave asystole" (Fig. 6-4). This P-wave asystole (a rare type of asystole) is one which may respond to TCP.

- **Vital signs:** Temperature, 36.5° C; heart rate, 80 beats per pacing; respirations, with bagging only; blood pressure, 90/60 mm Hg per Doppler ultrasound with pacing.

- **The cardiovascular quadrad:** *Tank (Volume)/ Resistance/Pump/ Rate:* Use this quadrad to ask, What is the nature of the problem? Beta blocker intoxication affects all four components of the cardiovascular quadrad through its negative inotropic, chronotropic, and vasodilator effects. You are addressing these with the medications noted earlier and with TCP.
  - *Is there a tank (volume) problem?* Yes. Beta blockers cause a vasodilation that will produce overexpansion of the tank relative to the blood volume. This overexpansion of volume lowers the blood pressure.

- *Is there a resistance problem?* Yes. The lowered resistance aggravates the tank (volume) problem.

- *Is there a pump problem?* Yes, because beta blockers produce negative inotropic effects that decrease the force of contraction.

- *Is there a rate problem?* Yes, because beta blockers cause a negative chronotropic effect and slow the heart rate.

- The normal saline bolus will expand the volume and diminish the tank problem. The epinephrine will produce vasoconstriction, thus reducing the tank and resistance problems. Epinephrine will also enhance the performance of the pump and speed up the heart rate.

- Glucagon improves function of two components: the pump, by enhancing myocardial contractility, and the rate, by improving heart rate and AV conduction.

- Calcium chloride can reverse the negative inotropic effects of beta blockers on the cardiac pump and the rate effects from the depressed automaticity of the beta blockers.

Vickie Wildebor

CASE 3 Continued

With rapid initiation of the interventions listed earlier, Mrs. Wildebor responded to the TCP and to the medications. She must be admitted and observed in the CCU until her condition is completely stabilized. Her physicians must determine whether she suffered any adverse neurologic sequelae from her cardiac arrest.

What were the major factors that made a difference in Mrs. Wildebor's successful resuscitation?

COMMENTS

- Mrs. Wildebor had the following advantages:

  - Her asystolic event was witnessed in the Emergency Department.

  - You knew the cause of her arrest: an overdose of beta blockers.

  - Her toxic effects of the beta blocker overdose left her with a myocardium that could easily respond to TCP. This is a well-known, effective use of TCP.

- If pacing is to be effective, it must be initiated early in resuscitation. If you decide to initiate pacing for asystole in particular clinical situations, you should do so early, simultaneous with administration of medications.

- The aggressive management outlined earlier was implemented quickly and was probably responsible for the lack of permanent neurologic sequelae.

- The emergency department clerk calls for a CCU bed, and Mrs. Wildebor is transferred to the CCU; the pacemaker is producing good mechanical contractions.

Gordon Parkinson

CASE 4

PACEMAKER FAILURE

Mr. Gordon Parkinson, a 72-year-old man living in a retirement home, is discovered unconscious in the library. No one knows how long he may have lain there. The staff calls 911 and reports a cardiac arrest. A licensed practical nurse (LPN) arrives and she begins CPR.

You are a member of the EMT first-responder team arriving with an automated external defibrillator (AED). The initial rhythm is asystole (but with some intermittent pacemaker spikes from his failed pacemaker) (Fig. 6-6). Appropriately, the AED does not recommend a shock. Respirations, heart rate, and blood pressure are all absent, so you continue with CPR while awaiting the arrival of the paramedics.

You then notice that Mr. Parkinson is wearing a state EMS–No CPR bracelet. On his bedside table is the signed documentation that goes with the bracelet. In your state this bracelet and document are recognized as a portable "No Code" document.

Do you need to continue resuscitation efforts and CPR at this time?

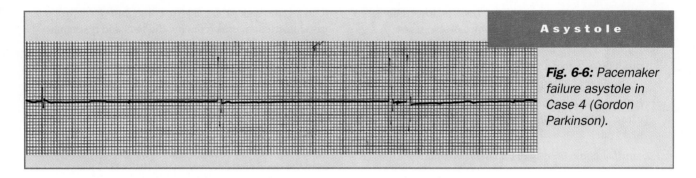

Asystole

Fig. 6-6: *Pacemaker failure asystole in Case 4 (Gordon Parkinson).*

COMMENTS

- Resuscitation efforts can be stopped once you discover clear evidence of the patient's wishes in regard to the care he or she wants to receive at the end of life.

- The 1992 AHA Guidelines concisely state that "rescuers who initiate basic life support (BLS) should continue until . . . a valid No-CPR order is presented to the rescuers. Ethically and legally there is no distinction between discontinuing CPR and not starting it in the first place."[*]

- One of the most significant changes in the 1992 AHA Guidelines was explicit acceptance of the concepts of patient self-determination, the patient's right to death with dignity, and the right of all competent people to make autonomous decisions related to health care.

- Medical directors of prehospital care systems must develop criteria by which emergency personnel, in coordination with medical control physicians, can stop resuscitation efforts in the field.

- Ceasing resuscitation efforts outside the hospital setting, according to a specific protocol, should be standard practice in all EMS systems. However, these same EMS systems must establish mechanisms for pronouncement of death and appropriate disposition of the body by community funeral homes or other approaches.

- In addition, EMS personnel should be trained to deal with family members and loved ones in a sensitive manner. Clergy and social workers can also assist with grief support for the living.

- Each system must obtain direction from its medical control physician, who carries, in most states, legal responsibility for these protocols and policies.

---

[*] Emergency Cardiac Care Committee and Subcommittees, American Heart Association: Guidelines for cardiopulmonary resuscitation and emergency cardiac care. VIII. Ethical considerations in resuscitation, *JAMA* 268:2282, 1992.

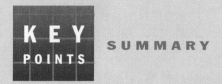

SUMMARY

- Apply the Five Quadrads to all asystolic arrests.

- Apply the Asystole Treatment Algorithm to all asystolic arrests.

- Search for a reversible cause if you want to reverse asystole, as follows:

  - Fundamental to treatment of asystole is the rapid and aggressive pursuit of a differential diagnosis.

  - This search is part of the Secondary ABCD Survey and part of the Asystole Treatment Algorithm.

- The major interventions for asystole are the following:

  - Continued CPR

  - Intubation

  - Early TCP

  - Epinephrine administration

  - Atropine administration

- These treatments are similar to the treatments recommended for PEA. Atropine is routinely given to all asystolic cardiac arrest patients, whereas it should be administered to patients with PEA only when slow electrical activity is present. Use TCP only for slow PEA.

- Work out a plan for when to stop resuscitation efforts if the rhythm is persistent asystole and there is a lack of response after the following standard interventions:

  - Successful intubation

  - Successful IV access with administration of appropriate medications

  - Persistent electrical "silence" (no electrical activity and continued asystole) for *at least* 10 minutes, but seldom longer

- Remember that asystole is also the "rhythm of death." A person in persistent asystole may simply be dead. That person has reached the end of his or her life. It is time for the resuscitation efforts to stop.

- Remember to deal sensitively with the living and with the people who have helped in the resuscitation attempt. Chapter 1 presents guidelines on telling the living, conveying the news of death to the survivors, organ and tissue donation, and critical incident stress debriefing.

- All of these issues must be learned and practiced effectively. These are skills that will be used in connection with most asystolic cardiac arrest patients.

Bradycardia

OVERVIEW

- *The bradycardia cases teach you an approach to patients with symptomatic bradycardia. You should remember the most critical question to ask about bradycardias: "Is this slow heart rate too slow for the clinical condition?"*

- *Just as with tachycardias, the word "too" forces you to think about patients and how they are doing clinically. You must learn to recognize when bradycardias are symptomatic because the presence of signs and symptoms drives most therapeutic decisions. The degree of symptoms determines what agents you select from your therapeutic arsenal, which includes the following:*

  - *Oxygenation*

  - *Ventilation support*

  - *Atropine*

  - *Transcutaneous pacing (TCP)*

  - *Catecholamines (dopamine, epinephrine, and isoproterenol)*

  - *Transvenous pacing*

- *Note that we have included oxygenation and ventilation support here as major therapeutic interventions for bradycardias. Remember that for adults, as for pediatric patients, hypoxia and hypoventilation are two of the major correctable causes of symptomatic bradycardia.*

- *We have markedly simplified rhythm identification. This is consistent with the AHA movement toward an emphasis on more practical rhythm identification.*

- *You must learn, however, to recognize bradycardia that is due to the major atrioventricular (AV) blocks. This is critical because the type of AV block forces the major decisions about transcutaneous and transvenous pacemakers.*

- *Learn the Bradycardia Algorithm (Fig. 7-1) in detail. The algorithm will help you organize your thinking about patients with bradycardia.*

MAJOR CONCEPTS TO MASTER

- **Learn the concept of "symptomatic" bradycardias. This means the heart rate is slow, your patient is symptomatic, and the symptoms are due to the bradycardia.**

- **Learn to recognize the major bradycardias, the heart blocks, and the therapeutic issues and approaches for each one, including the following:**

  - **When to use drugs**

  - **When to use TCP**

- **When to use transvenous pacing**

- **When to prepare for standby pacing**

- **When to engage in watchful waiting**

- **Learn the Why? When? How? and Watch out! for the major therapeutic interventions in symptomatic bradycardias, including medications (atropine, dopamine, epinephrine, and isoproterenol) and transcutaneous pacemakers (TCPs).**

Critical actions

The proper management of patients with symptomatic bradycardia requires the following critical actions:

- Follow the Universal Algorithm.
- Review the following **Five Quadrads:**
  - Primary ABCD Survey
  - Secondary ABCD Survey
  - Temperature/Blood Pressure/Heart Rate/Respiration
  - Oxygen/IV/Monitor/Fluids
  - Tank (Volume)/Resistance/Pump/Rate
- Take action immediately for any critical problem identified in the Primary or Secondary Surveys.
- Follow the Bradycardia Algorithm: Take action appropriately for hemodynamically significant bradycardias; understand, apply, and properly operate TCPs.
- Take a focused history.
- Perform a focused physical examination.
- Order a 12-lead ECG when appropriate.
- Order a portable chest radiograph when appropriate.
- Consider whether you need to apply the Acute Myocardial Infarction (AMI) Algorithm or the Shock/ Hypotension/Acute Pulmonary Edema Algorithm. The most serious bradycardias occur in patients with an AMI; furthermore, profoundly symptomatic bradycardia can produce a shock state.

Skills to learn

- You should know, in some detail, how to operate TCPs. In particular, you should know how to operate each and every TCP that you might have occasion to use in your clinical work.
- We do not cover the insertion and operation of emergency transvenous pacemakers in this chapter. Transvenous pacemakers require advanced, subspecialty skills. You should recognize, however, the indications for transvenous pacemakers—that is one of your major clinical responsibilities in the bradycardia cases.

Rhythms to learn

- Sinus bradycardia
- First-degree heart block
- Type I second-degree heart block (Mobitz type I)
- Type II second-degree heart block (Mobitz type II) with wide or narrow QRS complexes
- Third-degree heart block with a wide or narrow QRS complex

Medications to learn

- Oxygen
- Atropine
- Dopamine
- Epinephrine
- Isoproterenol

Jane Berg

CASE 1

You are on duty in the Emergency Department. Jane Berg, an eccentric lady whose age (90 years) equals her weight (90 pounds) is brought in by the paramedics. She had fallen on her porch while cleaning out the trap on her bug-zapper. She has an obvious fractured left hip with external foot rotation and foreshortening. The medics state that she "has a slow heart rate," and the nurses confirm a sinus bradycardia of 40 beats per minute (Fig.7-2). Her blood pressure is 180/100; respirations are 10 per minute. She is resting comfortably, chatting away about how nice "those handsome boys from the Fire Department" are and inviting them to her house for tea. She reports no pain and chats pleasantly with each person who approaches.

What do you want to do about her profound bradycardia?

COMMENTS

- First, ask the question, "Is this symptomatic bradycardia?" No, not in terms of the major symptoms and consequences that bradycardia can cause: an alteration in her blood pressure, mentation, and breathing.

- Does she need treatment for the bradycardia? No, not at this time. It is critical to realize that you should not treat asymptomatic sinus bradycardia. The major point is this: if the bradycardia is not producing symptoms, do not make the patient worse by giving inappropriate treatments.

- Could the bradycardia have led to her fall? Did she experience a brief period of hypoperfusion, get light-headed, fall, and break her hip? Certainly this is possible. A good clinician knows to consider arrhythmias as a possible cause of unexplained falls, "spells," syncopal episodes, and light-headedness. You can sort these questions out during her hospitalization for her hip fracture, although a monitored bed may be necessary.

- You should have asymptomatic bradycardic patients get up and walk around (assuming they have not broken a hip). Check the patient's heart rate and blood pressure. These will help you determine whether patients can achieve an appropriate increase in heart rate with exercise.

Overview of Rhythm Interpretation

- *For the ACLS provider all arrhythmias can be lumped into two categories:*
  - *Lethal (arrest) rhythms*
  - *Nonlethal (non-cardiac arrest) rhythms*
- *The Universal Algorithm reflects this classification because it forces the rescuer to identify the unresponsive, nonbreathing, and pulseless patient immediately. For the patient in a lethal cardiac*

arrest rhythm there are only four possible rhythms:
  - *Ventricular fibrillation (VF)*
  - *Ventricular tachycardia (VT)*
  - *Asystole*
  - *Assorted types of pulseless electrical activity (PEA), which include electromechanical dissociation (EMD), bradyasystolic, and pulseless idioventricular PEAs.*
- *In the clinical context of emergency cardiac care, there are only*

two non–cardiac arrest rhythms to consider:
  - *Too slow (less than 60 beats per minute)*
  - *Too fast (greater than 150 beats per minute)*
- *The adjective "too" focuses the ACLS provider on the next questions: How fast is "too fast"? and How slow is "too slow"? The answers depend on whether the rate problem is causing the patient to have clinical symptoms. The point is to not make decisions or take actions based*

Heart Block Identification in Bradycardias (Heart Rate Less Than 60 Beats per Minute)

- *Although the bradycardias are defined initially by rate, you must further classify the "slow" rhythms into the following categories of heart block:*
  - *First-degree heart block: PR interval longer than 0.2 seconds.*
  - *Type I second-degree heart block (Mobitz type I): The term "second degree" means that some QRS complexes are dropped following a normal P wave. The term "type I" means the PR interval progressively lengthens until eventually no conduction occurs and the P wave is not followed by a QRS complex (dropped beat).*
  - *Type II second-degree heart block (Mobitz type II) (with wide or narrow QRS complexes): The term "second degree" means that some QRS complexes are dropped following a normal P wave. In Type II second-degree heart block,*

however, the PR interval is fixed; a dropped QRS complex occurs intermittently.
  - *Third-degree heart block with a wide or narrow QRS complex: P waves and QRS waves occur regularly, but without a relationship between them.*
- *These blocks are easily identified by asking the following series of questions about the relationship between the P waves and the QRS complex:*
  - *Are there more P waves than QRS complexes?*
  - *Is the PR interval fixed?*
  - *Are the P waves and the QRS complexes independent?*
- *Finally you can determine information about the abnormality in the conduction system by looking to see whether the QRS complex is narrow (<0.12 seconds) or wide (>0.12 seconds).*
- *Wide QRS complexes indicate con-*

duction system disease at or below the AV node. This often indicates more severe conduction system disease, most often caused by coronary atherosclerosis. In the clinical context of an AMI, bradycardia with wide-complex type II second-degree heart block or wide-complex third-degree heart block indicates extensive anterior MI.
- *The inset below displays these critical questions in a decision tree format and indicates when to prepare for transcutaneous and transvenous pacing.*

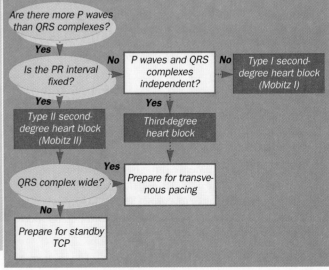

FIGURE 7-1

Bradycardia Algorithm

(For Patients not in Cardiac Arrest)

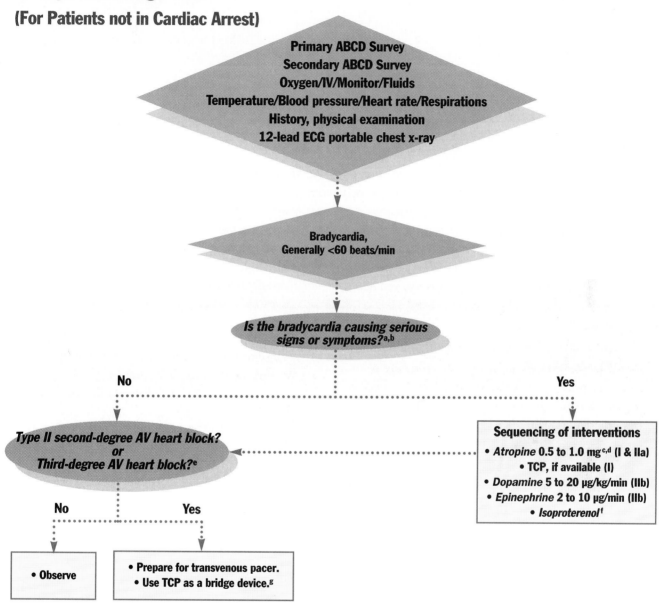

(a) The clinical signs or symptoms must be related to the slow rate. Clinical manifestations include the following:
- Symptoms (chest pain, shortness of breath, decreased level of consciousness)
- Signs (low blood pressure, shock, pulmonary congestion, congestive heart failure, AMI)

(b) Start TCP before atropine takes effect if patient is symptomatic.

(c) Transplanted hearts will not respond to *atropine*. Go at once to pacing, *catecholamine infusion*, or both.

(d) *Atropine* should be given in repeat doses every 3 to 5 minutes up to total of 0.03 to 0.04 mg/kg. Use the shorter dosing interval (3 min) in severe clinical conditions. *Atropine* is seldom effective in atrioventricular (AV) block at the His-Purkinje level (type II AV block and new third-degree block with wide QRS complexes) (Class IIb).

(e) A potentially fatal error is to treat third-degree heart block plus ventricular escape beats with lidocaine.

(f) Only use *isoproterenol* with extreme caution. At low doses it is Class IIb (possibly helpful); at higher doses it is Class III (harmful).

(g) Check that patients can tolerate TCP and that cardiac capture occurs. Use analgesia and sedation as needed.

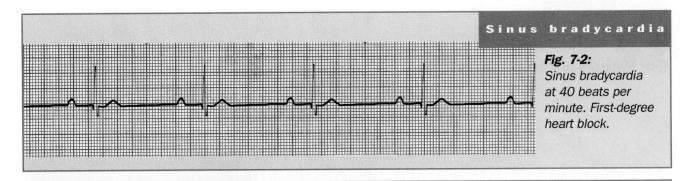

Sinus bradycardia

Fig. 7-2:
Sinus bradycardia at 40 beats per minute. First-degree heart block.

Laurice Weisfield

CASE 2

You are a family physician working in a busy group practice. You are seeing Laurice Weisfield, a 72-year-old woman who has been your patient for years. She complains of shortness of breath that has become progressively worse since she awoke this morning. She looks pale and tired, and displays labored breathing. Walking into the office "completely wiped me out." Beads of sweat gather on her forehead. The office nurse reports that her blood pressure is 100/60 and that "her heart rate is very slow" at 40 beats per minute. Respirations are 20 per minute; temperature is 36.5° C. How would you approach her immediate care?

COMMENTS

- *The patient in Case 2 appears ill. This observation should hit you strongly. Remember that you have a powerful, systematic tool that should always be applied to patients with potential cardiopulmonary emergencies—the "Five Quadrads":*

  - Primary Survey (ABCD)
  - Secondary Survey (ABCD)
  - Temperature/Blood Pressure/Heart Rate/Respirations
  - Oxygen/IV/Monitor/Fluids
  - Tank (Volume)/Resistance/Pump/Rate

- The Primary Survey can be done in seconds: she is not in cardiac arrest and does not need defibrillation.
- The Secondary Survey and her vital signs reveal problems with breathing, shortness of breath, tachypnea, and the slow heart rate.
- Oxygen/IV/Monitor/Fluids guadrad gives you the rhythm in Fig. 7-3 (type II second-degree block with a narrow QRS complex).
- **The three bradycardia questions.** The monitor tells

us that the rhythm is slow—bradycardia. Once the rhythm is identified as "bradycardia," the Bradycardia Algorithm (Fig. 7-1) directs us to ask the three bradycardia questions:

  - Are there serious signs and symptoms?
  - Is there a heart block? If there is a heart block, ask the following:
  - Does it appear to be Type II second-degree AV block (narrow or wide) or third-degree block (narrow or wide)?

- Are there serious signs and symptoms? You should memorize the list of signs and symptoms that "too slow" rhythms can produce. The list contains almost the same items as that for "too fast" rhythms, as follows:

  - *Symptoms:* Chest pain, shortness of breath, decreased level of consciousness, weakness, fatigue, exercise intolerance, light-headedness, dizziness, and "spells"

  - *Signs:* Low blood pressure, drop in blood pressure when standing upright, diaphoresis, pulmonary congestion on physical examination or chest x-ray, frank congestive heart failure or pulmonary edema, and acute coronary insufficiency (angina, other symptoms of AMI, and premature ventricular complexes [PVCs]).

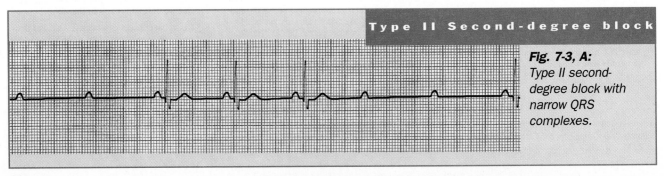

Type II Second-degree block

Fig. 7-3, A:
Type II second-degree block with narrow QRS complexes.

- In addition, watch for pause-dependent or bradycardia-dependent ventricular rhythms. During the long pauses of bradycardia in some patients ventricular escape beats develop that in turn might precipitate VT or even VF.

- In Mrs. Weisfield's case you have several serious signs and symptoms: shortness of breath that is getting worse, fatigue, exercise intolerance, diaphoresis, and she "just looks bad"—an important clinical observation. For Mrs. Weisfield the critical action for you to take is to recognize that she has symptomatic bradycardia and needs to be treated to speed up her heart rate. The first treatment listed in the following bradycardia intervention sequence is *atropine.* (NOTE: Oxygen is already being administered; see also the basic Bradycardia Algorithm [Fig. 7-1].)

> - **Atropine** *0.5 to 1.0 mg (Class I and IIa)*
> - **Transcutaneous pacing**
>   *(if available; Class I)*
> - **Dopamine** *5 to 20 µg/kg/min (Class IIb)*
> - **Epinephrine** *2 to 10 µg/min (Class IIb)*
> - **Isoproterenol** *2 to 10 µg/min (Class IIb)*

- The preceding intervention sequence, plus transvenous pacemakers, presents all the interventions you need to consider for symptomatic bradycardias. For Mrs. Weisfield, we should start with atropine.

Atropine

WHY?

- Atropine is a parasympatholytic drug, a vagolytic drug, and an anticholinergic drug.

- So what does that mean? The vagus nerve is the part of the parasympathetic nervous system that innervates the heart. The vagus nerve (and all parasympathetic drugs) discharges cholinergic neurotransmitters. Atropine blocks the effects of these cholinergic transmitters (i.e., it is an anticholinergic agent).

- Just remember that the parasympathetic nervous system (and the vagus nerve) *slow* the heart rate. Do you recall vasovagal attacks in which patients' heart rates slow down and they faint? These attacks usually are caused by a profound sudden discharge from the vagus nerve. The vagus nerve goes to the sinus node and to the AV node where vagal discharges *slow* the heart rate.

- "Lysis" or "lytic" means to dissolve—thus parasympatholytic or vagolytic agents "dissolve" or "lyse" the effects of vagal agents.

- Parasympathetic activity is often increased in the diseased myocardium; this activity may precipitate heart blocks and perhaps even asystole. (Some dispute this concept.) This explains why we use atropine in asystole: we are covering

the possibility that increased parasympathetic activity may be contributing to the clinical state of no cardiac automaticity.

- Atropine therefore produces benefits only in conditions in which there is excess vagal activity; atropine increases sinus node automaticity and AV conduction when they have been suppressed by abnormal parasympathetic or vagal discharges. Remember this when we discuss the role of atropine in the other bradycardias.

WHEN?

- *Symptomatic bradycardia:* Atropine is always appropriate to use when the bradycardia is causing the signs and symptoms.

- *Sinus bradycardia:* Make sure the patient is symptomatic from the bradycardia.

- *First-degree AV block:* Make sure the patient is symptomatic from the bradycardia.

- *Type I second-degree heart block (Mobitz type I):* Atropine is particularly effective in this block because Mobitz type I is almost always caused by excessive parasympathetic discharge (Fig. 7-3, *B*).

- *Type II second-degree heart block (Mobitz type II):* Remember that the QRS complexes in type II second-degree block can be either narrow (normal) or wide. Narrow complexes (Fig. 7-3, *A*) indicate an anatomically high AV node block (nodal or supranodal); wide complexes (Fig. 7-4) indicate a lesion lower in the AV node or even below the AV node (infranodal blocks). (Assume in these comments that bundle branch blocks are not causing the widened QRS complexes.)

  - The preceding discussion leads to an important but frequently misunderstood point: atropine is always appropriate to use for type II second-degree heart block (with both narrow and broad QRS complexes); however, it may be ineffective, especially if the QRS complex is wide, because lesions below the AV node (infranodal blocks) produce wide-complex type II second-degree block. Since atropine works only at the sinus and AV node, it produces little effect on infranodal lesions.

    NOTE: Several experts have made a great deal out of atropine producing a few cases of paradoxic slowing in hearts with infranodal blocks. In these unusual cases, the atropine speeds up the number of impulses from the sinus and AV node. This paradoxically reduces even further the number of impulses that get past the infranodal lesion. Do not let the possibility of this rare event cause you to withhold atropine from symptomatic patients with type II second-degree block. Just be aware that it can happen, although very rarely.

- *Third-degree heart block*: You can also use atropine for third-degree AV block, as the Bradycardia Algorithm recommends. As noted earlier, however, have low expectations that atropine will speed up the rate in these patients because the pathologic condition exists at an anatomic level where atropine has no effect. Because of the slight chance of success, and because of the rare possibility of even further slowing, many experts recommend omitting a trial of atropine for these patients. Certainly pacing is the treatment of choice here, just as the algorithm states. However, the question often comes up, whether atropine is acceptable for these patients. The answer is yes—with the caveats noted earlier, and as long as you are preparing for pacing.

- *Relative bradycardia:* In relative bradycardia the heart rate is somewhat above 60 beats per minute, but the rate is slow relative to the overall clinical condition. For example, a rate of 70 beats per minute in a patient with symptomatic hypotension is a relative bradycardia.
  - This condition most often occurs in AMI patients with excessive vagal activity. However, remember the cardiovascular quadrad in which you need to think of the Tank (Volume)/Resistance/Pump/Rate.
  - Do not give atropine to patients with slow heart rates and low blood pressure if the low blood pressure is a "low tank" problem. For that matter, do not give dopamine or epinephrine either. We discuss this further in Chapter 10.

Summary of Atropine Indications (When)

Rhythm	Clinical Situation	Atropine Use
Sinus bradycardia; First-degree heart block	Patient has symptoms, and the symptoms are due to the slow heart rate.	Acceptable; make sure patient has good oxygenation and ventilation.
Type I, second-degree heart block	Patient has symptoms, and the symptoms are due to the slow heart rate.	Highly recommended; make sure patient has good oxygenation and ventilation.
Type II, second-degree heart block; narrow QRS complex	Patient has symptoms, and the symptoms are due to the slow heart rate.	Recommended, especially in the setting of suspected AMI; likely to be effective.
Type II, second-degree heart block; widened QRS complex	Patient has symptoms, and the symptoms are due to the slow heart rate.	Acceptable; less likely to be effective with infranodal blocks. Prepare for pacing.
Type III heart block	Patient has symptoms, and the symptoms are due to the slow heart rate.	Acceptable; not likely to be effective. Prepare for pacing.
Asystole; bradyasystolic cardiac arrest; slow PEA	Full cardiac arrest	Recommended; given empirically. Assumption is a vagal component to the arrest.

HOW?

Here is what you should remember about the dosing of atropine:

- *The first dose of atropine for bradycardia is 0.5 to 1.0 mg.*
- *Repeat every 3 to 5 minutes up to a total of 0.03 to 0.04 mg/kg.*
- The end point with atropine is the clinical response: do not give repeat doses if the heart rate has responded satisfactorily.
- If the patient has not responded satisfactorily to 0.04 mg/kg, you need to move to the next interventions

in the sequence (pacing, dopamine, epinephrine, and isoproterenol).

- Do not give doses lower than 0.5 mg IV push.
- Give the higher dose and the shorter dosing interval when the clinical situation is more severe. For example, for full asystolic cardiac arrest give 1.0 mg every 3 minutes; for only mildly symptomatic bradycardia give 0.5 mg every 5 minutes.
- Remember "ALE" for endotracheal drug administration: atropine-lidocaine-epinephrine. Double the IV amount (1 to 2 mg) and dilute it in 10 mL of sterile water or normal saline.

WATCH OUT!

- Do not give doses lower than 0.5 mg because these can produce parasympathomimetic effects (that is, effects that "mimic" the parasympathetic nervous system). Such effects may paradoxically produce a slowing of the heart rate rather than speeding it up.

- Remember that you are giving atropine to increase the heart rate. You can increase the heart rate too much and produce an unwanted tachycardia. In patients with coronary artery or ischemic heart disease you can increase the angina and ischemic chest pain.

- The previously mentioned postatropine tachycardia can be so severe that it may precipitate VF or VT.

- In certain clinical situations, however, you must perform a careful balancing act. The most important dilemma is presented by the person with an AMI, cardiac ischemia, chest pain, and bradycardia. The conundrum is dramatically simple—leave the heart rate slow and the ischemia and chest pain get worse; speed the heart rate up and the ischemia and chest pain get worse. No easy answers here. This is discussed in detail in Bradycardia Case 4 (Dan Johnson) and in the AMI cases (Chapter 9).

- The guiding principle is to give atropine when you think you have the clinical indications and you are sure the symptoms and signs are due to the slow heart rate. However, use the lower, less frequent doses, and watch your patient carefully.

- Remember that atropine is an anticholinergic agent. Atropine can, therefore, precipitate the same anticholinergic syndrome that occurs in people who have taken an overdose of anticholinergic agents: delirium ("mad as a hatter"), decreased salivation ("dry as a bone"), flushed, hot skin ("red as a beet"), and blurred vision ("blind as a bat").

Laurice Weisfield
CASE 2 Continued

You obtain a rhythm strip and a 12-lead ECG on Mrs. Weisfield. The rhythm strip is displayed in Fig. 7-3, A (type II second-degree block with narrow QRS complexes). Mrs. Weisfield responds to two doses of atropine (1 mg IV followed by 0.5 mg 5 minutes later). Her heart rate increases to 65 beats per minute, her blood pressure to 110/75, and she feels much better. The dropped beats have vanished. You call 911, and the private ambulance company responsible for ALS care in your area arrives to transfer her to the Emergency Department of your local hospital. What were the critical actions that led to this positive outcome?

COMMENTS

- Case 2 is type II second-degree block with a narrow QRS complex.

- You recognized significant symptomatic bradycardia and the need to treat the bradycardia.

- You recognized type II second-degree heart block with a narrow complex. This indicates a block that should respond to atropine, since the problem is at or above the AV node.

Laurice Weisfield
CASE 2 Continued

You are now the physician on duty in the Emergency Department when Mrs. Weisfield arrives via ambulance. The medics report that the heart rate has slowed to 40 beats per minute during transport and that Mrs. Weisfield is now complaining of increasing shortness of breath, weakness, light-headedness, and some mild chest pain. Her blood pressure has dropped to 80/50, and she seems less alert. You obtain a rhythm strip and a 12-lead ECG. The rhythm strip is displayed in Fig. 7-4 (type II second-degree block with wide QRS complexes). What treatment would you initiate for this bradycardia?

COMMENTS

- You are faced with several clinical issues. First, Mrs. Weisfield now has gone into type II second-degree block with a wide (rather than a narrow) QRS complex. This indicates disease lower in the AV node. This should concern you more. Second, she is now less likely to respond to atropine, which helped so much in the prehospital setting.

Third, she is getting worse on clinical observation. You will have to take some action.

- One or two more doses of atropine would be acceptable here. She does not respond. You must move to the next intervention in the bradycardia intervention sequence, which is TCP.

- NOTE: You should already have been considering pacing as

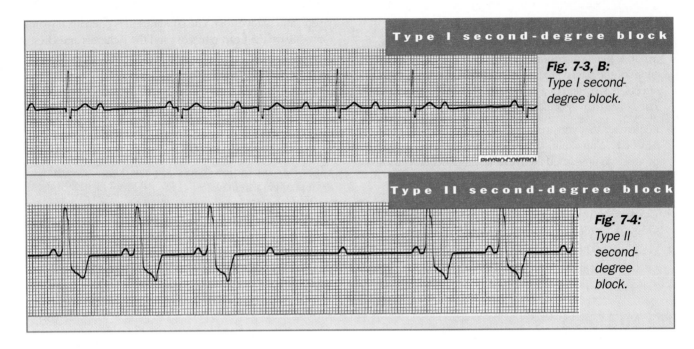

Type I second-degree block

Fig. 7-3, B: *Type I second-degree block.*

Type II second-degree block

Fig. 7-4: *Type II second-degree block.*

soon as the type II second-degree block was identified (see the Bradycardia Algorithm). Such patients, when symptomatic, often fail to respond to pharmacologic interventions and need pacing. In addition, in patients like Mrs. Weisfield, profoundly symptomatic complete heart block may suddenly develop, for which transvenous pacing (with TCP used as a bridge device to buy you and the patient more time) is the definitive treatment.

- We will next present the Why? When? How? and Watch out! for the remaining four interventions in the Bradycardia Algorithm.

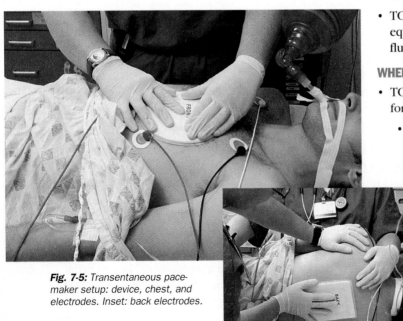

Fig. 7-5: *Transcutaneous pacemaker setup: device, chest, and electrodes. Inset: back electrodes.*

Transcutaneous Pacing

WHY?

- TCP provides direct-current stimulation to the myocardium. This stimulates a contraction that can maintain sufficient cardiac output for hours, even days.

- Use pacing to treat severe conduction system problems because pacing directly stimulates the myocardium, bypassing the defective conduction system.

- TCP is available immediately in most emergency departments and critical care units. Defibrillator manufacturers have added a TCP mode to most contemporary defibrillators and monitors.

- TCP, unlike transvenous pacing, requires no special equipment such as the fluoroscopy suite or portable fluoroscopy.

WHEN?

- TCP is a Class I intervention (acceptable, definitely helpful) for the following:

  - All symptomatic bradycardias. In particular, you should use TCP for bradycardias unlikely to respond to atropine (the infranodal blocks and the wide-complex blocks) and for complete heart block as follows:

    - Use TCP immediately if the symptomatic bradycardia is severe and unlikely to respond to atropine.

    - You can also use TCP for patients with bradycardia in whom pause-dependent or bradycardia-dependent escape rhythms develop, such as PVCs, bursts of VT, or even VF.

  - Use TCP for conditions besides symptomatic bradycardia, including the following:

- Overdrive pacing of refractory VTs or supraventricular tachycardias

- Asystolic or bradyasystolic cardiac arrest (see Chapter 6). Not used routinely; most likely to be of benefit with witnessed asystole or "P-wave asystole"

- Pulseless electrical activity (Chapter 5), especially if PEA is due to overdose (tricyclic antidepressants, phenothiazines, digoxin, calcium channel blockers and beta blockers, procainamide), electrolyte abnormalities, or acidosis

- NOTE: The concept of "pacing readiness" refers to anticipating the need for TCP in the setting of AMI when certain arrhythmias arise. These arrhythmias are a product of the AMI. If the ischemic injury worsens, you can anticipate that these arrhythmias might progress to more symptomatic bradycardia, even complete heart block, as follows:

  - Sinus node dysfunction that produces symptoms
  - Type II second-degree heart block
  - Third-degree heart block
  - New bundle branch block (left, right, alternating, or bifascicular block)

HOW?

- A variety of TCPs are on the market. Make sure you learn how to operate the TCP available where you manage

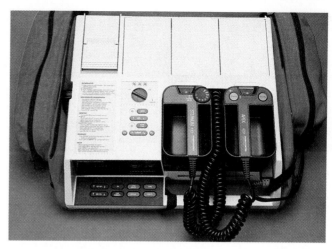

Fig. 7-6: Device face showing controls.

patients. Some TCPs are "free-standing" stand-alone units. Others are incorporated into defibrillators and monitors. This feature may not be readily apparent, so always *make sure you learn how to use your resuscitation equipment*. The generic steps common to all TCPs are described next.

- Attach the two pacing electrodes to the patient's chest (Fig. 7-5). One goes directly over the heart just to the left of the sternum, right over the apex. The other goes on the back, directly behind the front electrode. Place it outside the spinal column and inside the left scapula.

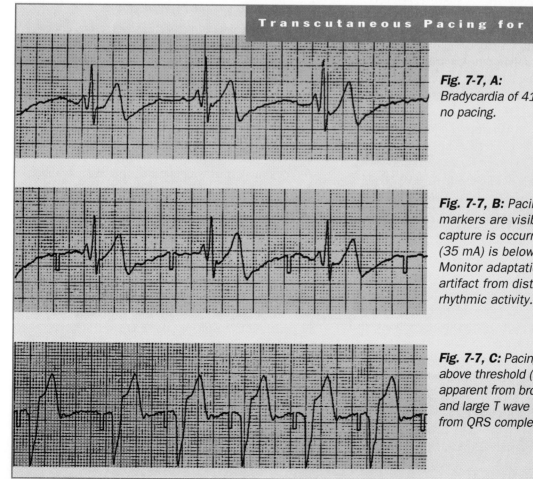

Transcutaneous Pacing for Bradycardia

Fig. 7-7, A: Bradycardia of 41 beats per minute; no pacing.

Fig. 7-7, B: Pacing stimulus markers are visible, but no ECG capture is occurring. Pacing current (35 mA) is below pacing threshold. Monitor adaptation prevents pacing artifact from distorting underlying rhythmic activity.

Fig. 7-7, C: Pacing stimulus now set above threshold (60 mA). Capture apparent from broad QRS complexes and large T wave in opposite polarity from QRS complex.

- Attach three-lead cardiac monitor electrodes (lead II position).
- Select a pacing rate, usually 80 beats per minute (Fig. 7-6).
- Select a pacing energy output, expressed in milli-amperes. For conscious patients start at a low energy output (e.g., 20 mA), and steadily increase the energy until capture is achieved.
- For bradyasystolic arrest start at maximal pacing output; if that achieves capture, reduce the output until capture is lost; then adjust slightly back up.
- Turn the power on. Observe for pacing pulse markers, indicating the device is discharging (Fig. 7-7, B).
- Observe for electrical and mechanical capture (Fig. 7-7, B and 7-7, C).
  - Electrical capture occurs when each pacer spike produces a broad QRS complex followed by a T wave that is opposite in polarity to the QRS (Fig. 7-7, C).
  - Mechanical capture occurs when the pacing produces a measurable hemodynamic response such as a palpable carotid or femoral pulse or a measurable blood pressure.
- NOTE: TCP produces jerking muscle contractions of the chest and shoulder girdle muscles. These movements can be confused with a palpable pulse; thus check for mechanical capture at the femoral or brachial arteries.

WATCH OUT!

- TCP causes physical discomfort to conscious patients, partly because of the electrical impulse but largely because of the stimulation of voluntary muscles. You may need to administer analgesia with a narcotic (morphine or fentanyl) or sedation with a short-acting benzodiazapine (midazolam or lorazepam [Ativan]), or more often, a combination of the two.
- Learn how to detect the characteristics of successful pacing through evaluating rhythm strips and pulses. The monitors that come with TCPs possess a dampening feature that prevents the pacing stimulus from grossly distorting the rhythm on the scope. If you monitor a paced patient through a nondampened monitor, you will see large distortions of the rhythm. These will obscure important underlying rhythms such as VF or VT.
- Failure to capture can mean you need to reposition the pacing electrodes, change the energy settings, dry off the patient's thorax if wet with sweat or water, or even shave or clip excessive body hair.
  - *Standby* or *bridge* pacing requires that you always test and make sure that the TCP is set up correctly and that it will indeed produce mechanical capture, as follows:
  - Do this by starting a brief period of pacing after first explaining to the patient that it will cause some discomfort.
  - Set the rate at slightly faster than the patient's intrinsic heart rate.
  - Slowly increase the energy output until you see the pacer spikes.

- Increase the energy further until you see the broad, slurred QRS complexes with prominent T waves that indicate mechanical capture.

Dopamine

WHY?

- Dopamine is an important adrenergic agent for emergency cardiac care.
- Dopamine is used to raise the blood pressure in patients without hypovolemia.
- Dopamine works on the "tank" portion (producing vasoconstriction and thus a smaller tank) and on the "pump" portion (leading to stronger cardiac action) of the cardiovascular quadrad.
- Atropine, on the other hand, works only on the "rate" portion of the cardiovascular quadrad.
- Depending on the dose, dopamine stimulates a series of adrenergic receptors; each group of stimulated receptors produces different effects: increased renal output, increased cardiac contractility, and increased blood pressures (see "How" section).

WHEN?

- Remember: *Use dopamine to treat symptomatic hypotension in patients without hypovolemia.*
- This is a simple indication that disguises several critical points. This statement brings together the following important concepts in emergency cardiac care:
  - Think of the patient (do they have symptoms?) before simply treating a number (heart rate or blood pressure).
  - Symptomatic hypotension is an important finding in patients with too-fast rhythms, too-slow rhythms, and hypotension or shock.
  - You cannot treat symptomatic hypotension without considering the cardiovascular quadrad of Tank (Volume)/Resistance/Pump/Rate.
- Thus the major use of dopamine in symptomatic bradycardia is to treat patients who also have hypotension or hypoperfusion as the major manifestation of their bradycardia.
- If dopamine is being used to raise the blood pressure in hypotensive bradycardic patients, make sure that they have a "full tank" and are not hypovolemic. If the patient is hypovolemic, dopamine will achieve only minimal effectiveness.
- Most commonly, the symptomatic hypotension is due to bradycardia (not hypovolemia), and dopamine is highly effective.
- Dopamine is also recommended to treat hypotension with signs and symptoms of shock when the systolic blood pressure is 70 to 100 mmHg. We discuss this in more detail in Chapter 10.

- Use dopamine in vasopressor doses (10 to 20 μg/kg per minute) to treat postresuscitation hypotension. (Transient *hyper*tension is the goal.)

- In cardiogenic shock and cardiac failure, dopamine can also be combined with vasodilators (like nitroglycerin and nitroprusside) to reduce preload and improve cardiac output. The vasodilators antagonize the arterial and venous constriction caused by high doses of dopamine.

HOW?

- Select the dose of dopamine based on the effects you are trying to achieve, as follows:

  - **Low doses of dopamine (1 to 5 μg/kg per minute)** have been called "renal doses." These doses produce a dopaminergic effect that dilates the renal, mesenteric, and cerebral blood vessels. This effect increases renal output. Do not use this lower dose in patients being treated for symptomatic bradycardia.

  - **Moderate doses of dopamine (5 to 10 μg/kg per minute)** have been called "cardiac doses." These doses produce beta-1-adrenergic and alpha-adrenergic effects that increase cardiac contractility and cardiac output and raise blood pressure. Start with this dose for patients with symptomatic bradycardia.

Overlap Syndromes in ACLS (Venn Diagram)

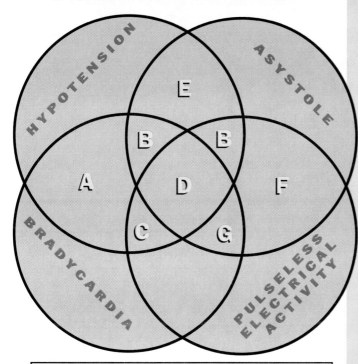

A—Symptomatic bradycardia (hypotensive)
B—"Mother of all bradycardias" (rate = zero; pressure = zero)
C—Slow PEA with profound hypotension (cardiac arrest)
D—Each problem at most critical
E—"Mother of all hypotension" (pressure drops to nothing)
F—PEA rate slows to zero
G—Profoundly hypotensive bradycardia (pressure = zero)

Epinephrine and the Cardiac Overlap Syndromes

(See Venn diagram on Overlap syndromes in ACLS on this page.)

- *Epinephrine is the fourth intervention to use for symptomatic bradycardia. At this point, the patient will usually be in dire clinical straits. The conduction system has not responded to atropine, the blood pressure has not responded to dopamine, and the myocardium has not responded to direct electrical stimulation from TCP. What do you do?*

- *You must appreciate a critical point here: You are approaching an "overlap" syndrome in emergency cardiac care. Often in cardiac emergencies patients present with combination or "overlap" problems—the fuzzy interface between two or more conditions and two or more treatment algorithms.*

- *Profoundly symptomatic bradycardia represents one of those areas. The blood pressure is low, and the heart rate is slow. Do you treat according to the algorithm for hypotension and shock or according to the Bradycardia Algorithm?*

- *The rate can get so slow that it is, in effect, asystole—the "mother of all bradycardias." Do you use the Asystole Algorithm? The blood pressure can diminish to a point of nondetectability: do you then consider the problem PEA and initiate CPR and the cardiac arrest protocols?*

- *Fortunately, epinephrine is an intervention guarding the narrow waist of the hourglass where all these conditions overlap and come together. Remember that epinephrine is the recommended agent for asystole, PEA, profound hypotension (at least in the form of norepinephrine), profoundly symptomatic bradycardia, and any pulseless or near pulseless clinical state (see Venn Diagram). The mechanism of action of epinephrine is such that epinephrine possesses great value for all these conditions.*

- **High doses of dopamine (10 to 20 µg/kg per minute)** have been called "vasopressor doses." Here the alpha-adrenergic effects produce strong arterial and venous vasoconstriction, which raises the blood pressure. Use these doses in patients with low blood pressure and signs and symptoms that suggest clinical shock.

- **Dopamine doses (over 20 µg/kg per minute):** At doses this high you get profound vasoconstriction—similar to effects of norepinephrine.

- Mix ampules (which come as 40 mg/mL in 5-mL ampules) (total = 200 mg) or 160 mg/mL (total = 800 mg) in 250 mL of normal saline, lactated Ringer's solution, or 5% dextrose in water (D_5W).

WATCH OUT!

- Watch out for excessive increases in heart rate (may induce supraventricular and ventricular arrhythmias).

- May aggravate pulmonary congestion in people with heart failure.

- May induce angina and ischemic changes in people with severe coronary artery disease.

- May cause tissue necrosis and sloughing if local skin infiltration occurs.

- Taper gradually (over several hours) to avoid a sudden drop in blood pressure.

- Reduce the dose to one tenth of the usual dose in people taking monoamine oxidase inhibitors (Eutonyl, Parnate, or Nardil), since these drugs will potentiate the effects of dopamine.

- Patients taking phenytoin (Dilantin) may have excessive hypotension with dopamine.

- Patients with pheochromocytoma may have hypertensive crisis when given dopamine.

- Do not mix with sodium bicarbonate or any alkaline solution, as this will inactivate dopamine.

Epinephrine

WHY?

There are two major reasons to give epinephrine in symptomatic bradycardia:

- First, epinephrine raises the blood pressure by constricting the peripheral blood vessels (pressor effect).

- Second, epinephrine increases the heart rate through increasing the electrical activity in the myocardium and the intrinsic cardiac automaticity (chronotropic effects).

WHEN?

- Use epinephrine for profoundly symptomatic bradycardia not responsive to atropine, dopamine, and TCP.

- Does this mean you cannot give epinephrine until after you have tried the other four interventions and they have

failed? Of course not. Sometimes the profoundly symptomatic bradycardic patients will be so close to shock, PEA, or even asystole, that you will need to go quickly to epinephrine—often at cardiac arrest doses (1 mg IV push) rather than bradycardia doses (2 to 10 µg/min)—and often almost simultaneously with atropine and dopamine. These patients are in such critical condition that you are not going to wait long for one drug to work before moving quickly to the next agent.

- Often clinicians speak of "starting a catecholamine infusion" for patients with symptomatic bradycardia. This phrase refers to the three postatropine agents dopamine, epinephrine, and isoproterenol. The phrase implies an equivalence among the three agents that is probably unjustified. Isoproterenol should be considered a last resort and is not in the same tier of acceptability as dopamine and epinephrine.

HOW?

- Add epinephrine 1 mg (1 mL of a 1:1000 solution) to 500 mL of normal saline or D_5W. This gives a concentration of 2 µg/mL.

- Start IV infusion at 1 µg/min. Titrate to hemodynamic effects of blood pressure and heart rate. You will probably end up with a rate of 2 to 10 µg/min.

- For profoundly symptomatic bradycardia patients approaching full cardiac arrest, do the following: add 30 mg (30 mL of a 1:1000 solution) to 250 mL of normal saline or D_5W to run at 100 mL/hour (again titrating to hemodynamic effects).

- If full cardiac arrest occurs, use the cardiac arrest doses of 1 mg IV push every 3 to 5 minutes (a bradycardic patient without pulses would be considered in PEA arrest).

WATCH OUT!

- Epinephrine, by raising the blood pressure and increasing the heart rate, can precipitate myocardial ischemia, increasing angina and chest pain.

- Be aware that by definition, people with symptomatic bradycardia who need epinephrine are people with a diseased myocardium, usually coronary artery disease.

- Even small doses of epinephrine (2 µg/min or 0.3 µg/kg per minute) can elevate the blood pressure and induce or exacerbate ventricular ectopy and VT or VF.

- Patients who are taking digitalis are much more likely to have toxic side effects resulting from epinephrine.

Isoproterenol

WHY?

- A pure beta-adrenergic agent, isoproterenol cause increased strength of cardiac contractions and increased heart rate but also peripheral vasodilation and venous pooling.

- Because of its powerful effects on speeding up the heart rate, isoproterenol has in the past been a favorite drug to use for symptomatic bradycardias.

- There are problems, however, with isoproterenol—it is also a vasodilator, causing a decrease in blood pressure. REMEMBER: Do not treat bradycardia unless the patient displays significant symptoms. Most often the major symptom is hypotension. Isoproterenol can make the heart beat faster, but it can also make the hypotension worse. The clinical axiom, "If you are sick enough to need isoproterenol you are too sick to tolerate it," is a useful rephrasing of this paradox.

- The denervated transplanted heart responds remarkably well to isoproterenol, and that is becoming the major remaining use for this agent.

WHEN?

- Isoproterenol is a third-line agent for temporarily increasing the heart rate in patients with symptomatic bradycardia.

- Use isoproterenol only after atropine, dopamine, TCP, and epinephrine infusion have failed.

- Many clinicians claim a long record of success with isoproterenol, increasing the heart rate satisfactorily without dropping the blood pressure excessively. They achieve this success first by using very low doses. Second, they watch carefully that the increase in heart rate raises the blood pressure enough to compensate for isoproterenol's vasodilatory effects.

- While you should respect the clinical experience many physicians have gained with isoproterenol, most experts now prefer other chronotropic and inotropic agents (dopamine, dobutamine, and amrinone).

- A second-line indication for isoproterenol is to achieve "pharmacologic overdrive pacing" of patients in the VT known as torsades de pointes. Note, however, that this should be attempted only after infusion of magnesium sulfate has failed.

HOW?

- Mix 1 mg of isoproterenol (comes in 1 mL ampules containing 1 mg) in 250 mL of normal saline, lactated Ringer's, or D_5W.

- Use a volumetric infusion pump to carefully control the flow.

- Infuse initially at low doses of 2 µg/min. Gradually titrate up to achieve a heart rate of 60 to 70 beats per minute.

- Limit the dose to 2 to 10 µg/min.

- When using isoproterenol to "break" torsades de pointes, titrate the dose up to increase the heart rate fast enough to suppress the VT.

WATCH OUT!

- Do not use isoproterenol during cardiac arrest. The vasodilatory actions reduce coronary perfusion pressure and increase mortality in laboratory studies. This is a Class III (harmful) use of the agent.

- Avoid isoproterenol in patients with ischemic heart disease. Isoproterenol may increase the heart rate and myocardial oxygen requirements so powerfully that disastrous myocardial ischemia results.

- The effects on symptomatic bradycardia patients with coronary artery disease may be catastrophic—they can have severe myocardial ischemia and worsening hypotension and can even have full cardiac arrest.

- Bradycardic patients may respond to isoproterenol with a severely symptomatic tachycardia, ventricular arrhythmias, and even VT, VF, and full cardiac arrest.

- The possibility of these scenarios should fill clinicians with apprehension every time they consider using isoproterenol.

- Avoid isoproterenol in patients with possible digitalis intoxication.

Laurice Weisfield

CASE 2 Continued

You ask the nurse to administer an additional dose of atropine 1 mg IV. This produces no change in the heart rate after 3 minutes, and Mrs. Weisfield continues to complain of weakness and shortness of breath. You decide to initiate TCP.

You ask the nurse to place the TCP pads on Mrs. Weisfield (anterior pad on the chest, over the apex; posterior pad on the back, midthoracic level, just to the inside of the scapula).

With the TCP rate set at 80 beats per minute and the pacing current at the lowest setting, you gradually increase the pacing current until you see pacing spikes (Fig. 7-7, B). The pectoralis muscles begin to slightly twitch. Mrs. Weisfield reports a tingling sensation and slight discomfort. You explain to her what is happening, and that the chest discomfort may increase. At a current level of 90 mA, the monitor screen suddenly changes to reveal that all the beats are broad complexes that look like PVCs. The T waves are slurred and are opposite in polarity to the QRS complexes (Fig. 7-7, C).

CONTINUED

> **Laurice Weisfield**
>
> **CASE 2 Continued**
>
> *You can now palpate a pulse at 80 beats per minute. The nurse measures a blood pressure of 110/80. You ask Mrs. Weisfield whether the pacing stimulus is too uncomfortable, and she replies that it certainly seems "to wake me up, however, I can tolerate it for now."*
>
> *Mrs. Weisfield's heart continues to be paced for 45 minutes while she is awaiting an available bed in the coronary care unit (CCU). You turn the pacing current down every 10 to 15 minutes to check the intrinsic rhythm. Each time the intrinsic rate is faster with fewer dropped beats. After 45 minutes of pacing you turn down the pacing current and notice that the intrinsic rhythm is sinus rhythm at 65 beats per minute with no dropped beats.*
>
> *The TCP remains in place but turned off, and the dopamine drip remains on standby. Mrs. Weisfield leaves the Emergency Department for further evaluation and treatment in the CCU.*
>
> *What were the critical actions that produced this successful outcome in Mrs. Weisfield? What is the role of the dopamine standby drip? Should you call the cardiologist to prepare for a transvenous pacemaker?*

COMMENTS

In Case 2 there were several important critical actions, as follows:

- You recognized the need to keep treating this symptomatic bradycardia after atropine failed.

- You used TCP in the proper manner, recognizing electrical and mechanical capture from the pacemaker.

- You prepared for TCP failure by preparing a standby dopamine drip.

- You alerted professionals responsible for transvenous pacemaker insertion of a patient with type II second-degree block.

- **Dopamine standby drip.** Whenever you plan to start TCP, always prepare for the possibility that it will not be effective or tolerated by the patient. Order a dopamine standby drip of 800 mg (one 5-mL ampule of 160 mg/mL)

in 250 mL of normal saline). If needed, start with at least 5 to 10 µg/kg per minute through a controlled infusion set.

- **Transvenous pacing.** Whenever you initiate TCP, contact the cardiologist or other specialist responsible for transvenous pacemakers. Remember the indications for TCP are also the indications for transvenous pacing. TCP has greatly reduced the need for emergency placement of temporary transvenous pacemakers. Several studies have demonstrated that the effectiveness of TCP approaches that of transvenous pacing in the emergency setting. In addition, the low morbidity and high practicality of TCP is far superior to emergency transvenous pacemaker placement.

> **Michael Brady**
>
> **CASE 3**
>
> *Mr. Michael Brady, a 45-year-old business executive, arrives at the Emergency Department at 9:30 PM. He began experiencing moderately severe substernal chest pain after a large dinner with his six children. After 2 hours, he began to feel weak and nauseated and began to sweat profusely on his forehead.*
>
> *His wife, Carol, insisted he come to the hospital, where you are evaluating him in Room 1. His vital signs: temperature, 37.2° C; heart rate = 50 beats per minute; blood pressure = 100/70; respirations = 12 per minute. He appears pale and uncomfortable. He has a normal ECG, but his rhythm strip displays a bradycardia (Fig. 7-4).*

COMMENTS

- Mr. Brady sounds suspiciously like he is having an AMI. He tells a typical story for a middle-aged man in terms of

the location and nature of his pain, and in terms of his delay in seeking care for over 2 hours.

- The clue here is the nature of the heart block: type I second-degree heart block (with narrow QRS complexes).

This rhythm abnormality is most often due to the parasympathetic discharge that can occur with AMI. This type of heart block responds well to atropine but often resolves spontaneously without specific treatment.

- The heart rate is slow, and Mr. Brady is symptomatic. The critical questions are whether the slowness is producing hypoperfusion and whether the hypoperfusion is aggravating the ischemia from the AMI.

- Mr. Brady needs to be admitted to rule out an AMI, despite the normal ECG. The story and risk factors are too suspicious.

- Initiate the AMI protocol with morphine-oxygen-nitroglycerin-aspirin. (This is the "MONA" mnemonic [see Chapter 9]). Watch the blood pressure and heart rate carefully. Chapter 9 presents the detailed management of AMI.

- At this point you would be wise to withhold atropine. Increasing the heart rate runs a high risk of increasing the cardiac ischemia. Besides, the symptoms here (the chest pain) are more likely the direct result of the suspected AMI than of the slow heart rate.

Dan Johnson

CASE 4

Dan Johnson is a 55-year-old products-liability attorney in town for a deposition. After a long day taking testimony from medical device manufacturers, he feels unusually fatigued and slightly nauseated, with vague chest discomfort. After an intense telephone conversation with his client he suddenly develops midsternal chest pain with left-arm radiation, nausea, and diaphoresis. He calls 911, and the paramedics arrive to evaluate him in his hotel room.

As a paramedic you find a pale, uncomfortable-appearing man sitting on the edge of the bed. He has blood pressure of 130/100, heart rate of 45 beats per minute, shortness of breath, and some rales at the bases. You start Oxygen/IV/Monitor/Fluids. You obtain a field 12-lead ECG and transmit it to the base hospital. The ECG reveals no acute ST-segment changes, but the rhythm strip is abnormal (Fig. 7-3, A).

You radio the base hospital and describe Mr. Johnson as "severely symptomatic" and you think the heart rate is "way too slow." Should you ask for permission to administer atropine 1 mg IV?

COMMENTS

- This is a tough one. Mr. Johnson is experiencing bradycardia and has a number of symptoms that could be due to the bradycardia. This may be "symptomatic bradycardia" that should be treated. However, he also has type II second-degree block, which frequently indicates more

severe conduction system disease and may be unresponsive to atropine.

- In your short report you emphasize the slowness of the heart rate and clearly convey that you think the shortness of breath, mild rales, and continuing chest pain are being aggravated by the bradycardia. You press your case for permission to administer atropine.

Dan Johnson

CASE 4 Continued

You obtain permission to give the atropine 1 mg and within 2 minutes observe a disappearance of the heart block and progressive acceleration of the heart rate to a sinus tachycardia of 110 beats per minute.

During transport to the Emergency Department Mr. Johnson begins to complain of a steady increase in the severity of his chest pain, stating that "it now feels like a heavy pressing weight on the center of my chest!" Upon arrival in the Emergency Department a second 12-lead ECG is obtained and now displays new 2 mm ST-segment elevation in leads V_1 to V_4 that were not present on the 12-lead obtained in the field 35 minutes previously.

COMMENTS

- Mr. Johnson appears to have suffered adverse consequences from the atropine. The atropine-induced acceleration of the rate further aggravated the myocardial ischemia and chest pain. The acute injury currents displayed in the 12-lead ECG in the hospital may be due to the rate-related ischemia.

- Did Mr. Johnson display enough indications to justify the atropine? Hard to say. The lesson here is to realize that "symptomatic bradycardia" is a real clinical challenge, especially when you have alternative reasons for the "symptoms" in a patient with bradycardia (in this case the primary AMI.)

- Most clinicians have experienced scenarios like this and have learned to be reluctant to use atropine to speed up the heart rate in people with probable ischemic heart disease, especially an AMI.

- One approach would have been to have started with a lower dose of atropine (0.5 mg, but no lower), but *only after* having initiated the usual AMI stabilization interventions: oxygen-nitroglycerin-morphine-reassurance. Mr. Johnson possessed a blood pressure that was high enough to tolerate the hypotensive effects of the nitroglycerin and the morphine. With hindsight we see that Mr. Johnson needed careful watching, not atropine.

Lydia Bingham, MD

CASE 5

Dr. Bingham is a 72-year-old retired pediatrician who arrives at the Emergency Department with complaints of severe fatigue over the past 24 hours. She is in good health with no chronic medical problems. She states that yesterday morning she suddenly began to feel "weak and dizzy" even when lying down or sitting. Walking short distances, such as trips to the bathroom or the kitchen, make her short of breath and light-headed "like I'm going to pass out."

You start Oxygen/IV/Monitor, 12-lead ECG, and chest x-ray. Vital signs: blood pressure = 80/60; heart rate 35 to 40 beats per minute; respirations = 20 per minute and labored; temperature = 37° C. The ECG reveals no acute ischemic changes, but there are Q waves in leads II, III, and av_F. The rhythm is third-degree heart block with a narrow QRS complex (Fig. 7-8, A).

Is Dr. Bingham suffering from "symptomatic bradycardia"? Is there a significant heart block? What treatments would you initiate?

COMMENTS

- Dr. Bingham's story of a relatively precipitous change in well-being with sudden onset of fatigue and exercise intolerance is "classic" for the onset of complete heart block. The ECG confirms some degree of coronary artery disease (the old inferior MI). Elderly women, in particular, may display this pattern of "silent" coronary artery disease.

- You ask the three bradycardia questions:
  - Are there serious signs and symptoms that are due to the bradycardia?
  - Is there a heart block? If there is a heart block, ask the following:
  - Does it appear to be type II second-degree AV block (narrow or wide) or third-degree block (narrow [Fig. 7-8, A] or wide [Fig. 7-8, B])?

- You can answer these questions rapidly: the symptoms are serious and are due to the bradycardia; she does have a heart block; and the heart block is narrow-complex third-degree.

- You make several decisions at once, based upon the Bradycardia Algorithm, as follows:

Atropine. You order atropine in an immediate effort to get the blood pressure and heart rate to increase, even though you know atropine is unlikely to have much effect on third-degree heart block. Atropine is not contraindicated.

TCP. You direct the house officer to attach the TCP pads to the patient (anterior pad on the chest, over the apex; posterior pad on the back, midthoracic level, just to the inside of the scapula), and you describe the sensation of pacing to Dr. Bingham.

Dopamine standby drip. You ask the nurse to mix up a dopamine drip of 800 mg (one 5-mL ampule of 160 mg/mL in 250 mL of normal saline). Ask him to prepare to start with 5 to 10 µg/kg per minute through a controlled infusion set.

Transvenous pacing. You know that patients with third-degree heart block often need a permanent, transvenous pacemaker. You also know that TCP may need to be "backed up" with a temporary transvenous pacemaker. Therefore the prudent clinician, even this early in the management of the patient, will call the cardiology service to identify who will have responsibility for placing either the temporary or permanent transvenous pacemaker, should you face that clinical necessity. If there is a high likelihood that a medical specialty service will be needed, call early rather than late. This is simple clinical wisdom and professional courtesy.

Lydia Bingham, MD

CASE 5 Continued

The nurse administers atropine 0.5 mg, but there is no response in heart rate or blood pressure. In 5 minutes you repeat the atropine, but at a higher dose of 1 mg. Again there is no response.

The nurse states, "Doctor, she is starting to throw PVCs." You glance quickly at the monitor screen (Fig. 7-9). The intern asks, "Shouldn't we give her a bolus of lidocaine to wipe out those PVCs?"

How do you respond?

C O M M E N T S

- Immediately check the pulse to determine whether the PVCs are "effective," which means the PVCs produce a mechanical contraction of the heart and this contraction produces a palpable pulse. In this setting you will generally observe that the PVCs are responsible for palpable pulses.

- Giving lidocaine at this point would be a serious error, perhaps even life threatening.

- With a heart rate this slow (35 to 40 beats per minute), ventricular escape rhythms begin because such rates approach the intrinsic automaticity rate of the ventricles. During the long bradycardic pauses, ventricular automaticity has time to emerge and produce the PVCs. PVCs are possible, as well as runs of VT.

- If you suppress these escape beats with lidocaine, you could reduce disastrously the number of cardiac beats that actually pump blood. For example, a person with a palpable pulse of 40 beats per minute and bigeminy would drop to a pulse of 20 beats per minute if lidocaine eliminated all the escape PVCs.

- PVCs or runs of VT are two of the signs of "symptomatic" bradycardia that mandate therapy. Dr. Bingham is symptomatic in several aspects and needed treatment even before she started having PVCs.

- The treatment at this point is to speed up the heart rate—to "overdrive" the intrinsic ventricular rate so that the PVCs will be suppressed.

- Since atropine was not effective, proceed with TCP as described earlier in the "How?" section for TCP.

- The critical actions required at this point in Case 5 are the following:

  - Recognize that PVCs can be one of the most serious signs in significant symptomatic bradycardia.

  - Recognize the need to speed up the heart rate to eliminate the PVCs.

  - Recognize the requirement to never treat third-degree heart block plus ventricular escape beats with lidocaine.

Lydia Bingham, MD

CASE 5 Continued

You set the TCP rate at 80 beats per minute and the pacing current at the lowest setting. You gradually increase the pacing current until you see the pacing-pulse marker (Fig. 7-7, B). You observe that the pectoralis muscles are twitching slightly on Dr. Bingham. She begins to notice a tingling sensation and slight discomfort. You explain to her what is happening and that the chest discomfort may increase. At a current level of 110 mA the monitor screen suddenly changes to reveal that all the beats are broad complexes that look like PVCs (Fig. 7-7, C). The T waves are slurred and are opposite in polarity to the QRS complexes.

You can now palpate a pulse at 80 beats per minute. The nurse measures a blood pressure of 110/80. The PVCs have stopped. Dr. Bingham looks more alert and vigorous, but this is partly due to the discomfort from the pacing. She is unsure whether the discomfort is the rather vigorous twitching of her chest and shoulder girdle muscles or the electrical current on her skin under the pacing electrodes.

You turn the current down to 90 mA and several pacing stimuli fail to capture and produce complexes. You turn the current back up to 95 mA, and get 100% capture. She is more comfortable, and you ask the nurse to administer morphine 2 mg IV, every 5 to 10 minutes to help diminish the pain.

C O M M E N T S

- Dr. Bingham had the desired response to TCP: pacing was effective in increasing her heart rate, eliminating the PVCs, and raising her blood pressure.

- Dr. Bingham also had a moderate amount of chest discomfort that required parenteral analgesia, but the pacing was not intolerable.

- If capture fails to occur, try repositioning the electrodes, particularly the posterior electrode. In men, shaving or clipping body hair may help.

- Clear, supportive explanations to patients receiving TCP help them accept the chest discomfort and may reduce the need for analgesics and sedatives.

- If too much discomfort remains, despite the analgesia, add a small dose of a sedative such as *lorazepam, midazolam,* or *diazepam.*

- Remember that the dopamine drip remains on standby and could be used for patients who cannot tolerate TCP or those for whom mechanical capture cannot be achieved.

- You can use TCP until the transvenous pacemaker specialist is ready to insert either a permanent or a temporary transvenous pacemaker. For some patients, TCP may provide support successfully for many hours, even several days.

- For patients who are not seriously symptomatic from their bradycardia you can place the TCP on "standby,"

admit them to the CCU, and keep the TCP ready to pace should an emergency arise. Remember to "test" the tolerance to pacing and the energy level at which capture occurs before the patient becomes severely symptomatic.

Lydia Bingham, MD

CASE 5 Continued

You question Dr. Bingham further about the events leading up to her sudden onset of weakness and exercise intolerance. She reveals that she may have had some vague chest discomfort, with radiation to both left and right sides, under her axilla. She also had pain in her mid-back region between her shoulder blades, but this was not severe.

On close second look at the 12-lead ECG you notice 1 mm ST-segment elevations in the inferior leads.

Did Dr. Bingham have a silent MI as the precipitating event for her complete heart block?

COMMENTS

- Certainly Dr. Bingham must be admitted to the CCU to rule out AMI in the standard fashion. The cardiologists will decide about when and whether to insert a permanent pacemaker.

- Dr. Bingham displays a common presentation for occult AMI in the elderly and in women. This text comments elsewhere about how the "classic" textbook description of AMI applies only to previously healthy, middle-aged men. We need to understand that AMI presents itself in different and unpredictable ways in the elderly, in

women, and in people with other chronic diseases, most notably diabetes and renal disease. Do not expect the full, textbook description of an AMI in such patients, even though they may well have subsequent ECG changes and enzyme changes that confirm an AMI.

- The ECG changes suggest that Dr. Bingham may have had an occult, minimally painful inferior AMI, one in which the major manifestation was the new onset of third-degree heart block.

Rhythm Strips

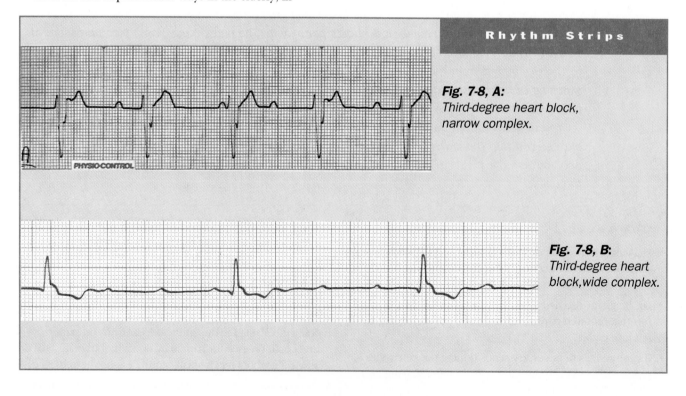

Fig. 7-8, A:
Third-degree heart block, narrow complex.

Fig. 7-8, B:
Third-degree heart block, wide complex.

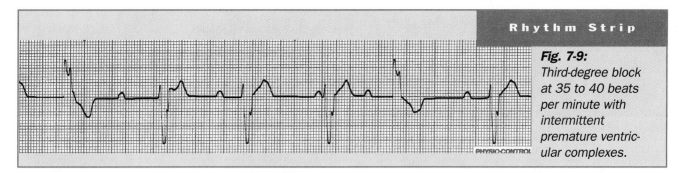

Rhythm Strip

Fig. 7-9:
Third-degree block at 35 to 40 beats per minute with intermittent premature ventricular complexes.

- The location of the infarct in patients with third-degree heart block associated with AMI gives some clues about the expected clinical course. In addition, consider the width of the QRS complex.

- Inferior AMIs produce third-degree heart block with a narrow QRS junctional escape rhythm. This conduction defect often resolves over several hours. Place a standby TCP on these patients (and test patient tolerance and capture) while waiting to see whether a transvenous pacemaker insertion will be needed or whether the block will resolve.

- The following are points to remember about third-degree heart block associated with AMI.

Anterior acute myocardial infarction

- Always prepare to insert transvenous pacemaker.

- Avoid atropine.

- Use TCP or catecholamine (dopamine or epinephrine) for more severe symptoms.

Inferior acute myocardial infarction

- Consider a trial of one or two doses of atropine 0.5 mg to determine responsiveness.

- Apply standby TCP. (Verify patient tolerance and mechanical capture.)

- Use dopamine or epinephrine if symptoms become severe.

CRITICAL CARE POINTS

- Recognize that AMI, even one without symptoms, must be ruled out in patients with the onset of third-degree heart block.

- Recognize that infarct location has clinical predictive value in patients with third-degree heart block.

Vincent Morrison

CASE 6

You are working in the CCU. Vincent Morrison, a 67-year-old used-car dealer, has been admitted with congestive heart failure, severe shortness of breath, and chest pain. The resident, pulmonary fellow, and anesthesiologist recommend rapid-sequence intubation to provide additional ventilation support.

You stand nearby, ready to help as they proceed to anesthetize and paralyze this patient. The resident asks if he can perform the intubation, and the anesthesiologist reluctantly agrees. You intensely watch the monitor screen as the resident begins the attempt to intubate. The initial rhythm is displayed in Fig. 7-10, A. With each 3-second sweep of the monitor screen the heart rate drops: 100, 95, 90, 85, 80, 75, 70 (Fig. 7-10, B and Fig. 7-10, C). The resident continues with somewhat clumsy attempts to intubate.

Does this rate of 70 beats per minute constitute "bradycardia"? What would you do or say now?

COMMENTS

- The physicians are failing to properly ventilate the lungs in this paralyzed patient during an intubation attempt. The intubation is taking too long. You should be extremely alarmed as you watch this man's heart rate slow down progressively. Without immediate intervention this man could go into cardiac arrest.

- Several critical points follow:

- The presentation is a relative bradycardia—even though the rate is 70 beats per minute, *relative* to what it was before the intubation attempt started, it is too slow!

- Case 6 presents the perfect "physiologic model" for what hypoxia and hypoventilation do to the heart rate: a heart starved for oxygen begins to slow down.

- This absolutely critical point is core information taught in Pediatric Advanced Life Support: progressive slow-

Bradycardias in Patients With Possible Acute Myocardial Infarction

MAJOR POINTS TO REMEMBER

Many important brady-cardias occur in the context of a possible AMI. Major points to remember about possible AMI in patients who have brady-cardia are listed here.

Slow Rhythms in Patients With AMI

- **Slow** rates may reduce coronary flow. Slow rates may increase ischemia and increase the development of ventricular escape arrhythmias. However:

- **Slow** rates protect against ischemia-induced arrhythmias. This is because faster rates put more demand on the ischemic myocardium. Therefore:

- Leaving symptomatic patients (pain is the most common symptom) in a **Slow** rate can be **bad,** *but:*

- Speeding up the heart rate of patients with AMI can be **very bad.** Faster rates induce strain, which leads to more ischemia; this leads to more ischemic damage, more irritability, and possibly lethal arrhythmias.

- The critical rule: Do not treat bradycardias in AMI unless forced by the patient's symptoms.

First-Degree Heart Block

- No treatment is necessary unless the patient is seriously symptomatic.

- Monitor for progression to other blocks or arrhythmias.

Type I Second-Degree Heart Block (Wenckebach or Mobitz I)

- This block is high in the conduction system and occurs at or above the AV node.

- This block is likely to indicate increased vagal stimulation.

- This block seldom indicates ischemic injury of the conduction system.

- No specific treatment is indicated unless the patient has symptoms that are due to the slow rate.

- Balance the options: Leave the rate slow and the ischemia may worsen or escape rhythms may occur; speed the rate up and you may make the ischemia worse and induce arrhythmias.

- Careful observation is usually the most prudent course.

Type II Second-degree heart block (Mobitz I or II)

- This block is lower in the conduction system, below the AV node.

- The block is either at the bundle branch level (frequent), or the bundle of His (less frequent).

- Remember that this block signals ischemic injury of the conduction system.

- Type II second-degree block has a high risk of progression to complete heart block.

- Complete block increases patient mortality.

- Critical point to remember: These patients have a severe injury to the conduction system at the infranodal region.

- Prepare for pacing (transcutaneous and transvenous). This means the following:

  - Alert the staff who will be responsible for insertion of transvenous pacer

  - Attach TCP **prophylactically.**

  - **Always,** give a brief test trial of TCP to make sure that it will capture (cause mechanical beats of the heart) and that the patient can tolerate it.

- Pain may be a major problem with TCP; therefore be generous with IV analgesics, muscle relaxants, and anxiolytics.

Third-degree heart block with normal-appearing QRS

- This block typically occurs at the level of the AV node.

- This rhythm has the following:

  - A normal-looking QRS

  - A rate between 30 and 50 beats per minute

- A normal-looking QRS indicates that a stable junctional escape pacemaker has taken over.

- This rhythm may be transient and usually has a good prognosis.

- While watchful waiting is often the best course, you should still anticipate the need for transcutaneous and transvenous pacing.

- Prepare for pacing (transcutaneous and transvenous) as noted earlier: Alert an appropriate consultant that you have a patient who may need emergency transvenous pacing.

Third-degree AV block with wide QRS complexes

- Block occurring below the AV node or at the level of bundle branches.

- The clues here are the wide QRS complex and a slow rate, usually less than 40 beats per minute.

- This is an infranodal block; therefore the only escape mechanism is from the ventricles below the block.

- Do **not** use lidocaine in these patients to suppress PVCs!!

- This block usually indicates that the AMI has extensively damaged the heart.

- This is **not** a stable rhythm—episodes of asystole are common.

- You should make immediate preparations for TCP and transvenous pacemaker.

Right ventricular infarction

- Right ventricular infarctions are notorious for producing relative hypovolemia and bradycardia, usually as a result of excessive parasympathetic tone.

- Hypotension often results, and these patients can appear to be in **impending cardiogenic shock.**

- A careful fluid challenge with normal saline may be lifesaving.

- The fluid challenge will increase the right ventricular filling pressures. This will increase the strength of the right ventricular contractions based on the Starling mechanism.

- Atropine, while not contraindicated, will be ineffective without the increase in volume.

ing of the heart rate usually indicates compromised ventilation.

- Adult ALS has not emphasized this point as much as Pediatric Advanced Life Support: When you are faced with *any* cardiac problem (such as symptomatic brady-cardia), always go back to the ABCDs of the Primary-Secondary Survey Approach. This way you will pick up problems like this bradycardia caused by absent ventilations.

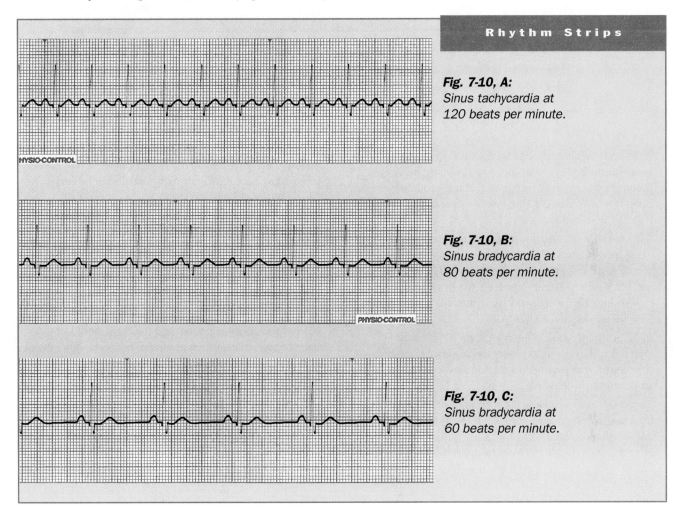

Fig. 7-10, A:
Sinus tachycardia at 120 beats per minute.

Fig. 7-10, B:
Sinus bradycardia at 80 beats per minute.

Fig. 7-10, C:
Sinus bradycardia at 60 beats per minute.

Vincent Morrison

CASE 6 Continued

As the attending physician you announce loudly, "Stop the intubation attempts. This man is going into cardiac arrest from hypoxia! Get that tube out of the way. Start bagging him with the ventilation bag. We need atropine 1 mg IV given if the heart rate does not return at once."
The rate continues to drop to 45, 40, and then 35 beats per minute. What else would you consider?

- You immediately order the intubation efforts to stop.
- This person needs immediate resuscitation from the intubation attempt. Use oxygen and positive-pressure ventilation.
- Begin immediate repositioning of the airway, insert the oropharyngeal airway (that should have been present before the intubation attempt).
- Bag vigorously with high-flow (10 to 15 L/min) 100% oxygen using a bag-valve-mask.

- Check blood pressure and pulse.
- Check the cardiac monitor.
- Check the oxygen saturation level.
- Administer **atropine, dopamine,** or **epinephrine** if there is not an immediate increase in the heart rate.
- When patient's condition appears stable, proceed with the intubation but with a more experienced operator.

Jack Scappini	You are a critical care nurse working on the neurology floor. Mr. Scappini was admitted early this morning with a dense middle cerebral artery stroke. He is unconscious and minimally responsive. He has loud cycles of Cheyne-Stokes breathing.
CASE 7	

After several hours on-shift you notice a change in the breathing pattern. It has become slower, much more like snoring. You check his pulse. It is 40; the blood pressure is 90/60. The intern enters the room and sees a sinus bradycardia of 40 beats per minute on the monitor. "This person is in severe bradycardia and needs atropine 1 mg, stat!"

What would you do or say now?

COMMENTS

- Case 7 is another example of the clinician inappropriately combining "symptoms" (in this case decreased blood pressure and altered mental status) and "slow heart rate" and thinking the combination equals "symptomatic bradycardia."

- Clinicians often make this mistake when dealing with chest pain patients who are having a heart attack and whose heart rates are either fast or slow. They fail to realize that it is the AMI that has made the heart beat too fast or too slow; they mistakenly think the rapid or slow heart rate has produced the chest pain.

- In Mr Scappini's case, a neurologic problem has produced respiratory compromise; the respiratory compromise in turn has produced a cardiac problem (bradycardia and hypotension).

- Certainly atropine will be the second most common drug you order for bradycardia, but the most important agent will be oxygen. However, the resident in this case has made a big mistake—he has simple-mindedly observed a bradycardia, noted some symptoms, and then ordered atropine. While atropine may not be harmful in this case, the resident should be thinking more in terms of the neurologic and respiratory problems, not simply in terms of a slow heart rate.

- What should the nurse do? As in so many clinical situations, nursing professionals should consider themselves full and equal partners on the health care team. The order for atropine here represents a potentially serious error. The nurse should politely yet clearly point out that atropine is not the first step here. "Let's try and improve the airway first, provide more oxygen and better ventilation, and then see what happens with the slow heart rate."

- All members of the Emergency Cardiac Care teams should learn from one another and respect the opinions and observations of others. Nothing is more important for good patient care than informed and caring team members.

- ACLS providers must understand the concept of symptomatic bradycardia—the bradycardia, not some other event such as neurologic disease, is the cause of the symptoms.

- All critical care teams should work together in an atmosphere of open, frank, but respectful communication. Recognize the value of observations from all members of the team.

KEY POINTS SUMMARY

Patients with slow heart rates can be evaluated and treated safely and effectively by following general principles and by asking several critical questions.

- *Always remember the most critical question to ask about bradycardias:* "Is this slow heart rate <u>too</u> slow for the clinical condition?"

- Learn the concept of "symptomatic" bradycardias. This means the heart rate is slow, the patient is symptomatic, *and* the symptoms are due to the bradycardia.

- Follow the *Five Quadrads* while evaluating and treating symptomatic bradycardia patients:

  - Primary ABCD Survey
  - Secondary ABCD Survey
  - Vital signs (Temperature/Blood Pressure/Heart Rate/Respirations)
  - Oxygen/IV/Monitor/Fluids
  - Tank (Volume)/Resistance/Pump/Rate

- Follow the Bradycardia Algorithm: Take action appropriately for hemodynamically significant bradycardias; know the Why? When? How? and Why not? for the Bradycardia Algorithm medications; understand, apply, and properly operate transcutaneous pacemakers.

- *The three bradycardia questions:* The Bradycardia Algorithm directs us to ask the following bradycardia questions:

  - Are there serious signs and symptoms?
  - Is there a heart block? If there is a heart block, ask the following:
  - Does it appear to be type II second-degree AV block (narrow or wide) or third-degree block (narrow or wide)?

- Finally, consider whether you need to apply the AMI Algorithm or the Shock/ Hypotension/Acute Pulmonary Edema Algorithm to patients with symptomatic bradycardia. The most serious bradycardias occur in patients with an acute AMI; furthermore, profoundly symptomatic bradycardia can produce a shock state. All of these conditions require careful thought and effective intervention.

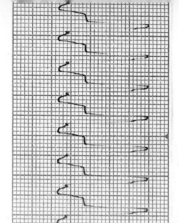

Tachycardia Cases
Stable Versus Unstable

O V E R V I E W

This chapter presents the tachycardia cases and the Tachycardia Algorithm. Many ACLS providers become intimidated by the apparent complexity of identifying and treating tachycardia rhythms. Certainly this is an area attracting a great deal of attention because of new medications and because of rapid advancements in the areas of automated rhythm analysis and automated external and implantable defibrillators and cardioverters.

In this chapter, however, we attempt to provide a simple, systematic approach to patients with tachycardias. This approach asks a series of clinical questions. The answers to these questions will lead the ACLS provider to the best therapeutic approach.

• After looking at the monitor, have you looked at the patient? Tachycardias provide the best example of the wisdom of the phrase, "Treat the patient, not the monitor." Here, just as with bradycardias, the patient's clinical condition—not the rhythm—determines both the therapeutic approach and the therapeutic urgency.

All patients with a rapid heartbeat require answers to the following specific questions:

• Is the patient's condition stable or unstable?

*• If **stable**, do you have time to identify the rhythm and treat with medications?*

*• If **unstable** from the rapid rhythm, do you need to perform immediate electrical cardioversion?*

• Are the signs and symptoms in a tachycardia patient produced by the tachycardia? Tachycardia interventions are not necessary if the tachycardia is not producing the problems.

• Is the heart rate less than 150 beats per minute? If so, cardioversion is seldom needed.

• Is the QRS complex broad or narrow? This criterion helps distinguish among supraventricular tachycardias and ventricular tachycardias. The distinction between the two often determines the need for urgency in controlling the rate and converting the patient.

• Is the blood pressure low? Is it normal? Elevated? These questions help determine the use of specific medications and the urgency of the clinical situation.

*The Tachycardia Algorithm, which may at first appear cluttered and complicated, should also be seen as a powerful **simplifying** tool. We use the term **simplifying** because **everything you need to know about treating tachycardias is introduced in this algorithm.** We admit that this is an immense oversimplification of a complex topic, but for a broad overview, like a large-scale map, it would be hard to find a better learning aid.*

MAJOR CONCEPTS TO MASTER

- Learn how to identify patients whose unstable condition is *due to their tachycardia.*
- Learn that if the patient displays serious signs and symptoms, *prepare for immediate cardioversion.*
- Know how to perform immediate cardioversion for patients in unstable condition because of their tachycardia (safely and painlessly).
- Learn that sometimes tachycardic patients can be in unstable condition, but their instability is not related to their tachycardia.
- Learn that immediate cardioversion is seldom needed for heart rates less than 150 beats per minute.
- Know to never shock normal sinus rhythm no matter how "unstable" the patient.
- Always remember: If the tachycardia complex appears wide, *treat the rhythm like ventricular tachycardia (VT).*

Critical actions

While managing each patient with tachycardia you should perform the following critical actions.

- Follow the *Five Quadrads* approach, as listed here:
  - Primary ABCD Survey
  - Secondary ABCD Survey
  - Oxygen/IV/Monitor/Fluids
  - Vital signs: Temperature/Blood Pressure/Heart Rate/Respirations
  - Cardiovascular quadrad: Tank (Volume)/Resistance/Pump/Rate
- During the Secondary Survey you will accomplish the following:
  - Obtain brief initial history.
  - Perform a focused physical examination.
  - Listen for carotid bruits before performing carotid sinus massage.
  - Start oxygen, obtain IV access, identify the rhythm.
  - Attach pulse oximeter and automatic blood pressure cuff when indicated and available.
  - Order and review ECG for rhythm diagnosis and exclusion of ischemia and infarction.
- Recognize atrial fibrillation, atrial flutter, paroxysmal supraventricular tachycardia (PSVT), wide-complex tachycardia (uncertain tachycardia vs. VT).
- Recognize cardiac ischemia if present.
- Perform proper carotid massage technique (or other vagal maneuvers) when indicated.
- Select correct drug for the arrhythmia and know the Why? When? How? and Watch Out! for each agent in the Tachycardia Algorithm.
- Correctly perform synchronized cardioversion at appropriate energy level.

Skills to learn

- How to operate a defibrillator
- How to perform electrical cardioversion
- How to perform a variety of vagal maneuvers

Rhythms to learn

- Atrial fibrillation
- Atrial flutter
- Paroxysmal supraventricular tachycardia
- Wide-complex tachycardia of uncertain origin
- Ventricular tachycardia

Medications to learn (Why? When? How? Watch Out!):

- Adenosine
- Anticoagulants
- Beta blockers
- Bretylium
- Digoxin
- Diltiazem
- Lidocaine
- Procainamide
- Quinidine
- Verapamil

Henry Armstrong
CASE 1

You are on duty in the Emergency Department at 9:30 PM. Henry Armstrong, a 55-year-old construction worker, has been persuaded by his fellow workers to come to the Emergency Department. Henry is in severe pain. "I'm hurtin' bad, Doc."

Henry states that he has had severe, crushing pain for 45 minutes. He says, "It is like an elephant stomping on my chest." He is sweating profusely and describes the pain as radiating down his left arm. He is slightly short of breath and very anxious.

How would you initially approach Mr. Armstrong?

FIGURE 8-1

Tachycardia Algorithm

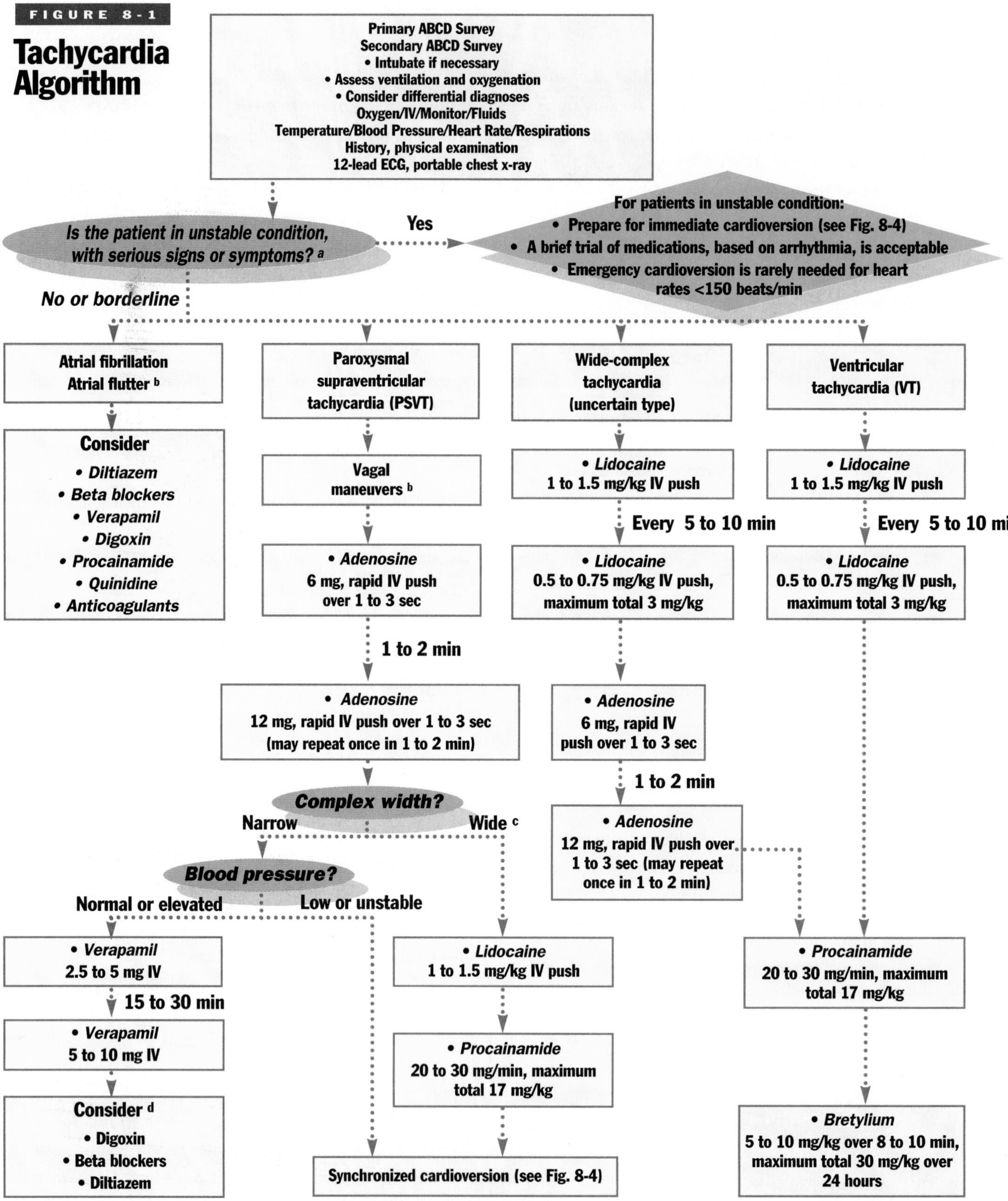

Primary ABCD Survey
Secondary ABCD Survey
• Intubate if necessary
• Assess ventilation and oxygenation
• Consider differential diagnoses
Oxygen/IV/Monitor/Fluids
Temperature/Blood Pressure/Heart Rate/Respirations
History, physical examination
12-lead ECG, portable chest x-ray

Is the patient in unstable condition, with serious signs or symptoms? [a]

Yes

For patients in unstable condition:
• Prepare for immediate cardioversion (see Fig. 8-4)
• A brief trial of medications, based on arrhythmia, is acceptable
• Emergency cardioversion is rarely needed for heart rates <150 beats/min

No or borderline

Atrial fibrillation
Atrial flutter [b]

Consider
• *Diltiazem*
• *Beta blockers*
• *Verapamil*
• *Digoxin*
• *Procainamide*
• *Quinidine*
• *Anticoagulants*

Paroxysmal supraventricular tachycardia (PSVT)

Vagal maneuvers [b]

• *Adenosine*
6 mg, rapid IV push over 1 to 3 sec

1 to 2 min

• *Adenosine*
12 mg, rapid IV push over 1 to 3 sec
(may repeat once in 1 to 2 min)

Complex width?
Narrow   **Wide** [c]

Blood pressure?
Normal or elevated   **Low or unstable**

• *Verapamil*
2.5 to 5 mg IV

15 to 30 min

• *Verapamil*
5 to 10 mg IV

Consider [d]
• *Digoxin*
• *Beta blockers*
• *Diltiazem*

Wide-complex tachycardia (uncertain type)

• *Lidocaine*
1 to 1.5 mg/kg IV push

Every 5 to 10 min

• *Lidocaine*
0.5 to 0.75 mg/kg IV push, maximum total 3 mg/kg

• *Adenosine*
6 mg, rapid IV push over 1 to 3 sec

1 to 2 min

• *Adenosine*
12 mg, rapid IV push over 1 to 3 sec (may repeat once in 1 to 2 min)

• *Lidocaine*
1 to 1.5 mg/kg IV push

• *Procainamide*
20 to 30 mg/min, maximum total 17 mg/kg

Synchronized cardioversion (see Fig. 8-4)

Ventricular tachycardia (VT)

• *Lidocaine*
1 to 1.5 mg/kg IV push

Every 5 to 10 min

• *Lidocaine*
0.5 to 0.75 mg/kg IV push, maximum total 3 mg/kg

• *Procainamide*
20 to 30 mg/min, maximum total 17 mg/kg

• *Bretylium*
5 to 10 mg/kg over 8 to 10 min, maximum total 30 mg/kg over 24 hours

---

(a) A patient's unstable condition must be caused by the tachycardia. Clinical signs and symptoms may include chest pain, shortness of breath, decreased level of consciousness, low blood pressure (BP), shock, pulmonary congestion, congestive heart failure, and acute myocardial infarction.

(b) Avoid carotid sinus pressure in patients with carotid bruits; avoid ice-water immersion in patients with ischemic heart disease.

(c) Wide-complex tachycardia known with certainty to be PSVT and BP that is normal or elevated, can be treated with verapamil.

(d) Avoid beta blockers after verapamil.

Adapted with permission, Journal of the American Medical Association, 1992, Volume 268, *Guidelines for Cardiopulmonary Resuscitation and Emergency Cardiac Care*, p. 2223, copyright © 1992, American Medical Association.

COMMENTS

- Always start with the Five Quadrads. While the Primary-Secondary ABCD Survey is most useful for patients in full cardiac arrest, the survey also guides you through a fairly complete initial assessment of the respiratory and cardiovascular status, as follows:
  - **Primary Survey:** No major problems are evident.
  - **Secondary Survey:** Some tachypnea plus shortness of breath and rales at each lung base are present. To pursue the differential diagnosis, you order 12-lead ECG, chest x-ray, and electrolyte studies.

- **Oxygen/IV/Monitor/Fluids:** You note the rhythm displayed in Fig. 8-2. The nurses, per routine, start oxygen via nasal cannula and an IV line.
- **Vital signs:** Temperature, 37.2° C; blood pressure, 180/110 mm Hg; heart rate, 140 beats/min; respirations 20 breaths/min.
- **Tank (Volume)/Resistance/Pump/Rate:** Mr. Armstrong displays increased blood pressure and heart rate. These appear to be due to his pain, anxiety, and distress.

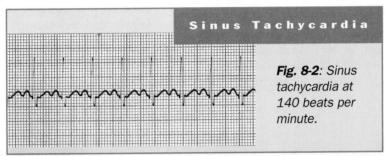

Sinus Tachycardia

Fig. 8-2: Sinus tachycardia at 140 beats per minute.

Henry Armstrong

CASE 1 Continued

You are beginning to suspect that Mr. Armstrong may have a significant rate problem. He has persistent sinus tachycardia of 140 beats/min associated with the severe chest pain, diaphoresis, radiating pain, and early pulmonary congestion.

Because of Mr. Armstrong's tachycardia, review the Tachycardia Algorithm (Fig. 8-1) and discuss the major clinical questions surrounding this algorithm.

COMMENTS

- The Tachycardia Algorithm emphasizes several major decision points. The most important question is contained in the oval that asks whether the patient is in "unstable conditions, with serious signs or symptoms."
- Notice that the *unstable condition* must be related to the tachycardia.
- The major serious signs or symptoms to look for with tachycardias are the following:
  - Low blood pressure
  - Shock
  - Pulmonary congestion
  - Congestive heart failure
  - Acute myocardial infarction (AMI)
  - Decreased level of consciousness
  - Shortness of breath
  - Chest pain
  - Continued premature ventricular complexes (PVCs) in the setting of possible AMI
- Mr. Armstrong certainly appears to be in unstable condition and severely symptomatic, with severe, crushing chest pain, diaphoresis, pulmonary congestion, and possible early congestive failure. The unwary provider would be tempted to say "yes" here—this patient is in unstable condition, with serious signs or symptoms; therefore we should prepare for immediate cardioversion, as indicated on the right side of the algorithm.

- Do not be distracted, however, by the tachycardia. Do not let a rapid rate alone interfere with your clinical judgement. Note the following important warning:
  - Immediate cardioversion is seldom needed for a heart rate less than 150 beats per minute.
- Our 55-year-old patient's heart rate is 140, and this should give us pause to consider whether cardioversion is indeed the right approach.
- In fact, Henry is having an acute myocardial infarction. That condition alone could lead to the tachycardia plus the signs and symptoms. The AMI occurred first, producing the severe pain of infarction. The pain led to anxiety, catecholamine discharge, and subsequent elevated blood pressure and heart rate. You could severely harm this individual if you made the mistake here of attributing his symptoms to the tachycardia and performing electrical cardioversion.
- Furthermore, this patient's rhythm is sinus tachycardia. We must ask, "What good would it do to shock someone in normal sinus rhythm?" The purpose of a cardioversion shock is to *produce* a sinus rhythm. Since the patient is already in a sinus rhythm, cardioversion makes no sense and adds nothing therapeutically. *This mistake—shocking rapid sinus rhythm in a patient whose condition is "unstable and symptomatic"—can be fatal, producing VT or VF.*

Henry Armstrong	Mr. Armstrong continues to appear extremely uncomfortable and anxious, becoming pale and more diaphoretic and clenching his jaw in quiet suffering.
CASE 1 Continued	

Since you decide not to specifically treat the rapid tachycardia of Mr. Armstrong, what are you going to do?

COMMENTS

- The proper therapeutic approach would be to treat the AMI that appears to be Mr. Armstrong's major problem.

- Use the agents recommended for AMI treatment: oxygen, morphine, nitroglycerin, aspirin, thrombolytic agents, beta blockers, heparin, and magnesium. (These are discussed in Chapter 9.) You should not specifically treat the tachycardia.

SUMMARY OF MAJOR POINTS IN CASE 1

- Make sure the signs and symptoms in a patient with tachycardia are produced by the tachycardia before starting the tachycardia interventions.

- Immediate cardioversion is seldom needed for a heart rate less than 150 beats per minute.

- Sinus tachycardia is a sign of something else being wrong. It is like a fever during a serious infection: treating the fever does not get rid of the infection.

- *Never* shock sinus tachycardia!

Theoda Evans	*UNSTABLE VENTRICULAR TACHYCARDIA*
CASE 2	*Two personnel from the Good Shepherd Ambulance Company are transporting Theoda Evans, a 48-year-old woman, to your hospital's catheterization laboratory for a planned coronary angiogram. They*

detour to your Emergency Department with the patient on a gurney because the patient told them she is beginning to feel dizzy and light-headed.

You greet the ambulance personnel in the corridor of the Emergency Department. They call your attention to the monitor screen on the portable monitor/defibrillator placed on the stretcher between the patient's feet. The monitor displays the rhythm in Fig. 8-3.

You glance over at the patient and note that she has a glazed look in her eyes and does not respond to your question, "How are you doing?" You quickly check for a carotid pulse. You can feel the carotid artery, but the pulse is very rapid and weak. You instruct the ambulance personnel to move her rapidly into Room 1.

What would be your immediate approach once she is in Room 1?

COMMENTS

First, quickly perform the Primary-Secondary Survey.

Primary Survey

- *Airway:* Open, air is moving.
- *Breathing:* Moving air and gasping ventilations are present.
- *Circulation:* Pulse is barely palpable.
- *Defibrillation:* You are beginning to think of electrical cardioversion.

Secondary Survey

- *Airway and Breathing:* If the patient's condition deteriorates further, she may need intubation. You confirm nasal oxygen administration at 4 L/min.

- *Circulation:* Heart rate is 180 beats/min; systolic blood pressure is 70 mm Hg. You attach your Emergency Department monitor to the cables from the ambulance personnel monitor/defibrillator. The 18-gauge IV is running well.

Ventricular Tachycardia

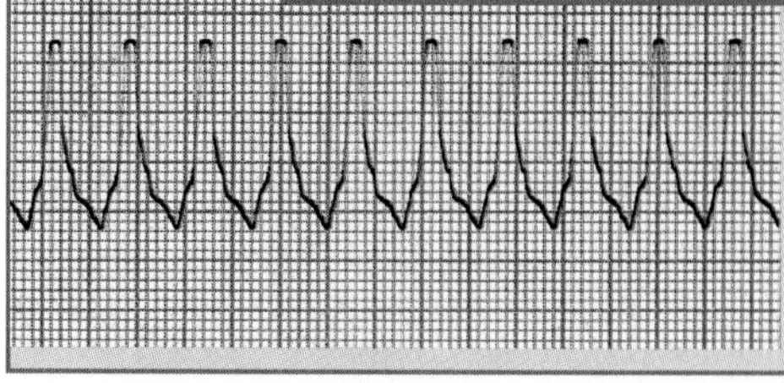

Fig. 8-3: Ventricular tachycardia. Broad complex at 180 beats per minute.

- *Differential diagnosis:* She is responsive to painful stimuli, her blood pressure is 70 mm Hg systolic. This patient has a "too fast" rhythm. She is in VT. You must now review the Tachycardia Algorithm and ask the following critical tachycardia questions:

  - *Is she in unstable condition?* Yes. She is unquestionably in unstable condition, with compromised blood pressure that appears to be affecting her level of consciousness.

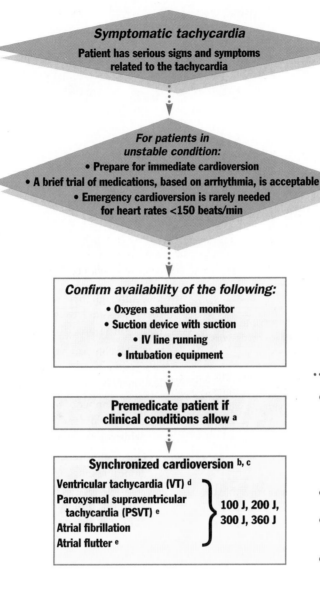

FIGURE 8-4

Electrical Cardioversion Algorithm

(Patient Is Not in Cardiac Arrest)

Symptomatic tachycardia
Patient has serious signs and symptoms related to the tachycardia

For patients in unstable condition:
• Prepare for immediate cardioversion
• A brief trial of medications, based on arrhythmia, is acceptable
• Emergency cardioversion is rarely needed for heart rates <150 beats/min

Confirm availability of the following:
• Oxygen saturation monitor
• Suction device with suction
• IV line running
• Intubation equipment

Premedicate patient if clinical conditions allow [a]

Synchronized cardioversion [b, c]
Ventricular tachycardia (VT) [d]
Paroxysmal supraventricular tachycardia (PSVT) [e]
Atrial fibrillation
Atrial flutter [e]

} 100 J, 200 J, 300 J, 360 J

[a] Many experts recommend anesthesia if service is readily available. Effective pre-medication regimens have included a sedative (e.g., **diazepam, midazolam, barbiturates, etomidate, ketamine, methohexital**) with or without an analgesic agent (e.g., **fentanyl, morphine, meperidine**).

[b] You often need to resynchronize the defibrillator after each cardioversion.

[c] If synchronization is delayed and clinical conditions are critical, perform unsynchronized shocks.

[d] Treat polymorphic VT (irregular form and rate) like ventricular fibrillation: 200 J, 200 to 300 J, 360 J.

[e] PSVT and atrial flutter often respond to lower energy levels (start with 50 J).

Adapted with permission, Journal of the American Medical Association, 1992, Volume 268, *Guidelines for Cardiopulmonary Resuscitation and Emergency Cardiac Care*, p. 2224, copyright © 1992, American Medical Association.

• *Are the symptoms and signs related to her tachycardia?* Yes. The patient has had a change in the ECG rhythm; she has VT with a ventricular rate greater than 150 beats per minute. This is unstable and has led to an associated change in blood pressure and in mentation.

Theoda Evans	Mrs. Evans has unstable tachycardia with significant signs and symptoms related to the tachycardia. The Tachycardia Algorithm directs us to "prepare for immediate cardioversion" and to see Fig. 8-4, (Electrical Cardioversion Algorithm).
CASE 2 Continued	

What are the major issues around the decision to perform electrical cardioversion?

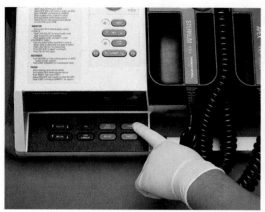

Fig. 8-5: Right, Setup for synchronized cardioversion. Below, Control panel of defibrillator monitor showing sychronized cardioversion.

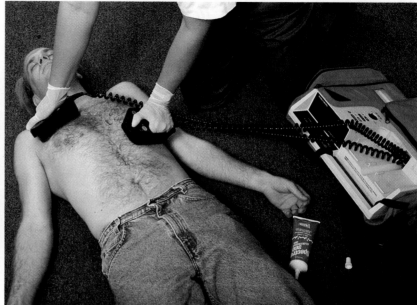

COMMENTS

• In Case 2, electrical cardioversion is the intervention of choice. For the hemodynamic instability use cardioversion before antiarrhythmic therapy.

• Inexperienced ACLS providers sometimes misinterpret the preceding approach and think that antiarrhythmics are prohibited in unstable conditions in patients with a pulse. Delay is the issue. Clinicians should move rapidly to perform cardioversion, especially when it may take several minutes to locate, prepare, and administer medications.

• When patients with symptomatic tachycardia are able to maintain a pulse and measurable blood pressure, you should perform cardioversion in a calm, controlled man-

ner. Although there should be no unnecessary delays, there does not have to be a frantic rush to shock the patient in a hurried, ill-prepared manner.

• Once the clinician has made the decision to perform cardioversion, however, he or she may still administer medications if the medications are immediately available.

   • One member of the resuscitation team can, for example, administer lidocaine (1.0 to 1.5 mg/kg IV push) while another member prepares the defibrillator.

   • Once cardioversion succeeds, you are going to start a lidocaine infusion, so why not go ahead and load with lidocaine before the shock? Sometimes this antiarrhythmic infusion, even for patients in unstable condition, may succeed in pharmacologic cardioversion.

Theoda Evans	You quietly yet firmly announce to the Emergency Department team that Mrs. Evans will need to have electrical cardioversion as quickly as possible. You stand at the foot of the stretcher. A great deal of activity is underway.
CASE 2 Continued	

Can you describe the major care elements that you will immediately review in preparation for the cardioversion? Describe how to perform electrical cardioversion.

COMMENTS

• The Electrical Cardioversion Algorithm (Fig. 8-4) lists several of the care elements that you should review. Check that the following items are available:

   • Oxygen saturation monitor
   • Suction device (ready to operate)
   • IV line (in place)
   • Intubation equipment (ready if needed)

• Since you have followed the Five Quadrads and the Universal Algorithm, the patient is already attached to a monitor and an oxygen source. An IV line is available. (Remember the third quadrad, "Oxygen-IV-Monitor-Fluids," as one word.)

• If time and clinical condition permit, give patients some combination of analgesia plus sedation. If you are in a hospital setting, have qualified personnel provide assistance with airway and anesthesia.

• A variety of premedication regimens are acceptable, including sedatives (diazepam, midazolam, barbiturates, etomidate, ketamine, and methohexital), with or without an analgesic agent (fentanyl, morphine, or meperidine). Some experts recommend near general anesthesia before cardioversions. The clinical goal is to alleviate the pain and suffering of the procedure without causing adverse effects.

Steps for Synchronized Cardioversion

- *See Electrical Cardioversion Algorithm (Fig. 8-4) for sedation options.*
- *Turn on defibrillator.*
- *Attach monitor leads to the patient ("white to right, red to ribs, what's left over to the left shoulder"), and ensure proper display of the patient's rhythm.*
- *Engage the synchronization mode by pressing the "sync" control button.*
- *Look for markers on the R-waves indicating sync mode.*
- *If necessary, adjust R-wave gain until sync markers occur with each QRS complex.*
- *Select appropriate energy level (see Fig. 8-4, Electrical Cardioversion Algorithm).*
- *Position conductor pads on patient (or apply gel to paddles).*
- *Position paddles on patient (sternum-lateral).*
- *Announce to the team members "Charging defibrillator—stand clear!"*
- *Press charge button on lateral paddle (right hand).*
- *When paddle is charged, begin the final "clearing chant." State firmly in a forceful voice the following chant before each shock:*

- *"I am going to shock on 3. One, I'm clear." (Check and make sure you are clear of contact with the patient, the stretcher, and equipment.)*
- *"Two, you're clear." (Make a visual check to ensure that no one near the patient is touching either the patient or stretcher.)*
- *"Three, everybody's clear." (Check all around one more time before pressing the shock buttons. In particular, do not forget about the person providing ventilations. He or she should not have hands on the ventilatory adjuncts, including the endotracheal tube!)*
- *Apply 20 to 25 pounds of pressure on both paddles.*
- *Press and hold both discharge buttons simultaneously. Watch for the muscular contractions that usually occur with the energy transfer of the shock. It may take several seconds before the shock is actually delivered.*
- *Check the monitor. If tachycardia persists, increase the energy level (J) according to the Electrical Cardioversion Algorithm.*
- ***Reset the sync mode after each synchronized cardioversion because most defibrillators default back to unsynchronized mode.*** *This default to unsynchronized mode is to allow an immediate defibrillation if the cardioversion produces VF.*

- The sidebar "Steps for Synchronized Cardioversion" reviews the operation of a defibrillator/monitor in "sync" mode to perform cardioversion. See also Fig. 8-5.
- For ease of recall, the Electrical Cardioversion Algorithm recommends a standard sequence of energy levels for synchronized cardioversions: 100 J, 200 J, 300 J, 360 J.

- Although the proceeding energy sequence is acceptable, many experts recommend a lower initial energy level for atrial flutter and PSVT (50 J) and a higher initial energy level (start with 200 J) for polymorphic VT (irregular morphologic appearance and rate).

Theoda Evans

CASE 2 Continued

While attending to the various preparation steps noted earlier, you ask the lead nurse in the room to administer a small dose of midazolam 2 mg IV followed by meperidine 25 mg IV. She responds, "Don't you think she is a bit too unstable to tolerate those medications?" Mrs. Evans has now decreased in her level of consciousness to a point where she responds to painful stimuli only with weak withdrawal. You concur with the nurse and hold the sedative and analgesic order.

You ask her to administer a loading dose of lidocaine 1.5 mg/kg IV push. This takes about 30 seconds, and you are ready to deliver the cardioversion.

You ask the medical student on rotation in the Emergency Department to take the defibrillator paddles and proceed with the cardioversion. The medical student, under your direction, follows the exact procedure outlined in the box above. The cardioversion shock is delivered at 50 J and converts the patient's rhythm to a sinus rhythm at 85 beats per minute. Her blood pressure quickly rises to 110/90, and she begins to regain a full level of consciousness. You ask the clinic assistant to obtain a bed in the coronary care unit (CCU) and to page the on-call cardiology attending.

What would be the next medication to administer?

Once the patient has had successful cardioversion, you should load them with lidocaine and then follow with a maintenance infusion, as follows:

- *Lidocaine loading dose:* (1.0 to 1.5 mg/kg IV push; repeat at 0.5 to 0.75 mg/kg every 5 to 10 minutes, to a maximum total of 3 mg/kg)
- *Lidocaine maintenance infusion:* 2 to 4 mg/min (30 to 50 µg/kg per minute)

Bruno Torelli

CASE 3

ATRIAL FIBRILLATION

You are on duty in the Emergency Department. Mr. Bruno Torelli, a 71-year-old, well-tanned, vigorous and healthy ex-professional golfer comes into the Emergency Department. He states that he noticed his pulse was 140 when he took his blood pressure with his personal automated blood pressure machine. He is on a diuretic and calcium channel blocker for long-standing hypertension. His wife, however, thinks his rapid heart rate was actually present 3 days ago when she checked his blood pressure. "It was fast, and very irregular."

You follow the routine of the Five Quadrads. You determine the following: blood pressure = 130/90; heart rate = 110 to 140 beats/min; chest, clear; normal chest x-ray and chest exam. You attach nasal oxygen cannula, start an IV, and place him on the monitor. His rhythm strip displays the following (Fig. 8-6):

What is the particular tachycardia rhythm? What are the main features that allow for identification?

How would you treat this rhythm according to the Tachycardia Algorithm?

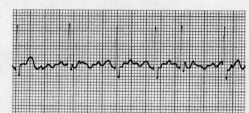

Fig. 8-6: Atrial fibrillation at 110 beats per minute.

- The rhythm in Case 3 is **atrial fibrillation**. The key characteristic of atrial fibrillation follows: *it is irregularly irregular.*

- Look for two features: variation in the RR interval and variation in the amplitude of the R-wave. Atrial fibrillation is the only arrhythmia that produces irregular R-R intervals *plus* different R wave amplitudes. If you see these two features, the rhythm is atrial fibrillation.

- *Do not* try to diagnose atrial fibrillation by the presence of fibrillatory waves on the baseline. *Do not* make the common mistake of thinking the baseline must display these fibrillatory waves. In some studies more than half the patients with atrial fibrillation have flat monitor baselines without fibrillatory waves. Most monitor baselines that look like fibrillatory waves are due to artifacts and bad lead connections.

- The Tachycardia Algorithm does not make specific recommendations on how to approach the patient with atrial fibrillation or atrial flutter. The box states, "Consider" and then lists the following medications to "consider":
  - Diltiazem
  - Beta blockers
  - Verapamil
  - Digoxin
  - Procainamide
  - Quinidine
  - Anticoagulants

- In the 1992 ACLS Guidelines the word "consider" often indicated a situation where the experts could not make up their minds. Even in 1992, however, a consensus was rapidly growing that diltiazem offered the best safety-effectiveness profile for rate control in rapid atrial fibrillation or atrial flutter.

- By 1995 diltiazem appears to be the most widely accepted "drug of choice" for rate control in acute atrial fibrillation or atrial/flutter.

Bruno Torelli

CASE 3 Continued

Mr. Torelli looks as healthy as the active golfer that he is. He is clearly in stable condition, and without serious signs or symptoms. His heart rate, however, is rapid at 110 beats per minute.

Given the completely asymptomatic nature of his atrial fibrillation, what are some of the major treatment considerations to keep in mind?

COMMENTS

- *Do not make this patient in Case 3 worse with your treatments!* Both atrial fibrillation and atrial flutter can be stable and may not need treatment. In the absence of serious signs and symptoms, observation may be the best immediate approach. Remember, treat the patient, not the monitor!

- Although he is not bothered now, you cannot help but think that his 71-year-old heart cannot sustain this rate of 110 to 140 beats per minute much longer without becoming symptomatic. You are thinking that he may need some agent to control his ventricular response.

- He has underlying hypertension (which may be the cause of his atrial fibrillation) and is on a regimen of cardiovascular drugs. Keep this in mind if you choose to treat his atrial fibrillation.

- The history does not answer the question of how long Bruno has been in atrial fibrillation. Mrs. Torelli seems the type to pay close attention to her husband's health, and when she says she thinks he had an irregular, rapid heartbeat 3 days ago, you suspect that she is right.

- You should remember that patients with atrial fibrillation more than several days in duration may have developed intraatrial emboli. The common guideline that many clinicians follow is 48 hours—consider emboli present if the new-onset atrial fibrillation has been present for more than 48 hours.

- There is a risk of arterial embolization (especially cerebral emboli leading to devastating neurologic damage) when cardioversion is performed. Therefore these patients should be given anticoagulation therapy before attempts at pharmacologic and especially, before electrical conversion.

Bruno Torelli

CASE 3 Continued

As you discuss the situation with Mr. and Mrs. Torelli, they begin to ask a series of questions. How would you respond when they ask the following questions?

COMMENTS

WHAT CAUSED THE ATRIAL FIBRILLATION?

- Consider acute conditions that might cause the atrial fibrillation or atrial flutter: AMI, hypoxia, pulmonary embolism, electrolyte abnormalities, toxic effects of medication (particularly digoxin or quinidine), and thyrotoxicosis. One scheme to use as a memory aid for the causes of atrial fibrillation is as follows:

  - Causes from outside the body: Cocaine, caffeine, other recreational drugs, alcohol, or cardiovascular medications like digoxin or quinidine

  - Causes inside the body but outside the heart: Either pulmonary causes such as chronic obstructive pulmonary disease or pulmonary embolism or endocrine causes such as hyperthyroidism

  - Causes inside the heart: Hypertension, coronary artery disease, valvular disease, congenital heart disease, cardiomyopathy, or pericarditis

DOES MR. TORELLI NEED TO BE ADMITTED?

- New-onset atrial fibrillation can indicate a silent ischemic event, particularly in the elderly. Obtain a 12-lead ECG and meticulously question Bruno about any symptoms that might indicate an AMI. Remember that a normal ECG does not eliminate the possibility of an AMI.

- Many, although not all, clinicians would admit a patient like Bruno simply to rule out an AMI with serial enzyme studies and ECGs. His need for anticoagulation therapy would also justify admission.

DO YOU NEED TO TREAT MR. TORELLI'S RAPID HEART RATE?

- You should be concerned at the rapid ventricular response to the atrial fibrillation. On closer questioning, you learn that Mr. Torelli does get short of breath when exerting himself, such as when climbing quickly in and out of his golf cart with his golf clubs. This suggests that the 140-beats-per-minute rate is close to cardiac decompensation and that when he exercises and increases his rate even more, he cannot tolerate it. Without better rate control he may suddenly have decompensation with angina, pulmonary edema, or an AMI.

- Since he is already receiving a calcium channel blocker for his hypertension, he demonstrates that he can tolerate this class of agents. Administer **diltiazem** IV to slow the ventricular response, since it is now considered to have the best effectiveness with the least amount of side effects.

- Examine the ECG carefully for the indicators of Wolff-Parkinson-White (WPW) syndrome. You should not give calcium channel blockers such as diltiazem and verapamil to patients with WPW syndrome plus rapid atrial fibrillation.

- Spontaneous conversion to normal sinus rhythm often occurs once medications have achieved rate control. If not, specific therapy can be given to produce pharmacologic conversion.

SHOULD HE ALSO RECEIVE TREATMENT TO CONVERT HIS ATRIAL FIBRILLATION TO NORMAL SINUS RHYTHM?

- Yes. Patients do better when atrial fibrillation is converted to normal sinus rhythms. Their hearts function more effectively, and problems of stroke and pulmonary emboli associated with clots breaking loose from their dysfunctional atria are avoided.

- Patients should receive the following:
  - First, an agent for rate control
  - Second, anticoagulation therapy with heparin
  - Third, an agent for pharmacologic cardioversion
- In summary, you face the following major treatment issues with atrial fibrillation:

  (1) *Electricity.* Is the ventricular response so rapid that the patient is deteriorating and needs immediate electrical cardioversion?

  (2) *Rate control.* In less urgent situations you can slow a rapid ventricular response with pharmacologic means: calcium channel blockers such as diltiazem and verapamil or beta blockers such as esmolol, metoprolol, atenolol, and propranolol are recommended. Most experts now favor **diltiazem** as the agent of first choice.

  ONE CAUTION TO REMEMBER: IV propranolol should not be given soon after IV verapamil. You can cause profound bradycardia and even asystole when these two agents are given close together (less than 30 minutes apart). You should learn and become comfortable with a specific therapeutic sequence for atrial fibrillation and atrial flutter.

  (3) *Pharmacologic cardioversion.* For pharmacologic conversion, most experience has accumulated with **procainamide** and **quinidine.** Experts have questioned the role of digoxin for urgent treatment of atrial fibrillation and flutter, and it has fallen into disfavor, especially with the success of the calcium channel blockers and the beta blockers.

  (4) *Immediate anticoagulation.* Always worry about the blood clots that form in the walls of fibrillating atria. Within 48 hours of the onset of atrial fibrillation, potentially lethal clots have formed in many patients. Conversion to normal sinus rhythm, either electrical or pharmacologic, can dislodge these clots into the pulmonary and cerebral vessels. There the clots can cause pulmonary infarction and disabling, even fatal strokes. Start **heparin** for atrial fibrillation in patients to whom you plan to give cardioversion to normal sinus rhythm. The patients should be given effective anticoagulation therapy for 24 to 48 hours before efforts are started to achieve pharmacologic cardioversion. Heparin doses are as follows:
  - Bolus IV: give 80 international units (IU)/kg.
  - Continue 18 IU/kg per hour.
  - Then adjust to maintain activated partial thromboplastin time: 1.5 to 2 times the control values.

  (5) *Long-term anticoagulation.* Patients who remain in atrial fibrillation need anticoagulation therapy to prevent the consequences of emboli and stroke. These include patients who are not candidates for electrical cardioversion or who fail to have conversion pharmacologically, or patients who keep reverting to atrial fibrillation after successful cardioversion.

BOX 8-1

Key Points
When Dealing With
Atrial Fibrillation and Atrial Flutter

- *Think of treatable conditions that might be causing the fibrillation or flutter.*
- *Atrial fibrillation and atrial flutter are often stable rhythms and do not need treatment. Atrial flutter, however, is less stable than atrial fibrillation.*
- *Admit most patients with new-onset atrial fibrillation or atrial flutter.*
- *Use electrical cardioversion if the patient displays serious signs and symptoms.*
- *The first priority of treatment should be to slow the ventricular response with IV diltiazem. You can also use verapamil or beta blockers. This rate slowing alone will often result in conversion to normal sinus rhythm.*
- *After the immediate efforts to slow the ventricular*
*response, use **procainamide** or **quinidine** to convert the heart to normal sinus rhythm.*
- *Initiate anticoagulation therapy before cardioversion if the atrial fibrillation has been present for more than 24 to 48 hours.*
- *Maintain long-term anticoagulation for patients who remain in atrial fibrillation.*
- *Think of treatable conditions that might be causing the arrhythmia.*
- *Admit most patients with new-onset atrial flutter you do not suceed in cardioverting.*
- *Atrial flutter is likely to respond to vagal maneuvers, at least in terms of slowing the ventricular response.*
- *Atrial flutter is noticed soon after onset by most patients. They seek care quickly, so intraatrial emboli and the need for anticoagulation are less often concerns.*
- *Atrial flutter commonly requires less energy for electrical conversion; therefore start with 50 J for the first synchronized shock.*

Bruno Torelli

CASE 3 Continued

IN STABLE ATRIAL FLUTTER
To make some additional clinical points, consider the management of Mr. Torelli if he presented himself in exactly the same manner as described earlier, but with the rhythm noted in Fig. 8-7.
What is this rhythm? What are the differences between the management of this rhythm and atrial fibrillation?

COMMENTS

• The rhythm is atrial flutter. Atrial flutter is less stable than atrial fibrillation and often requires even more careful clinical attention. In particular, a rapid ventricular response indicates a potentially unstable clinical situation.

• You should heighten your sense of urgency if the tachycardia can lead to deleterious effects such as precipitating angina in patients with ischemic heart disease. This is a distinct possibility in an older person like Mr. Torelli, even though his condition appears quite stable.

• Unlike in atrial fibrillation, vagal maneuvers may serve a diagnostic purpose in atrial flutter. Carotid

sinus massage may render the flutter waves more apparent and thus confirm the diagnosis. Case 4 (PSVT) presents several additional cautions and comments about carotid sinus massage and vagal maneuvers.

Atrial Flutter

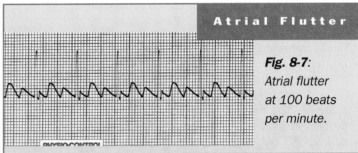

Fig. 8-7: Atrial flutter at 100 beats per minute.

Nigel Hawthorne

CASE 4

PSVT
You are reviewing x-rays near the Emergency Department write-up area. The 52-year-old head of the dental clinic, Dr. Nigel Hawthorne, walks up beside you and says, "Excuse me, but I think I'm having a bit of a tachycardia."

He reports that a few minutes ago in the cafeteria he was drinking his second double-espresso coffee when suddenly he became aware that his heart was beating rapidly. He walked calmly to the Emergency Department without shortness of breath or chest pain. You ask him to recline on a nearby stretcher, signaling the head nurse to come help.

Vital signs are as follows: Temperature = 37°C; blood pressure = 135/85; heart rate = 140 beats/min; respirations = 12 breaths/min. Lungs are clear; cardiac examination results are normal. He takes no medications other than a daily aspirin and the espressos. The 12-lead ECG reveals no acute changes other than the rhythm strip to the right (Fig. 8-8).

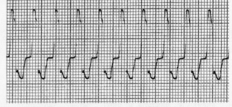

Fig. 8-8: Paroxysmal supraventricular tachycardia.

What is this rhythm, and what is the general treatment sequence to follow?

COMMENTS

• The Tachycardia Algorithm displays the general treatment sequence for this rhythm which is **PSVT.**

• General treatment sequence is as follows:
  • Vagal maneuvers
  • **Adenosine** 6 mg
  • **Adenosine** 12 mg (may repeat once in 1 to 2 minutes)
  • **Verapamil** 2.5 to 5 mg (if complex width is narrow and blood pressure is normal)
  • **Verapamil** 5 to 10 mg

• Of the vagal maneuvers, remember that carotid sinus pressure is contraindicated in patients with carotid bruits,

and avoid ice-water immersion in patients with ischemic heart disease.

• The following are the major things to remember about patients with PSVT:
  • Always be alert for clinical instability or deterioration.
  • Try vagal maneuvers first.
  • Adenosine is the drug of choice for PSVT that is stable.
  • Make sure you know how to use adenosine correctly.
  • *Never* use verapamil if the supraventricular complex is wide.
  • *Never* use verapamil if the blood pressure is low or unstable.

Nigel Hawthorne	Dr. Hawthorne's condition is stable, and immediate cardioversion is not necessary. Start oxygen, IV, and a monitor. Obtain a 12-lead ECG while taking a history. Perform a problem-oriented physical examination. Therapy for PSVT aims to interrupt a cycle of impulses that goes from above the ventricles, to ventricles, back to the atrioventricular (AV) node.
CASE 4 Continued	

from above the ventricles, to ventricles, back to the atrioventricular (AV) node. Describe in detail the sequence of interventions you will now use to treat Dr. Hawthorne.

COMMENTS

Treat patients with stable PSVT in the following manner.

VAGAL MANEUVERS

- Vagal maneuvers increase parasympathetic tone and slow conduction through the AV node. Patients with recurrent PSVT have usually tried many vagal maneuvers and will know already which ones work. Ask the patient with recurrent PSVT what he or she has found that worked in the past. There are many vagal maneuvers in the arsenal against PSVT and atrial flutter. Emergency care physicians seem to be attracted to the bizarre and have filled the letters-to-the-editor sections of many emergency care journals with creative efforts to discover vagal sensors on virtually all body parts and orifices, including the following:

  - Carotid sinus massage
  - Forced breath-holding
  - Facial immersion in ice water
  - Coughing
  - Nasogastric tube placement
  - Gag reflex stimulation by tongue blades, fingers, and oral ipecac
  - Eyeball pressure
  - Deep-knee squatting
  - MAST garments
  - Trendelenburg's position
  - Foley catheter insertion
  - Circumferential digital sweep of the anus
  - Catapulsion from an aircraft carrier

- One of the more effective and socially acceptable of these techniques is simple forced breath-holding. Rather than supply the time-honored instruction, "Bear down hard like you are trying to push out a big, hard stool," put your hand firmly on the patient's abdomen and ask the patient to try and push your hand away with the abdominal muscles while holding his or her breath.

- Perform carotid sinus massage carefully, with ECG monitoring, and avoid its use in older patients. Start an IV line, and have atropine sulfate and lidocaine available for immediate use. Several problems can occur in association with carotid sinus massage, including cerebral emboli, stroke (embolic and occlusive), syncope, sinus arrest, asystole, increased degree of AV block, and paradoxic tachyarrhythmias in digoxin-toxic states.

- *Technique:* Turn the patient's head to the left. Perform a firm massage of the carotid sinus for 5 to 10 seconds. Repeat several times after brief pauses. If there is no change, massage the left carotid bifurcation near the angle of the jaw. *Never* attempt simultaneous, bilateral massage.

ADENOSINE VERSUS VERAPAMIL

- Both adenosine and verapamil are highly effective in converting PSVT to normal sinus rhythm. Clinical studies have confirmed that adenosine is as effective as verapamil in initial conversion of PSVT. Adenosine does not produce hypotension to the level that verapamil does, and it has a short half-life. Most clinicians consider adenosine the safer agent. Even patients later identified as having VT have remained in stable condition when given adenosine.

- **Adenosine.** Adenosine is the first drug to use for hemodynamically stable PSVT. Think in terms of a sequence of agents for persistent PSVT: adenosine-adenosine, then verapamil-verapamil (if the complex remains narrow and the blood pressure has not dropped). You must, however, know how to administer adenosine. Success depends on proper administration, as follows:

  - Make sure you have a good IV line with a large-gauge needle. (Antecubital vein is preferred.)
  - Start supplemental oxygen through nasal prongs.
  - Have lidocaine, atropine, and a monitor/defibrillator immediately available.
  - Verify that defibrillator gel or pads are present.
  - Place the patient flat in bed, preferably in slight reverse Trendelenburg's position.
  - Sit down next to the patient. Speak to the patient directly; say that he or she may feel funny, maybe frightened, and may feel some brief chest pain for a few seconds. This pain is similar to ischemic chest pain.
  - Reassure the patient that you are going to be right with him or her.
  - Start the strip chart recorder on the monitor.
  - Administer adenosine 6 mg by *rapid* (1 to 3 seconds) IV push.
  - Run the IV line wide open after the push.
  - There should be some change in the rhythm in 10 to 15 seconds; most conversions occur in less than 30 seconds.

- If necessary, after 1 to 2 minutes a 12-mg dose should be administered in the same rapid manner.
- If necessary, in 1 to 2 minutes another 12-mg dose can be administered.

- When conversion occurs, the patient's heart may display several seconds of asystole followed by resumption of normal sinus rhythm. This can be up to 10 to 15 seconds in duration and result in presyncopal symptoms (which is why the reverse Trendelenburg's position helps).
- Be ready to move to verapamil if the complex remains narrow and the blood pressure remains acceptable.

VERAPAMIL

- The tachycardia algorithm directs you to always ask the following questions before using verapamil for persistent PSVT after adenosine:
  - First, is the complex still narrow?
  - Second, is the blood pressure still reasonably normal? If the answer to either of these questions is "no," do not use verapamil.
- Remember the following additional points about using verapamil:
  - Administer verapamil more slowly than adenosine.
  - Use 2.5 to 5 mg IV given over 2 minutes.
  - Give smaller amounts (2 to 4 mg) over longer periods of time (3 to 4 minutes) for the elderly or when the blood pressure is in the lower range of normal.
  - A second dose of 5 to 10 mg can be given in 15 to 30 minutes if the PSVT persists or recurs and if the blood pressure remains acceptable.
  - Verapamil often produces a significant decrease in blood pressure that can be reversed with calcium chloride, 0.5 to 1.0 given slowly IV.

- Many clinicians pretreat patients with an IV infusion of calcium chloride over 5 to 10 minutes before administration of verapamil. You can do this to help patients with questionable hemodynamic suitability for verapamil.
- If hemodynamic compromise develops and the PSVT continues, perform cardioversion immediately.

- There are several clinical situations where you should *not* use verapamil, or at least use it with extreme caution. These include the following:
  - Patients with low blood pressure
  - Patients with wide-complex tachycardias
  - Patients who have recently been given IV beta blockers
  - Patients who take oral beta blockers
  - Patients with WPW syndrome plus atrial fibrillation
  - Patients with sick sinus syndrome
  - Patients with AV block without a pacemaker

AFTER ADENOSINE AND VERAPAMIL

- If the patient does not respond to vagal maneuvers, two or three doses of adenosine, and two or three doses of verapamil, consider any of the following:
  - Diltiazem
  - Digoxin
  - Beta blockers
  - Sedation and rest
  - Overdrive pacing
  - Elective cardioversion (see Tachycardia Algorithm)
- Patients who remain in PSVT after this point must be admitted, or consultation with cardiology is required.

Dr. Orville Stanford
CASE 5

A 64-year-old retired college professor presents himself to the Emergency Department with the chief complaint of palpitations and rapid heartbeat of 24 hours' duration. Dr. Orville Stanford has been cruising the San Juan Islands in his 36-foot sailboat and is active and vigorous, without complaints of chest pain, shortness of breath, or fatigue.

A young graduate student accompanies him, and she confirms that "he is in better shape than most younger men." He has a normal physical examination with heart rate of 140 beats/min, blood pressure of 130/95, and respirations of 12 breaths/min. The monitor shows the tracing to the right (Fig. 8-9).

What is the most important initial question to ask about people in tachycardia? What is the rhythm on this tracing?

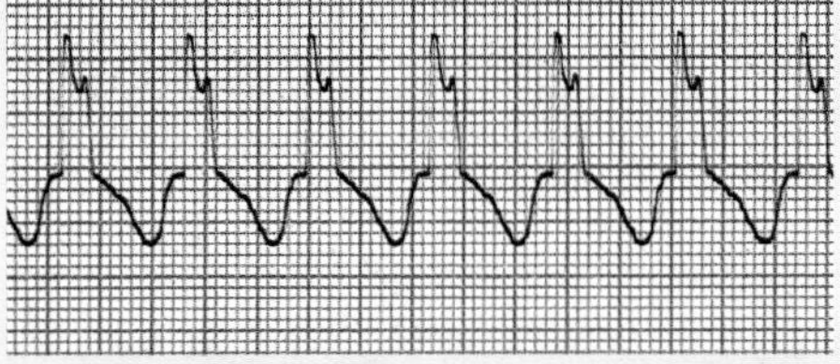

Fig. 8-9: Wide-complex tachycardia of uncertain type.

COMMENTS

- The Tachycardia Algorithm directs us to ask one basic question for all tachycardias (and bradycardias): Is the tachycardia "too fast?" (or "too slow?" in the case of bradycardias).

- This question translates into the question, "stable or unstable, with serious signs and symptoms?" If the answer is "unstable," you will need to move at once to cardioversion.

- Dr. Stanford, however, is unquestionably in stable condition and does not need immediate cardioversion.

- His tachycardia is wide-complex; it is not clear on initial analysis whether it is VT or some other type of **wide-complex tachycardia**. Your clinical challenge now is to try and decide what type of wide-complex tachycardia he has and then, which medications to use to achieve safe conversion.

Dr. Orville Stanford

CASE 5 Continued

You decide that Dr. Stanford's tachycardia is stable and that immediate cardioversion is not indicated.

Since stable VT has the potential to become unstable and to produce clinical deterioration, how would you decide whether this wide-complex tachycardia of uncertain origin is VT?

COMMENTS

- Wide-complex tachycardias of "uncertain" origin can be of the following types:

  - The patient has ventricular tachycardia.

  - Supraventricular tachycardia with aberrancy: This means that a functional bundle branch block kicks in, usually at higher rates (rate-related).

  - The patient has a preexistent bundle branch block, so wide complexes occur even in sinus rhythm.

  - The patient has WPW syndrome with conduction from the atrium to the ventricle that utilizes the accessory pathway.

- Some clinicians have a misconception that a patient in VT will always appear unstable and distressed and display a more rapid heart rate or a lower blood pressure than normal. This is a mistake.

- Patients with VT can be just as stable and comfortable as our professor. Do not think that VT is ruled out just because the patient appears stable. Do **not** use *clinical* criteria to distinguish between PSVT with aberrant conduction and VT.

- Many textbooks and articles present lengthy, detailed guidelines to help distinguish between VT and supraventricular tachycardias with aberrancy. *The prudent clinician, faced with urgent care of an ill patient, should ignore these detailed criteria for ECG analysis and attend to the patient.* As one aphorism puts it, "Beware the person bearing calipers—they may pay more attention to the rhythm strip than to the patient."

- A useful rule to ensure safety: you should **not** use *electrocardiographic* criteria to distinguish between aberrant conduction and VT. Many clinicians, however, become enamored of esoteric criteria on the ECG to help distinguish VT from aberrancy. Their detailed distinctions are too cryptic and unreliable to be useful in the emergency setting, and they would not change the recommended therapy (which is, *do NOT use verapamil*).

Dr. Orville Stanford

CASE 5 Continued

You decide to continue to consider Dr. Stanford's tachycardia as "uncertain" regarding supraventricular tachycardia versus VT. Since he remains in quite stable condition on clinical examination, you have time to consider a pharmacologic approach.

What are the medications recommended for wide-complex tachycardia, and what are the major points to consider about these medications?

COMMENTS

- The Tachycardia Algorithm recommends the following treatment sequence for wide-complex PSVT or tachycardias of uncertain origin:

  - Lidocaine 1 to 1.5 mg/kg IV
  - Lidocaine 0.5 to 0.75 mg/kg IV
  - Adenosine 6 mg IV
  - Adenosine 12 mg (repeat in 1 to 2 minutes if needed)
  - Procainamide 20 to 30 mg/min

- Notice an important point about the construction of the Tachycardia Algorithm: You cannot get to a recommendation for **verapamil** for wide-complex tachycardias of uncertain type for VT.

  - Administration of **verapamil** to a patient with VT can be a **lethal error.** Patients in VT who are in stable condition usually have achieved that "stability" by maximum myocardial contactility and vasoconstriction. Verapamil, as a vasodilator, can cause decompensation and hemodynamic collapse.

- In addition, verapamil can accelerate the heart rate even further and decrease the blood pressure in all patients, but especially in patients with WPW syndrome. *Do not give verapamil to patients with a wide-complex tachycardia unless the tachycardia is known with certainty to be supraventricular in origin.*

- An "always" and a "never" follow:
  - *Always* treat wide-complex tachycardias of uncertain type as if the rhythm is VT.
  - *Never* treat wide-complex tachycardias with verapamil.

- The Tachycardia Algorithm recommends, first, two loading doses of **lidocaine** as the agent to use for all wide-complex tachycardias *not known with certainty to be supraventricular in origin.* (See special memory aid box.)

- Follow with **adenosine** in two rapid administrations if the wide-complex tachycardia persists. Note that:
  - **Adenosine** has also been effective as a diagnostic antiarrhythmic for uncertain wide-complex tachycardias.
  - **Adenosine** produces little harm in patients who have VT and will often "convert" patients with wide-QRS-complex tachycardia.

- NOTE: **Procainamide** is acceptable to use for people with VT, and it is certainly acceptable for wide-complex tachycardias of uncertain type. However, **procainamide** takes longer to administer and to take effect, and has a greater potential for lowering the blood pressure, than does adenosine.

- Note how the Tachycardia Algorithm has been carefully constructed to restrict the use of **verapamil** to only

---

SPECIAL MEMORY AID

Treatment of PSVT, VT, and Wide-complex Tachycardias

Here is an easy way to remember the treatments for paroxysmal supraventricular tachycardia (PSVT), wide-complex tachycardias of uncertain type, and ventricular tachycardia (VT):

- *VT:* Lidocaine-lidocaine-**procainamide**-bretylium
- *PSVT:* **Vagal**-adenosine-adenosine-**verapamil**-verapamil
- *Wide-complex tachycardia:* Since you are not sure whether to treat the condition like VT or like PSVT, you waffle between the two choices and take the first two drugs from VT and second two from PSVT, as follows: Lidocaine-lidocaine-adenosine-adenosine.

---

patients with narrow-complex PSVT plus normal or elevated blood pressures. Verapamil can convert wide-complex tachycardias that are supraventricular in origin. You can use verapamil if the blood pressure is normal or elevated and if the wide-complex tachycardia is known with certainty to be PSVT. Some experts, however, argue that you can confirm this diagnosis only by means of electrophysiologic stimulation testing.

- For patients with tachycardia, lidocaine and procainamide are Class I agents (acceptable and definitely effective); adenosine is a Class IIa agent (acceptable and probably effective); and verapamil is a Class III agent (possibly or probably harmful).

Rusty Kincaid

CASE 6

You are making rounds on Saturday morning in the CCU. A former junior-college football coach, Rusty "No-Neck" Kincaid, was admitted last night with complaints of chest pain. The nurse reports that his enzyme levels were mildly elevated at 12 hours and that he displayed 1 to 8 PVCs/min during the evening.

Coach Kincaid tries to persuade you to let him go home before the "big game" kickoff at noon. During this increasingly intense conversation, you notice the coach go into the rhythm shown in Fig. 8-10.

You quickly glance at Coach, who is detailing the importance of the afternoon game. He has not missed a beat and continues to speak with energy and passion. You check his heart rate, which is 160 beats/min and vigorous, and the nurse checks a blood pressure at 140/95. "Coach, are you feeling OK?" you ask. "Not unless you get me out of this damn den of wimpy nerds!" You decide quickly that the rhythm is probably VT and that Coach's obvious mental instability is chronic and not due to altered cardiopulmonary function.

What is the first thing you would do? What are the general approaches to the treatment of patients with this arrhythmia?

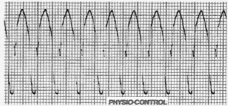

Fig. 8-10: Ventricular tachycardia

- The rhythm in Case 6 is VT. The first step is to confirm that Coach Kincaid is awake and alert, that his condition is stable without serious signs or symptoms.

- Verify that a defibrillator/monitor is in the room and that it is a brand and model that you know well. He is certainly at risk for clinical deterioration.

VENTRICULAR TACHYCARDIA (STABLE)

- General treatment sequence is as follows:
  - **Lidocaine** 1 to 1.5 mg/kg IV
  - **Lidocaine** 0.5 to 0.75 mg/kg IV
  - **Procainamide** 20 to 30 mg/min
  - **Bretylium** 5 to 10 mg/kg

- Remember, from the clinical perspective, that in patients with VT the condition can present itself in one of three ways:
  - Full cardiac arrest
  - Hemodynamic instability (but not full cardiac arrest)
  - Clinical stability

FULL CARDIAC ARREST

- Always remember that persistent VT without a pulse, with signs of a full cardiac arrest, must be treated like VF. (See the Universal Algorithm and the VF/VT Algorithm for full cardiac arrest in Chapter 4.) To review, the treatment sequence is as follows:
  - Three unsynchronized, stacked **shocks** (200 J, 300 J, and 360 J)
  - Intubation and starting an IV line
  - Epinephrine-**shock** (every 3 to 5 minutes)
  - Lidocaine-**shock** (twice)
  - Bretylium-**shock** (twice)
  - Procainamide-**shock**
  - Magnesium, sodium bicarbonate per special situations

VENTRICULAR TACHYCARDIA WITH HEMODYNAMIC INSTABILITY (NOT FULL CARDIAC ARREST)

- If your patient with VT has low blood pressure, shortness of breath, chest pain, altered consciousness, or pulmonary edema, prepare for **immediate cardioversion,** as discussed earlier.

VENTRICULAR TACHYCARDIA WITH CLINICAL STABILITY

- Use **lidocaine** as the drug of choice in VT with clinical stability.

- Follow with **procainamide** as necessary.

Rusty Kincaid

CASE 6 Continued

Since Coach Kincaid is in clinically stable condition, you have time to provide medications to help convert the VT.

What are the three major medications used in the pharmacologic treatment of VT? And what are the major points to remember about them?

Major points to remember about the three medications used to treat stable VT (if unstable, use electricity!) are listed here.

LIDOCAINE

- Use lidocaine as the first-line agent for stable VT (and for any wide-complex tachycardia of uncertain origin).

- Lidocaine requires an initial loading dose of 1 to 1.5 mg/kg; when necessary, a second dose of 0.5 to 0.75 mg/kg can be administered 5 to 10 minutes later. The total loading dose is 3 mg/kg. If lidocaine appears to convert the arrhythmia, continue a lidocaine drip of 2 to 4 mg/min.

- There are many approaches for lidocaine administration. All the preceding approaches are acceptable and effective (Class IIA).

- Be aware, though, that you must balance carefully between two extremes: ineffective medication levels and toxic effects.

PROCAINAMIDE

- Use procainamide as the second-line agent for stable VT.

- Procainamide is *not given* as a bolus but as a steady IV infusion.

- The Tachycardia Algorithm recommends an infusion rate of procainamide at 20 to 30 mg/min, to a total dose of 17 mg/kg. This odd, and difficult-to-remember dose of 17 mg/kg appears, on pharmacologic study, to be the best loading dose. This will result in more accurate dosing than the former recommendation of "a total loading dose of 1000 mg" given without reference to the patient's size.

- If procainamide suppresses the VT, start a continuous infusion at 2 to 4 mg/min to maintain the suppression.

- The endpoints of procainamide therapy are as follows:
  - Hypotension
  - More than 50% widening of the QRS complex
  - A maximum dose of 17 mg/kg
  - Suppression of the arrhythmia

BRETYLIUM

- Use bretylium as the third-line agent for the treatment of sustained VT.

- Bretylium displays more effectiveness as an antifibrillatory agent than as an antiarrhythmic agent for tachycardias.

- Administer bretylium 5 mg/kg, not as a bolus as with VF, but in 50 mL normal saline and infused over 8 to 10 minutes.

- If bretylium appears to convert the arrhythmia, complete the loading dose (5 mg/kg) and begin a continuous infusion at a rate of 1 to 2 mg/min. The maximum 24-hour total dose should be 30 mg/kg.

Rusty Kincaid

CASE 6 Continued

You administered lidocaine 1.0 mg/kg IV push to Coach. The rhythm did not convert. With a second 0.5- to 1.0-mg/kg dose of lidocaine given 5 minutes later, however, you did achieve conversion to a normal sinus rhythm at 85 beats per minute. You followed this with a third bolus to achieve a full loading dose of 3.0 mg/kg and then started an infusion of 4 mg/min for approximately 6 hours.

Coach began to experience paresthesias in his hands and feet and numbness around his mouth. You decide to check a serum lidocaine level and to stop the infusion as well. The paresthesias disappeared in 30 minutes, and there was a continuously stable rhythm.

Coach's condition remained stable during his hospital stay except for a brief episode of VT during his cardiac catheterization. He had a stenosis of his left anterior descending coronary artery that was treated with an atherectomy, and he was discharged pain free and feeling good.

KEY POINTS

SUMMARY

We must emphasize again that the major point to remember about evaluating patients with tachycardias is that you must evaluate the patient. The clinical condition determines most of the therapeutic approach. A focus on rhythm analysis to the exclusion of patient evaluation will not serve the best interests of the patient.

You determine the clinical condition by first following the Five Quadrads approach:

- The Primary-Secondary Survey will lead you to the answer of the first and most critical tachycardia question: *Is this patient's condition unstable with serious signs and symptoms?*

- A "yes" answer moves you immediately to electrical cardioversion, which should be performed efficiently, effectively, and painlessly.

- A "no" answer lead you to a consideration of the four major classes of tachycardia: atrial fibrillation or atrial flutter, PSVT, wide-complex tachycardias of unknown type, and VT.

- The four classifications, while an oversimplification, will guide you to consider the major therapeutic interventions to use *in the patient with stable tachycardia.*

As a final comment, we cannot emphasize enough that the most critically ill tachycardia patients will require the emergency intervention of electrical cardioversion or electrical defibrillation. Chapters 3 and 4 have stressed the need to learn about and know your defibrillator with intimate familiarity. This same advice holds true for tachycardia patients. Know your defibrillator well, and you will serve your patients well.

Acute Myocardial Infarction

O V E R V I E W

The Acute Myocardial Infarction (AMI) cases instruct ACLS providers to take a systematic approach to patients with possible acute myocardial infarction. The AMI cases teach a greater awareness of timely action and interventions within the following areas:

- *Community*

- *EMS system*

- *Emergency Department (ED)*

- *Hospital*

This chapter does not, however, review all the information necessary to manage people with possible AMI. These cases do cover the most critical concepts, actions, skills, rhythms, and medications needed to begin understanding this complex topic and to start participating effectively in the care of such patients.

MAJOR CONCEPTS TO MASTER

- **Learn the AMI Algorithm. Pay particular attention to the issues related to the community, the EMS system, and the ED. These are the settings where ACLS providers must make many critical decisions.**

- **Learn the major signs and symptoms of an AMI.**

- **For thrombolytic therapy, the key points to learn, as follows, are when to give it and when not to give it:**

  - **Clinical *indications* for thrombolytic therapy**

  - **Absolute contraindications**

  - **Relative contraindications**

- **There are 10 medications and interventions to consider in the initial management of the AMI patient. You will not use all of the medications on each patient. Learn the "Why?" "When?" "How?" and "Watch Out!" for each one.**

- **Learn the ECG criteria for the "Triple Is" approach: Ischemia, Injury, and Infarction.**

- **Learn the ECG criteria for thrombolytic therapy (injury).**

- **Learn to recognize and manage the most frequent AMI complications—arrhythmias, hypotension, and hypertension.**

Critical actions

While managing the AMI cases you should always do the following:

- Recognize that the best way to decrease morbidity and mortality is for *patients* to recognize early the signs and symptoms of AMI and to seek care in a timely fashion.

- Learn how suspected AMI patients are managed in your community's EMS system, even if you work in the ED or the in-hospital setting. Community management by EMS systems may include the following:

  - Procedures for rapid transportation of patients to ED

  - Prehospital screening of patients to receive thrombolytic therapy

  - Prehospital 12-lead ECGs

  - Prehospital protocols for administration of thrombolytics

- Know how possible AMI patients are managed in your ED, especially if that is the major setting for your work; understand in particular how the ED is informed of a possible AMI patient.

- Recognize the major features of effective ED management of possible AMI patients. These are as follows:

  - A "door-to-drug" team approach is used that emphasizes rapid triage of all patients with chest pain.

  - *Standing orders* are in place for nurses to start Oxygen/IV/Monitor, as well as vital signs, oxygen saturation, and at times, nitroglycerin, aspirin, and pain relief with narcotics, and to order a 12-lead ECG.

  - A 12-lead ECG machine is in the department, and a specific person is trained and designated to operate the device. The ECG technician should not have to travel from elsewhere to get to the ED or go outside the ED to get the ECG machine.

  - Identified in advance is the physician who must decide to give thrombolytic therapy (ED physician, cardiologist, or other); this person must determine whether there are clinical indications for thrombolytic therapy, plus the *absence* of the absolute and the relative contraindications for thrombolytic therapy. Hospital clinical policy should support this person, who will usually be the ED attending as the decision maker.

- Develop protocols for chest x-rays, blood studies, and indicated consults, as well as for obtaining a brief, targeted history and physical examination.

Skills to learn

- Learn the ECG criteria for the "Triple I's"—Ischemia, Injury, Infarction.

- Learn the ECG criteria for thrombolytic therapy (injury).

Rhythms to learn

The most common arrhythmias that may occur with AMI and their initial treatment are the following:

- Normal sinus rhythm, sinus bradycardia, and sinus tachycardia

- Atrioventricular (AV) blocks: first-degree, second-degree (types I and II), and third-degree blocks

- Multiple premature atrial complexes (PACs), atrial tachycardia, atrial tachycardia with block, and atrial flutter with various degrees of block

- Premature ventricular complexes (PVCs) (Learn whether to provide suppression treatment for ventricular ectopy.)

- Ventricular fibrillation (VF) and ventricular tachycardia (VT)

Medications (and one intervention) to learn

- Morphine
- Oxygen
- Nitroglycerin
- Aspirin
- Thrombolytic agents
- Heparin
- Magnesium

- Beta blockers
- Lidocaine
- Magnesium sulfate
- Coronary angioplasty (percutaneous transluminal coronary angioplasty [PTCA])

Avery Lancaster

CASE 1

A 55-year-old attorney named Avery Lancaster rushes about his home in the early morning. He has just gulped two cups of coffee between smoking two cigarettes when a severe cramp under his sternum makes him pause. He becomes aware that he is short of breath and that his left arm feels like the circulation has been cut off.

What are the major risk factors for an AMI that Mr. Lancaster displays?

RISK FACTORS

- He bears the cardiovascular misfortunes of being middle-aged, North American, and male.

- In addition, he is addicted to cigarettes.

- The aggressive "type A" person, always under a sense of time pressure, may be at risk for acute cardiac events, although few data support this widely held stereotype.

- The caffeine in the coffee has acquired a negative reputation, but no well-designed studies have demonstrated an independent association between coffee consumption, caffeine, and coronary artery disease.

- Some studies have shown associations between cardiac events and early morning hours.

GENDER

- Cardiovascular disease remains the leading cause of death in both women and men in the United States. Most textbook descriptions of AMI and coronary artery disease describe men, which is understandable, since 70% to 80% of AMI patients are men.

- New research suggests that women experience an AMI differently from men. Women experience their AMIs in ways that are subtly different—they have less "crushing" chest pain, and they have less precise pain localizations, with symptoms frequently felt in the back, between the shoulder blades, and in the upper abdomen.

- Chest pain in women turns out to be an AMI less often than in men. However, the workup and evaluation must be gender blind. Never discount the possibility of an AMI just because the patient is a woman (particularly a young woman).

Avery Lancaster

CASE 1 Continued

Mr. Lancaster sits down in the living room. His chest pain seems to worsen, and the ache in his arm throbs steadily. His wife notices how pale he looks and the large drops of sweat on his face. His breaths come in long, deep sighs. Despite his wife's immediate concerns and questions, he does not admit to any unusual symptoms, stating, "Just a little indigestion, Honey. I'll be all right in a minute."
What do you think is going on now?

THE EARLY SYMPTOMS

Cardiologists would love to know exactly what events are taking place in Mr. Lancaster's coronary arteries at this point. He clearly has compromised flow to a major coronary artery. The following questions arise:

- Has the atheromatous plaque ruptured and the associated thrombus enlarged to completely occlude the artery?

- Is the thrombus getting bigger and narrowing the flow to the extent of producing just myocardial ischemia?

- Is actual injury occurring and myocardial tissue dying?

- Is one of the coronary arteries going in and out of vasospasm with no mechanical blockage from an atheromatous plaque and enlarging thrombus?

All of the preceding conditions or processes are possibilities.

PATIENT DELAY

- The major issue right now, however, is *delay*. Mr. Lancaster is trying to explain his symptoms as "indigestion." Many people would now accuse him of denial. He is ignoring or "denying" symptoms that most lay people have learned are "warning signs" of possible AMI.

- The other explanation is that the chest pain of an AMI really can feel like indigestion.

- Or Mr. Lancaster may be thinking, "Is this the big one?" and he is playing little mental games with himself—"Oh man, this may be it. If it keeps up for a few more minutes, I'll call 911."

Avery Lancaster

CASE 1 Continued

His wife wants him to go to the hospital. He refuses. She asks if she can call 911, but he again refuses. "I don't want all those damn flashing red lights and sirens, and the neighbors looking to see what's going on." The pain eases somewhat but does not disappear, and he looks better. He is irritable and uncomfortable and makes his wife leave the room. One hour and 30 minutes pass.
What is going on now?

COMMENTS

TIME IS MUSCLE

- Mr. Lancaster has now failed to seek care and evaluation in a timely fashion. This problem of "delay in seeking care," multiplied nationwide, represents a terrible tragedy. Both patient-caused and health care–caused delays present a major obstacle to the effective treatment of AMIs. The more time that passes, the more myocardium that is lost.

- The National Heart Attack Alert Program has noted patient delays in seeking help to be the major barrier to achieving the maximum possible effectiveness of thrombolytic agents. Numerous studies have examined the average length of time between the onset of symptoms and arrival at an ED. "Three to 4 hours" appears so often in these studies that it may be a behavioral constant.

VARIABLE SYMPTOMS PATTERNS

The following factors have contributed to the unfortunate delay in Case 1.

- First, he seems to have gotten better. Several researchers have observed this "stuttering" or "intermittent" pattern of pain in AMI patients.

- Next, he possesses the common stereotype of not wanting to attract attention, not wanting to "be a bother." The embarrassment of having "flashing red lights and sirens" from a 911 call, with all the associated neighborhood attention, is understandable.

- In addition, many cardiologists and other physicians still give the outdated advice of having patients with acute chest pain drive to the hospital via private vehicle. This is a potentially tragic practice and reflects the ignorance of physicians and patients about the adverse events that can occur in the early hours of an AMI, and about the effective advanced therapy available with an EMS response.

DECISION MAKERS

- The additional problem here is that Mr. Lancaster has insisted on retaining the role of decision maker. Despite his symptoms and their alarming nature, he refuses to transfer decision making to his wife, and she has not yet insisted on assuming that responsibility. The psychological aspects of these delays are complex.

Avery Lancaster

CASE 1 Continued

Suddenly, the pain becomes much more severe. "It feels like someone has just put their foot on my chest and now he won't get off!"

He tells his wife to get the car, that he will go to the hospital. Instead she wants to call 911. He refuses.

The wife looks at her pale, sweating husband, now lying collapsed on the sofa. "I don't care what you say, I'm going to call 911 right now! Be quiet, be still, and don't move from that sofa!"

Why is it so important to have Mr. Lancaster call 911 and not go to the Emergency Department by private vehicle? What are the important aspects of prehospital care for AMI patients?

COMMENTS

PRIVATE VEHICLES VERSUS 911

- Almost half the patients with documented AMIs fail to call 911 and instead drive themselves or have family or friends drive them to the ED. Many patients report that their physician actually told them, "Well, you better drive on to the hospital and get your chest pain checked out."

- Certainly, many factors contribute to this irrational behavior: concern over embarrassment, "causing trouble," reluctance to attract neighborhood attention by summoning emergency vehicles, and not wanting to "call for an ambulance when I don't really need it."

- In addition, many patients are unaware of two extremes of good and bad—the good that EMS personnel can do and the bad events that can occur in the early minutes of an AMI.

THE ADVANTAGES OF 911

- By calling 911 and getting an Advanced Life Support (ALS) ambulance unit, the patient has early access (within 10 minutes usually) to oxygen, monitoring, IV medications for pain relief, arrhythmia and blood pressure control, and especially early defibrillation should VF/VT occur.

- In addition, in a growing number of communities the ALS prehospital unit will obtain a 12-lead ECG and may even administer thrombolytic therapy before transporting the patient to a hospital.

EMS THERAPIES

EMS systems should have AMI protocols that address the following topics:

- Oxygen/IV/Monitor/Fluids

- Vital signs

- Nitroglycerin (sublingual or spray)

- Pain relief with narcotics

- Arrhythmia and blood pressure control

- 12-lead ECG with immediate computer analysis and possible transmission to ED

- Prehospital screening for administration of thrombolytic therapy (In some locations thrombolytic agents are administered in the field, but this remains under evaluation.)

- Notification to ED of possible AMI patient

- Rapid transport to ED

CRITICAL POINTS TO REMEMBER ABOUT EMS THERAPIES

- Not all of the preceding approaches are used in every community.

- Advanced Life Support units can initiate important elements of treatment much faster than would occur if patients took the time to transport themselves to the ED (oxygen, nitroglycerin, and pain relief). In addition, medics can treat the VF/VT that can occur in up to 30% of patients with definite AMI.

- Advanced Life Support personnel can begin gathering the information related to inclusion or exclusion criteria for thrombolytic therapy.

- Advanced Life Support personnel can use 12-lead ECG with computerized analyses to "alert" the ED that an AMI patient is en route to the hospital. Studies have demon-

strated that this "alerting phenomenon" can dramatically decrease the time from the call for help to the administration of thrombolytic therapy.

- EMS systems have not observed a benefit from prehospital thrombolytic therapy when the following are in place: prehospital "alerting" of possible AMI patients; ambulances that have short patient transport time intervals (less than 15 minutes); and EDs that have short "door-to-drug" time intervals (less than 30 minutes).

- However, communities where the EMS vehicles have long transport time intervals, or where the EDs do not evaluate chest pain patients quickly should consider prehospital administration of thrombolytics.

YOUR COMMUNITY

Not every community EMS system will provide all of the interventions listed earlier. The standard of care today, however, is that every EMS system *must at least* have considered these options. Every ACLS provider should know what happens in his or her community. If you were to call 911 right now for a possible AMI in your next-door neighbor, what would arrive in the first EMS vehicle? What equipment and medications will it be carrying? You should know the answers for your community.

Franklin Grover McNeily

CASE 2

A 55-year-old businessman is brought to the hospital by his wife in the family car. He has been experiencing severe chest pain, shortness of breath, and diaphoresis for 1½ to 2 hours. He walks up to the registration clerk appearing very uncomfortable. His wife states, "I think my husband is having a heart attack."

In a well-prepared Emergency Department, what should happen next?

COMMENTS

- Every Emergency Department, Urgent Care Center, walk-in clinic, or outpatient clinic that might encounter patients with AMIs needs to develop a response plan. The AHA, as well as the National Heart Attack Alert Program, recommends a response plan known as the "door-to-drug" team approach.

- The "door-to-drug" team approach requires the following:

  - Rapid triage of patients with chest pain

  - Established clinical decision-maker (emergency physician, cardiologist, or other)

  - Thirty- to 60-minute interval to thrombolytic therapy when indicated

- Emergency Departments should consider that all patients with chest pain may be having an AMI. These patients are "myocardially infarcting." Remind the reception area and other staff members about how they react to patients who

begin to have grand mal seizures. The same sense of urgency applies for AMI. There must be designated roles for personnel to follow whenever a person with "chest pain" is triaged.

- The clinical decision-maker is the person who assumes responsibility for the patient, especially the decision to initiate thrombolytic therapy when indicated. We have long since passed any "cardiology versus emergency medicine" conflict. The principle is that the person of first contact should focus as quickly as possible on ECG eligibility criteria, presence of indications, and absence of contraindications.

- In most situations the emergency physician will be the decision maker, often in a collegial consultative relationship with cardiologists. Hospital care groups should prospectively establish who makes the final decision regarding thrombolytic therapy. Clinical decision-makers will vary from hospital to hospital and setting to setting.

FIGURE 9-1

Acute Myocardial Infarction Algorithm

Early Management of Patients with Chest Pain and Possible Acute Myocardial Infarction (AMI) in Three Management Settings

COMMUNITY

All Communities should emphasize:
- Early recognition of AMI signs and symptoms
- Call fast and Call EMS (911)
- EMS transport, not private transport

EMS SYSTEM

All EMS systems should have protocols for:
- Oxygen/IV/Monitor/Fluids
- Temperature/Blood Pressure/Heart Rate/Respirations
- As needed use of nitroglycerin
- As needed use of pain narcotics
- Early alerting of Emergency Department (ED)
- Prehospital 12-lead ECGs with computerized analysis
- 12-lead ECG transmission and remote analysis
- Prehospital thrombolytics when indicated

EMERGENCY DEPARTMENT

Chest pain protocols in place
- Emphasis on short "door-data-decision-drug" intervals (30 to 60 minutes)
- Thrombolytic decision-maker identified in advance (most often emergency attending)

"Door-data decision-drug" interval in ED

Immediate ED assessment:
- Oxygen/IV/Monitor/Fluids
- Temperature/Blood Pressure/Heart Rate/Respirations
- 12-lead ECG
- Review ECG for indications for thrombolytic therapy
- Review history and physical exam for indications and contraindications for thrombolytic therapy
- Order chest X-ray
- Order blood studies for cardiac enzymes and coagulation and electrolyte studies

Immediate treatments for almost all AMI candidates:
- *Oxygen* at 4 L/min
- *Morphine* IV
- *Nitroglycerin*, sublingual paste or spray
- *Aspirin* by mouth

If indicated and no exclusions:
- *Thrombolytic* agents

Other treatments to consider with AMI patients:
- *Heparin* IV
- *Nitroglycerin* IV
- *Beta blockers* IV or po
- *Lidocaine* IV
- *Magnesium sulfate* IV
- *Coronary angioplasty or angiography*

30 to 60 minutes to thrombolytic therapy

Adapted with permission, Journal of the American Medical Association, 1992, Volume 268, *Guidelines for Cardiopulmonary Resuscitation and Emergency Cardiac Care*, p. 2220 copyright © 1992, American Medical Association.

Franklin Grover McNeily

CASE 2 Continued

The triage nurse quickly escorts Mr. McNeily to Exam Room 1. His vital signs are rapidly obtained: blood pressure = 160/105; heart rate = 110 beats/min; respirations = 14 breaths/min. He reports a history of elevated blood pressure, but he is on no treatment regimen. He had a bleeding peptic ulcer 2 months ago, requiring 2 days of hospitalization. Because of expense, he stopped taking his H2-blocker ulcer medication 1 week ago. Tonight his stool specimen is faintly guaiac positive.

What are the first things you do?

COMMENTS

All EDs should have written protocols for the immediate care of possible AMI patients.

IMMEDIATE ASSESSMENTS

- Oxygen/IV/Monitor/Fluids. "Oxygen-IV-Monitor-Fluids" should be thought of as one word in Emergency Cardiac Care. These are always appropriate actions to take.

- Obtain Temperature/Blood Pressure/Heart Rate/Respirations.

- Obtain 12-lead ECG within 5 minutes. There should be a designated person to obtain ECGs without delay in every ED.

- Perform brief targeted history and physical examination.

- Decide on eligibility for thrombolytic therapy.

- You should use the Five Quadrads as an aide-memoire for this early assessment. The Five Quadrads help you remember 20 different actions. You should consider all items within the first few minutes of treating anyone with a possible cardiopulmonary emergency.

ASSESSMENTS TO BE MADE SOON

- The following ED assessments, while not immediate, should be obtained soon after the patient's arrival:
  - Chest x-ray
  - Blood studies (of electrolytes, enzymes, and coagulation)

- Avoid arterial punctures (because of possible thrombolytic agents later).

- CAUTION: Never delay your progress toward a thrombolytic therapy decision while obtaining chest x-rays, laboratory tests, or requesting technical staff to obtain ECGs.

Franklin Grover McNeily

CASE 2 Continued

The man is placed on a stretcher and given oxygen at 4 L/min; an IV line is started, and monitor leads are attached. The clinic assistant enters to begin attaching the leads for a 12-lead ECG. The nurse gives the patient one aspirin to chew and swallow and places a sublingual nitroglycerin tablet under his tongue. This does not relieve the pain. She begins to draw up some morphine.

You note that all of these actions are proceeding smoothly, almost automatically, with no orders from you. What is a system you can use to review the medications that you should consider in AMI?

COMMENTS

TEN TREATMENTS TO CONSIDER IN AMI

- The algorithm for AMI (Fig. 9-1) lists 10 treatments to consider in management of a person with possible AMI. If the ECG meets the criteria for treatment with thrombolytic agents, move thrombolytics to the top of your list.

- Do not, however, neglect the other interventions, especially oxygen, nitroglycerin, morphine, and aspirin. These are almost always indicated in the patient with acute chest pain that you suspect to be ischemic in origin. In most EDs and critical care units (CCUs) these four agents are part of a routine, standing protocol. The other six interventions are administered depending on specific indications.

- Here are the medications (and one intervention) to consider in the treatment of AMI patients:
  - Morphine
  - Oxygen
  - Nitroglycerin
  - Aspirin
  - Thrombolytics
  - Heparin
  - Beta blockers
  - Magnesium sulfate
  - Lidocaine
  - Acute angioplasty (PTCA)

- The preceding list can be easily memorized for future recall by means of the facetious mnemonic of "Mona Thrombo Has Big, Magnificent Lips for Pizza." The first letter of each word in the mnemonic stands for the agent (see box below).

Morphine	M
Oxygen	O
Nitroglycerin	N
Aspirin	A
Thrombolytics	Thrombo
Heparin	Has
Beta blockers	Big
Magnesium	Magnificent
Lidocaine	Lips
PTCA (pronounced "Pizza")	Pizza

- The preceding mnemonic has an advantage in that it lists *almost* all the agents in the order they should be considered and administered. (Oxygen should really come first.) REMEMBER: **You are thinking about thrombolytic therapy from the moment you hear that a patient is having chest pain.** The list, however, tells us the four medications (MONA) you should order immediately. Assuming no contraindications, the MONA agents are nearly always given. Only selected chest pain patients will receive the agents recalled later in the mnemonic.

Learning pharmacologic treatment of AMI

- In this book we emphasize the following features to learn about every medication:
  - Why? (Actions)
  - When? (Indications)
  - How? (Dosing)
  - Watch Out! (Precautions)
- Consider **"MONA"** as the first interventions: MorphineOxygenNitroglycerinAspirin.

Oxygen used in AMI

WHY?

- Supplemental oxygen increases oxygen in the blood flowing to ischemic tissue.

WHEN?

- ALWAYS use when AMI is suspected.
- Remember one word: "Oxygen-IV-Monitor-Fluids."

HOW?

- Start with nasal cannula at 4 L/min.
- Use oxygen saturation levels to "titrate" oxygen administration.
- Check that the oxygen saturation exceeds 97% to 98%.
- If unable to achieve such a level, increase the delivery of oxygen to 6 L/min.
- Switch to Venturi mask if oxygen saturation still remains low.
- Switch to nonrebreather mask if Venturi mask does not achieve 97% to 98% oxygen saturation.

WATCH OUT!

- Very rarely: chronic obstructive pulmonary disease patients with hypoxic ventilatory drive will experience hypoventilation with oxygen administration.

Nitroglycerin Used in AMI

WHY? (Actions)

- Decreases the pain of ischemia
- Increases venous dilation
- Decreases venous blood return to heart
- Decreases cardiac preload
- Decreases myocardial oxygen consumption
- Dilates coronary arteries
- Increases cardiac collateral flow
- COMMENT: The preceding actions make nitroglycerin an extremely important drug for AMI patients. Several studies have observed IV nitroglycerin to affect mortality to a degree statistically similar to that for thrombolytics.

WHEN? (Indications)

- Continued suspected ischemic chest pain
- Unstable angina (change in angina pattern)
- Acute pulmonary edema (if systolic blood pressure is greater than 100 mm Hg)
- Elevated blood pressure in setting of AMI (especially with signs of left ventricular failure)
- COMMENT: Controversy surrounds the question of whether nitroglycerin should be routinely administered to patients with suspected AMI. Many physicians administer routine nitroglycerin infusions in people with high suspicion of AMI. Some studies have demonstrated a significant benefit on several outcome measures; however, more recent megatrials have not.

HOW? (Dosing)

- Spray inhaler: One spray, repeated every 5 minutes.
- Sublingual tablets: Give 0.30 to 0.40 mg. Repeat every 5 minutes.
- Paste: Apply 1 to 2 inches with backing pad.
- IV infusion: 10 to 20 µg/min; increase by 5 to 10 µg/min every 5 to 10 minutes. Titrate to effect.

- In patients with evidence of AMI limit systolic blood pressure drop to 10% if patient is normotensive (e.g., 120 to 110 mm Hg systolic) or to 30% if patient is initially hypertensive (e.g., 180 to 120 mm Hg systolic).

- Some drop in blood pressure is desirable in terms of altering hemodynamics and myocardial ischemia; however, excessive falls compromise remaining coronary perfusion.

- COMMENT: The clinical goals in nitroglycerin administration (particularly IV infusion) are not just to relieve pain but also to produce altered hemodynamics. Changes in blood pressure are desired and indicate that these altered hemodynamics are taking place.

WATCH OUT! (Precautions)

- Use with extreme caution if systolic blood pressure is less than 90 mm Hg.

- Limit systolic blood pressure drop to 10% if patient is normotensive.

- Limit systolic blood pressure drop to 30% if patient is hypertensive.

- Watch for headache, excessive drop in blood pressure, syncope, and tachycardia.

- Instruct patient to sit or lie down.

Morphine sulfate used in AMI

WHY? (Actions)

- Reduces pain of ischemia

- Reduces anxiety

- Increases venous capacitance

- Decreases systemic vascular resistance

- The preceding actions lead to reduced oxygen demands on the heart.

- Reduced oxygen demands lead to less ischemia and less infarct extension.

- COMMENT: Pain can be severe in patients who are "myocardially infarcting." Patients in pain produce much greater levels of catecholamines. These increase blood pressure, heart rate, and the oxygen demands on the heart. You must reduce these demands on the infarcting heart. Morphine is a key agent for this purpose. Both morphine and nitroglycerin have a purpose beyond pain relief. They each alter hemodynamics in a positive manner and are indicated even if the ischemic pain is minimal.

WHEN?

- Continuing chest pain

- Evidence of vascular congestion (acute pulmonary edema)

- Systolic blood pressure greater than 90 mm Hg

- No hypovolemia

- COMMENT: Some experts are placing less emphasis on morphine as an important agent to use in acute pulmonary edema (Class IIb, possibly helpful). They question the

rationale for giving a strong respiratory depressant to people who, in effect, are clinically drowning.

HOW?

- Give 2 to 5 mg IV slowly; give 1 mg/min every 5 minutes for 30 minutes.

- Goal is to eliminate the pain while watching for excessive blood pressure drop or respiratory depression.

- COMMENT: Most EMS systems, EDs, and CCUs use a "titrated to pain relief" approach. This approach directs the paramedic or nurse to evaluate whether the pain is sufficiently relieved and when the next dose should be administered.

WATCH OUT! (Precautions)

- Drop in blood pressure, especially with the following:
  - Volume-depleted patients
  - Patients with increased systemic resistance
  - Patients receiving beta blockers

- Depression of ventilation

- Nausea and vomiting (common)

- Bradycardia

- Itching and bronchospasm (uncommon)

- COMMENT: Use Trendelenburg's position as first response to moderate-to-severe blood pressure drops. (Use caution in obese patients.) Use naloxone 0.4 to 2 mg IV (repeat every 5 to 10 minutes as needed, to 10 mg) to reverse respiratory depression.

Aspirin used in AMI

WHY? (Actions)

- Blocks formation of thromboxane A_2

- Thromboxane A_2 causes platelets to aggregate and arteries to constrict.

Therefore these actions will have the following effects:

- Reduction in overall mortality in AMI

- Reduction in incidence of nonfatal reinfarction

- Reduction in incidence of nonfatal stroke

- COMMENT: The ISIS-2 Study revealed that aspirin alone, started within 24 hours of the onset of symptoms, reduced overall mortality the same degree as did thrombolytic therapy alone (streptokinase). For AMI and unstable angina, aspirin is the most cost-effective agent available.

WHEN?

- As soon as possible!!

- Standard therapy for all patients with new pain suggestive of AMI

- Given within minutes of arrival at the Emergency Department

- COMMENT: The AHA and the American College of Cardiology both now make this recommendation. Consider whether aspirin is given early and routinely in your EMS system or ED.

HOW?

- 160- to 325-mg tablet taken as soon as possible
- COMMENT: Some EMS systems have paramedics administer aspirin in the prehospital setting. Many EDs keep containers of aspirin in the examination and treatment rooms to allow immediate administration.

WATCH OUT! (Precautions)

- Relatively contraindicated in patients with active ulcer disease or asthma
- Contraindicated in patients with known hypersensitivity to aspirin
- Higher doses can interfere with prostacyclin production and interfere with positive benefits

---

Franklin Grover McNeily

CASE 2 Continued

The ED clinical assistant has obtained the 12-lead ECG (Fig. 9-2) and hands it to the nurse. The two of you review the recording together. The nurse asks, "Does he get admitted? Does he get thrombolytics?" Given this history, examination, and ECG, would you admit this patient to rule out a possible AMI? How do you make the diagnosis of AMI and make the decision to give thrombolytics?

COMMENTS

The following major decisions have to be made at this point:

- Does this person need to receive thrombolytic therapy?

- Does this person need to be admitted to rule out an AMI?

- Is this person "myocardially infarcting?" Is he actually having an AMI?

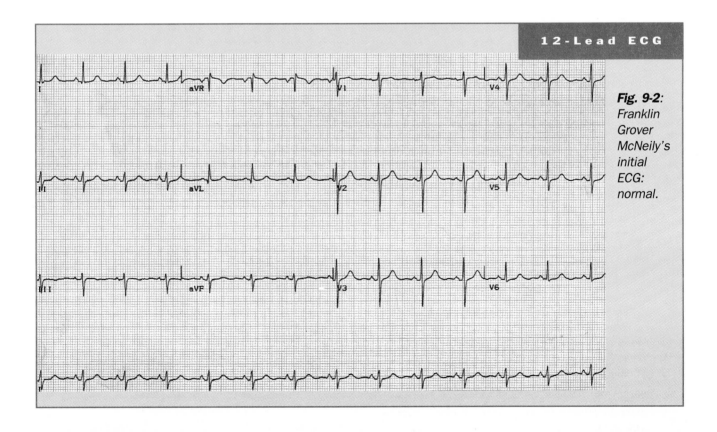

12-Lead ECG

***Fig. 9-2**: Franklin Grover McNeily's initial ECG: normal.*

Decisions regarding AMI in the acute care setting (before enzyme studies)

- **The decision to admit the patient and rule out AMI is based on history as follows:**

  - Characteristic pain of more than 15 minutes (crushing, substernal)

  - Unrelieved by rest

  - Unrelieved by nitroglycerin

  - Radiation to arms (ulnar), neck, or jaw

  - Associated signs of diaphoresis, shortness of breath, anxiety, or impending doom

- **The decision to administer thrombolytic agents is based on ECG (plus history) as follows:**

  - Anterior leads (leads V_1 to V_4): must have ST-segment elevation greater than 2 mm in at least two leads.

  - Inferior leads (II, III, and aV_F) must have ST-segment elevation greater than 1 mm in at least two leads. (However, AMI is not ruled out by a normal ECG!)

- **The decision as to whether an AMI actually occurred is based on all three—history, cardiac enzymes, and ECG evolution—as follows:**

In this rapidly evolving area, new cardiac enzyme analyses are under evaluation. Furthermore, thrombolytic agents themselves have a profound influence on the entire question of whether an AMI occurred, for acute infarctions are often prevented by thrombolytic intervention. Enzyme diagnosis of AMI will not be covered in this handbook.

- *The following critical points must be appreciated and understood regarding the diagnosis of AMI:*

  - A "normal" ECG (Fig. 9-2) does not rule out AMI. Mr. McNeily's normal ECG will prevent him from receiving thrombolytic agents, but he will still need to be admitted based on his history, physical examination, and risk factors.

  - Patients can present themselves with many variations in the "classic" story.

  - "Atypical" presentations occur with unique subsets of patients. For example, individuals with diabetes or renal disease, especially the elderly, often present themselves with an "occult" or "asymptomatic" or "painless" or "atypical" AMI. Remember these different terms. You must consider AMI in these patients when they seek medical care with a variety of vague and often painless symptoms. Young people (20 to 30-year-olds) with classic chest pain may be using cocaine.

  - Remember that coronary artery disease is the leading cause of death in women, just as it is in men. While the incidence of AMI in women is lower than in men, AMI remains the major consideration in women presenting with signs and symptoms suggestive of AMI.

  - Do not forget to obtain serial ECGs in the ED, especially if the initial ECG is nondiagnostic and the pain continues. Consider the dynamic nature of AMI, and note that ECGs as well can be dynamic. With continuing pain, a second ECG may begin to show ST-segment elevations even when the initial ECG was normal.

Franklin Grover McNeily

CASE 2 Continued

For learning purposes, however, let's change the initial ECG to one that is abnormal. Consider what you would do if the ECG looked like the tracing in Fig. 9-3: classic anterior MI.

COMMENTS

The ECG in Fig. 9-3 displays marked anterior ST-segment elevations of 2 to 8 mm.

- Remember to measure ST-segment elevation in the proper location (Fig. 9-4), as follows:

  - Measure vertical ST-segment deviation 0.04 seconds (1 mm) after the J point. The J point marks the end of the QRS complex and the beginning of the ST segment. Use the PR line as the baseline for measuring the vertical deviation.

- Many people use the following "Triple I" approach to evaluating ECGs:

  - Ischemia: Produces T-wave inversions

  - Injury: Produces ST-segment elevation

  - Infarction: Produces pathologic Q waves in atypical leads

ECG criteria for anterior AMI

- Key: Anterior leads (leads V_1 to V_4) must have greater than 2 mm ST-segment elevation in at least two leads (Fig. 9-3).

- Reciprocal changes are not always present.

- Q waves or T wave-inversion increases sensitivity.

- The ST-segment in leads V_5 and V_6 may be elevated.

- Key point for you to remember: *These are the patients who are most likely to benefit from thrombolytic treatment.*

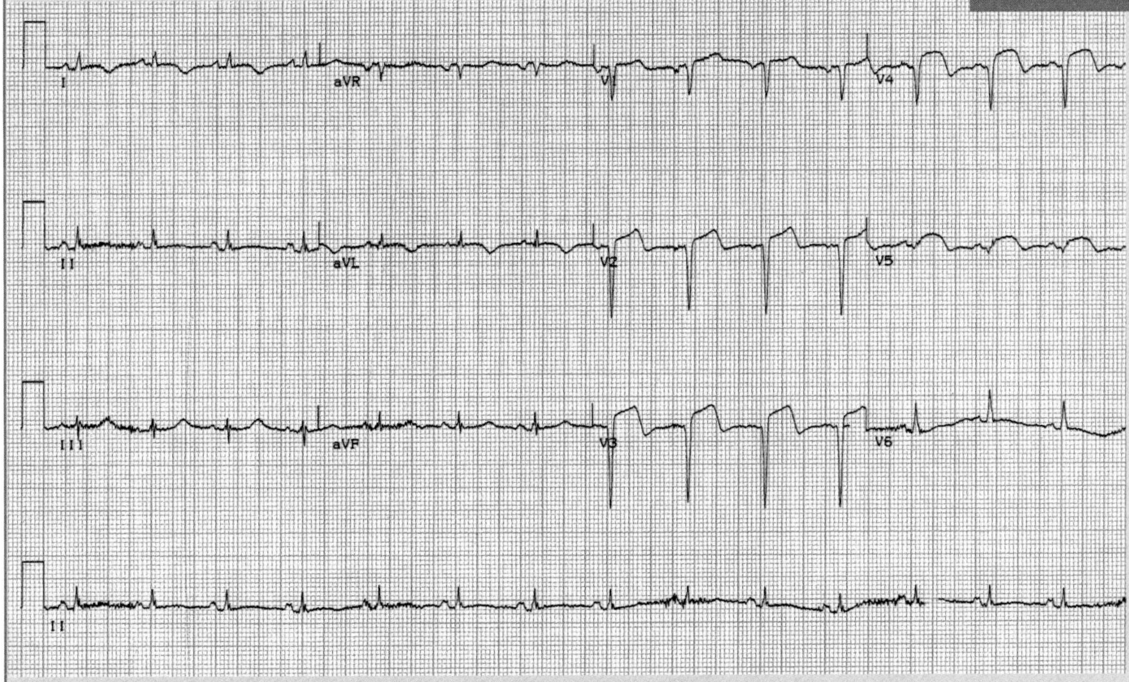

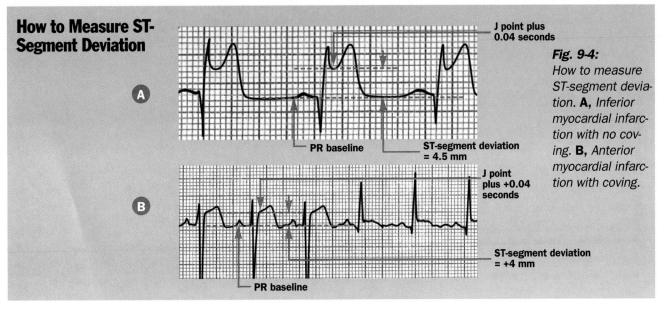

Fig. 9-3: Electrocardiogram of anterior myocardial infarction.

How to Measure ST-Segment Deviation

Ⓐ

Ⓑ

J point plus 0.04 seconds

PR baseline

ST-segment deviation = 4.5 mm

J point plus +0.04 seconds

ST-segment deviation = +4 mm

PR baseline

Fig. 9-4: How to measure ST-segment deviation. **A,** Inferior myocardial infarction with no coving. **B,** Anterior myocardial infarction with coving.

ECG Criteria for Inferior AMI

- Key: Inferior leads (leads II, III, and aV_F) must have greater than 1 mm ST-segment elevation in at least two leads.

- Measurement is as follows:

- Measure ST-segment deviation 0.04 seconds after the J point.

- Measure relative to the PR segment.

- Lead aV_L will always display T-wave inversion or ST-segment depression.

- Leads V_5 and V_6 may be elevated.

Franklin Grover McNeily

CASE 2 Continued

You conclude that this patient, based on the ECG in Fig. 9-3, is having a large anterior AMI.

The critical question now is: Does he qualify for thrombolytic therapy? (See Fig. 9-5.)

COMMENTS

- In treating patients with AMI, you should ask the following sequence of questions:
  - Is the history (pain) consistent with AMI?
  - Is the ECG consistent with acute injury (ST-segment elevations)?
  - Does the patient have any absolute contraindications to thrombolytic therapy?
  - Does the patient have any relative contraindications to thrombolytic therapy?
- Review the lists of contraindications for thrombolytic therapy (see "Eligibility Criteria" below). REMEMBER: No set of contraindications can anticipate every clinical circumstance.
- In addition, the lists of absolute and relative contraindications are changing dynamically as we gain more experience in treating people with MI. For example, many patients who have received thrombolytics soon went into cardiac arrest and received prolonged CPR. The experience with these patients has taught us that prolonged CPR should not be an absolute contraindication to thrombolytic therapy.

Eligibility criteria for thrombolytic therapy

ABSOLUTE CONTRAINDICATIONS

- Active internal bleeding
- Suspected aortic dissection
- Known traumatic CPR (fractured ribs, fractured sternum, hemothorax, or pneumothorax)
- Severe, persistent hypertension, despite pain relief and initial drugs (blood pressure higher than 180 mm Hg systolic or higher than 110 mm Hg diastolic)
- Recent head trauma or known intracranial neoplasm
- History of cardiovascular accident (CVA) in past 6 months
- Pregnancy

RELATIVE CONTRAINDICATIONS

- Recent trauma or major surgery in the past 2 months
- Initial greater than 180 mm Hg systolic or greater than 110 mm Hg diastolic that is controlled by medical treatment

FIG. 9-5

Example Review List for Thrombolytic Therapy

All of the "yes" boxes and all of the "no" boxes must be checked before thrombolytic therapy can be given. (Modified from the Myocardial Infarction and Triage Trial, Seattle–King County EMS Division.)

YES	CRITERION	NO
☐	Oriented, can cooperate, appropriate	
☐	Ongoing chest pain	
☐	ECG = Two leads with ≥2 mm ST-segment elevation in anterior (V_1 to V_4) leads OR two leads with ≥1 mm ST-segment elevation in inferior leads (II, III, and aV_F)	
☐	Pain for >15 minutes and <6 hours	
☐	Age (34 to 74 years)	
☐	Systolic blood pressure difference = >60 and <180 mm Hg	
☐	Systolic blood pressure right arm vs. left arm = <20 mm Hg	
☐	Diastolic blood pressure = <110 mm Hg	
	Stroke, seizures	☐
	Brain surgery, head trauma	☐
	Central IV lines within last 2 weeks	☐
	Trauma within last 2 weeks	☐
	Percutaneous transluminal coronary angioplasty within last month	☐
	Previous thrombolytic therapy	☐
	Takes warfarin or Coumadin	☐
	Known bleeding problem	☐
	Gastrointestinal bleed in last 2 months	☐
	Surgery in last 2 months	☐
	Jaundice, hepatitis, kidney failure	☐
	Colitis, Crohn's enteritis	☐

- History of CVA, tumor, injury, or brain surgery
- Known bleeding disorder or current use of warfarin
- Significant liver dysfunction or renal failure
- Prior exposure to streptokinase or anistreplase during the preceding 12 months
- Known cancer or illness with possible thoracic, abdominal, or intracranial abnormalities

- Prolonged CPR without known trauma (greater than 15 to 20 minutes, especially with endotracheal intubation)

- Many EDs and EMS systems have developed checklists to use to review the clinical indications and contraindi-

cations for thrombolytic therapy. Fig. 9-5 presents a sample review list of indications and contraindications for thrombolytic therapy. Before proceeding with thrombobolytic therapy, all of the "yes" boxes must be checked off, plus all of the "no" boxes.

Rhythm Strip

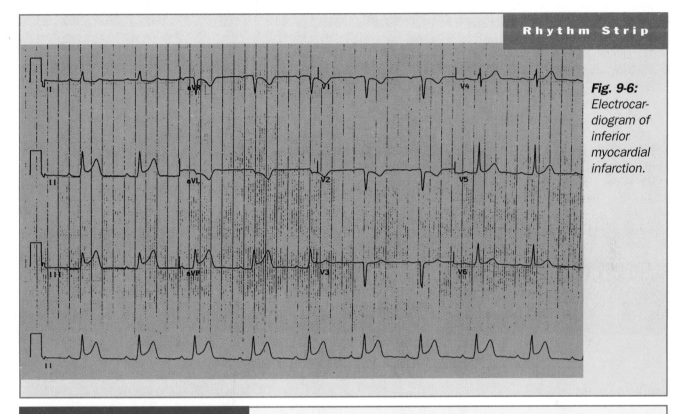

Fig. 9-6: *Electrocardiogram of inferior myocardial infarction.*

Franklin Grover McNeily

CASE 2 Continued

For this patient we note the following:
- *History is consistent with AMI.*
- *ECG is consistent (Fig. 9-6).*
- *Diastolic blood pressure is too high (relative contraindication).*
- *There is recent history of bleeding ulcer (relative contraindication).*
- *There is guaiac-positive stool specimen (relative contraindication).*

The patient's blood pressure drops to 150/95, the pulse is 100 beats per minute after rest, morphine, and nitroglycerin; however, the pain remains uncontrolled and severe.

What is the balance of indications and contraindications for Mr. McNeily? Would you give him a thrombolytic agent at this point?

COMMENTS

- This patient is "myocardially infarcting" with ECG signs of a large anterior MI. The drop in his blood pressure would be considered by many experts to have eliminated one contraindication.

- We still must balance the risks versus the benefits. The risks are stroke because of the hypertension, and gastrointestinal bleeding because of the ulcer history and positive

stool specimen. The benefits come from the fact that this man falls in the category of patients who will most benefit from thrombolytic therapy and who would face high risk of mortality and morbidity. Most clinicians would recommend treating this patient with thrombolytic agents.

- There is no absolute age limit for thrombolytic therapy. Thrombolytic therapy conveys the most benefit for patients greater than 70 years of age; however, the risk of intracerebral bleeding also increases with age.

- Most benefits from thrombolytic therapy occur for patients with anterior and multiple-location infarctions, and when the ECG displays ST-segment elevation or new left bundle branch block.

- The guiding principle is "The sooner the better."

- Although thrombolytic therapy is most beneficial when the duration of chest pain is less than 6 hours, it is also beneficial when duration of chest pain is greater than 6 hours if chest pain is intermittent or ST-segment elevation persists.

- In giving thrombolytics, there is no outer limit for the duration of symptoms. Some clinical centers are exploring the value of giving thrombolytics 12 or more hours after onset of symptoms. Initial studies have been positive.

- The final decision to order thrombolytic therapy is a clinical decision based on the following:

- History
- Age
- ECG findings
- Location of infarction
- Duration of symptoms
- Estimate of risks versus benefits

CURRENTLY AVAILABLE THROMBOLYTIC AGENTS

- Streptokinase
- Recombinant tissue plasminogen activator (r-TPA)
- Anisoylated plasminogen-streptokinase activator complex (APSAC)

Local practice often determines which agent is used in a particular practice setting. The key point is to know whether thrombolytic agents are indicated and the various contraindications.

Franklin Grover McNeily

CASE 2 Continued

You decide to proceed with administration of a thrombolytic agent. If you choose to use r-TPA, you will need to also administer heparin (although there is some controversy around this point).
What are the "Why? When? How? and Watch Out!" for heparin?

Heparin used in AMI

WHY?

- Coronary thrombi develop from thrombus formation over ruptured plaque.

- Even after thrombolysis there remains residual thrombus in addition to the original vascular injury (active surfaces).

- These active surfaces stimulate more thrombus formation.

- Heparin prevents recurrence of thrombosis after thrombolysis takes place. The cardiologists' phrase for this phenomenon is that heparin "maintains patency of the infarct-related artery (IRA)."

- Heparin prevents mural thrombus formation in patients with a large anterior AMI.

- Heparin forms part of the "thrombolytic package" that is given to patients.

- Aspirin is the other agent almost always given in combination with thrombolytic therapy.

- Much of the debate associated with the multiple thrombolytic clinical trials stems from when, how, and whether heparin was used.

- Patients with large anterior AMIs are at risk for thrombi in the ventricular wall and cerebral emboli. American College of Cardiology and AHA Guidelines recommend heparin in such cases (Class IIa).

WHEN?

- Option 1: Use at same time as thrombolytic agent.

- Option 2: Use upon completion of thrombolytic infusion.

- Option 3: Use on empirical basis in patients with large anterior AMIs without thrombolytics.

- Option 4: Use on empirical basis in patients with unstable angina. (Heparin is standard therapy for patients admitted with unstable angina.)

- COMMENT: Specific directions for when to use heparin should be established by responsible staff in every hospital and ED. Many clinicians use echocardiography to determine which patients should get heparin to prevent mural thrombi; if echocardiography shows a large hypokinetic area of the ventricles, give heparin. (These hypokinetic areas provoke thrombus formation.)

HOW?

- Bolus IV: 80 international units (IU)/kg.

- Continue: 18 IU/kg per hour.

- Then adjust to maintain activated partial thromboplastin time (PTT): 1.5 to 2.0 times the control values.

- COMMENT: The 80 IU/kg bolus replaces the former bolus of 5000 IU, which does not achieve therapeutic levels as quickly and uniformly as an 80 units/kg bolus.* The maintenance dosage of 18 IU/kg per hour replaces the former

---

* From *Ann Intern Med:* 119:874-881, 1993.

dosage of 1000 IU/hour for 24 hours. This explains why a control PTT is one of the laboratory tests you obtain early. Almost all patients should receive **aspirin** 160 to 325 mg along with the heparin.

WATCH OUT!

- Heparin has virtually the same contraindications as for thrombolytic therapy, as follows:
  - Active bleeding
  - Recent intracranial, intraspinal, or eye surgery
  - Severe hypertension
  - Bleeding tendencies
  - Gastrointestinal bleeding
- COMMENTS: If the patient qualifies for thrombolytic therapy, he or she qualifies for heparin (but whether you actually give heparin depends on the thrombolytic agent; currently r-TPA is the thrombolytic agent that is always combined with heparin).

Franklin Grover McNeily

CASE 2 Continued

Before giving the heparin and r-TPA consider how you would approach this patient if the following events occurred: after 4 L/min oxygen, four sublingual nitroglycerin tablets, and morphine (12 mg IV) the pain diminishes but does not completely disappear. He remains diaphoretic. His blood pressure is 170/110, and his heart rate is 105 beats/min. What would you consider now?

COMMENTS

You now are treating a person with a probable AMI and the following:

- Persistent, uncontrolled **pain**
- **Elevated blood pressure**
- **Rapid heart rate**
- The preceding combination of signs and symptoms presents strong indications for **beta blockers.**

Beta blockers used in AMI

WHY?

- To decrease automaticity and arrhythmias
- To reduce sinus node discharge
- To lower blood pressure
- To lower myocardial contractility
- To block catecholamine stimulation
- To reduce myocardial oxygen consumption
- COMMENT: The value of beta blockers lies in their ability to reduce the size of infarction. Remember the concept of "myocardial salvage." You are attempting to keep as much of the threatened myocardium as possible from dying.
- Remember as well the balance between "supply" and "demand." The myocardium in the area supplied by the infarcted artery must balance its blood supply from the "infarct-related artery" (often termed the IRA) with its metabolic demands. The doomed infarcting tissue is surrounded by an area of threatened ischemic tissue. Whether this ischemic tissue evolves into dead, infarcted tissue depends on this supply-and-demand balance.
- The beta blockers in this situation reduce demand on the threatened myocardium. Beta blockers reduce oxygen consumption by lowering heart rate and blood pressure and help prevent ischemic tissue from becoming infarcted tissue. This "salvages" myocardium and reduces infarct size.

WHEN?

- AMI (anterior) with evidence of excess sympathetic activity (elevated heart rate and blood pressure)
- Large MIs treated early (less than 6 hours of pain)
- Refractory chest pain or tachycardias that are due to excessive sympathetic tone
- Many EDs, in collaboration with their cardiology service, routinely administer a beta blocker to patients admitted with possible AMI.
- COMMENT: Administration of IV beta blockers to patients with AMI can have significant side effects. Start IV beta blockers with caution. Usually consult with the cardiologists who will assume care of the patient in the CCU.

HOW?

- Here are three common "recipes" to use for giving beta blockers to AMI patients:
- **Metoprolol:** 5 mg IV infusion (slow), every 5 minutes to a total of 15 mg, or the following:
- **Atenolol:** 5 mg IV infusion (over 5 minutes). Wait 10 minutes, then give second dose of 5 mg IV (over 5 minutes), or the following:
- **Propranolol:** 1 mg IV (slow) every 5 minutes to a total of 5 mg.
- COMMENTS: Metoprolol possesses an advantage of a short half-life (30 minutes). If it lowers the blood pressure or slows the heart rate too much, you can stop the infusion and the effects will soon fade away. Esmolol, which many clinicians prefer, has this same advantage, plus it has an even shorter half-life (less than 10 minutes).

WATCH OUT!

Contraindications to IV beta blockers include the following:

- Congestive heart failure or pulmonary edema
- Bronchospasm, asthma, or lung disease
- Bradycardia (heart rate less than 50 to 60 beats/min)
- Hypotension (systolic blood pressure less than 100 mm Hg)
- Heart block or conduction delays
- COMMENTS: The conditions listed as contraindications can get worse in response to beta blockers. Beta blockers also cause marked myocardial depression and thus should be used with respect and close observation.

Calcium channel blockers used in AMI

- COMMENTS: Calcium channel blockers are an interesting agent to consider for AMI. The pharmacologic properties of the agents suggest that they would produce considerable benefits. Nevertheless, multiple large-scale, multicenter trials have not confirmed a reason to use them in the early hours of an AMI. The AHA does *not* recommend the use of calcium channel blockers in the initial management of AMI. We include them here to provide a comprehensive review and because ACLS providers will continue to hear discussions about calcium channel blockers in the AMI patient.

WHY?

- To dilate coronary arteries
- To dilate peripheral arteries
- To depress AV and sinoatrial node activity
- To increase flow to ischemic areas
- To slow heart rate
- To reduce afterload
- Overall: To reduce ischemia and infarction
- COMMENTS: The pharmacologic effects just listed explain why, theoretically, calcium-channel blockers should improve certain outcomes following AMI. By producing an overall reduction in ischemia and size of infarction, calcium channel blockers should reduce long-term mortality and morbidity. This tempting pharmacologic profile led to many clinical trials of calcium channel blockers for evolving AMI. The trial results have been disappointing and inconclusive. Supporters of calcium channel blockers, however, have pointed out that most of these trials were done in the prethrombolytic era and thus may not apply now. Their argument is that calcium channel blockers may be valuable after the infarct-related artery is opened by thrombolytics.

WHEN?

- Unstable angina (Class I recommendation)

- Postinfarction angina (should be combined with nitrates) (Class IIb recommendation)
- Consider for persistent chest pain when there is no relief from IV nitrates
- Consider as cardioprotective agent in non-Q-wave infarction (Class IIa recommendation)
- COMMENTS: Despite the lack of evidence that we should give calcium channel blockers routinely in AMI, the specific indications listed earlier were recommended by the task force on early management of AMI of the AHA and the American College of Cardiology.* While the issue remains under intense study, the current consensus is that calcium channel blockers are *not* routine therapy for all AMI patients but just for the subsets noted earlier.

HOW?

- Diltiazem 30 to 60 mg by mouth three times a day (for cardioprotective effects)
- Diltiazem 0.25 mg/kg IV over 2 minutes; repeat as needed in 15 minutes at 0.35 mg/kg, over 2 minutes (for atrial fibrillation or atrial flutter conversion)
- COMMENTS: The most commonly used calcium channel blockers all possess different pharmacologic profiles, including actions and side effects, as follows:
  - Nifedipine is a powerful arterial dilator that is used for hypertensive urgencies; however, poor control of response makes it relatively contraindicated in AMI.
  - Verapamil is a potent AV nodal depressor that is used for paroxysmal supraventricular tachycardias (PSVTs).
  - Diltiazem is also a potent AV nodal depressor that does not cause the blood pressure drop of the others.
- Diltiazem is the only calcium channel blocker used for cardioprotective effects in AMI. The others produce too much depression of myocardial function. Intravenously, diltiazem is used for Afib and Aflutter conversion.

WATCH OUT! (Precautions)

- Hypotension
- Bradycardia
- Decreased left ventricular contractility
- Patients receiving beta blockers
- Avoid in patients with any signs of left ventricular failure or dysfunction.
- COMMENTS: Although the pharmacologic effects of calcium channel blockers suggest that they would be useful for AMI patients with hypertension and tachycardias, beta blockers are probably better for those indications. The major precaution is to avoid calcium channel blockers in people with clinical signs suggesting that their left ventricle is not working correctly (shortness of breath, fatigue, limited exercise capacity, rales, and pulmonary congestion on chest x-ray). These patients could get much worse.

---

* From *Circulation* 82:679, 1990.

Franklin Grover McNeily

CASE 2 Continued

Before administering thrombolytics, the nurse taking care of Mr. McNeily states that she has been observing one to two PVCs per minute on the monitor. She asks whether she should give him a bolus of lidocaine and follow it with a continuous infusion.

What would you advise?

COMMENTS

- Lidocaine, AMI, and PVCs: how do you manage this combination? The arrival of thrombolytic therapy has produced major changes in our approach to PVCs in patients with AMI. You must first understand the following different uses of lidocaine:

    - Prophylactic lidocaine (to prevent arrhythmias before they start)

    - Therapeutic lidocaine (to suppress arrhythmias after they start)

- Ventricular "irritability" can range from less than one PVC per minute to multiple PVCs to continuous PVCs. This irritability must be viewed in the context of a patient with AMI and continued pain.

- A single PVC should stimulate observation, not treatment. However, continuous PVCs, one right after another (that is, VT), must be treated aggressively. Where do you draw the line in this familiar example of "fuzzy thinking" in Emergency Cardiac Care? Where is the division between "not too many PVCs?" and "probably too many PVCs"?

- We face the same "fuzzy thinking" problems with tachycardias (how fast is too fast?); bradycardias (how slow is too slow?); and hypotension (how low is too low?).

- The answer depends on the clinical situation and how the patient is doing. As one wit stated, "As a last resort look at the patient." Restated correctly: "As your first resort—look at the patient."

Lidocaine used in AMI

WHY?

- Lidocaine works through the following mechanisms:

    - Raises VF threshold

    - Suppresses ventricular irritability

    - Decreases excitability in ischemic tissue

- The net effect of these mechanisms is that you prevent some patients from going into VF/VT.

COMMENTS

- A clear rationale supports the use of lidocaine for PVCs. Consequently the overuse of lidocaine in the past is easy to understand. Lidocaine certainly can reduce and eliminate PVCs. PVCs may in turn stimulate "reentry" VT, which can degenerate into fatal VF. Nevertheless, routine prophylactic lidocaine is no longer recommended, since there are the following problems with lidocaine use:

    - There is a new recognition of a slight risk of fatal asystole.

    - Many randomized trials have demonstrated that lidocaine does not reduce mortality.

    - Lidocaine can cause seizures and other neurologic problems, hypotension, and fatal asystole.

    - Lidocaine indications are confusing (prophylaxis versus treatment).

    - Lidocaine pharmacokinetics are complex; administration protocols vary.

WHEN?

- Give lidocaine *treatment* for *AMI* patients with new-onset **symptomatic** ventricular ectopy.

- Prophylactic lidocaine to prevent VF/VT is *not* recommended for AMI patients.

- Prophylactic lidocaine prior to thrombolytic therapy is *not* recommended.

COMMENTS

- The key principle to understand is that the *more severe* the AMI plus the *more* signs of irritability, plus the *more* severe symptoms lead to *more* indications for lidocaine. PVCs are a sign of the AMI—it is the AMI, not the PVCs that needs treatment. People who are "myocardially infarcting" and who display symptomatic ventricular irritability *may* benefit from *treatment* with lidocaine. Do not be a "PVC" warrior. The proper treatment of PVCs in AMI is to properly treat the AMI, as follows:

    - Morphine
    - Oxygen
    - Nitroglycerin
    - Aspirin
    - Beta blockers
    - Thrombolytic agents

- As a general rule, you should have considered each of the preceding agents (and used them if indicated) before administering lidocaine.

The "warning arrhythmias" concept

For a number of years ACLS personnel have learned a list of so-called "warning arrhythmias" in AMI. If any of the following occurred, the patient was thought to need lidocaine suppression:

- Six or more PVCs/min
- Closely coupled PVCs
- R on T (PVC on T wave)
- PVCs in pairs
- PVCs in runs (short bursts of three or more)
- Multifocal PVCs

- These indications for lidocaine, no matter how well-intentioned, led to overtreatment with lidocaine. Lidocaine does not address the root cause of the PVCs—ischemic and injured myocardium.

- Remember that treating PVCs with lidocaine is like treating fevers with aspirin—you are treating a sign of the problem, not the problem itself.

- We now possess more direct treatments for AMIs than in the past. PVCs, in a patient who appears to be having an AMI, serve as an alarm bell and are a warning that other AMI treatments (remember "MONA Thrombo") need to be applied quickly and effectively.

HOW?

- The following is how to administer lidocaine if you decide to use it in AMI:
  - Bolus dose: 1 to 1.5 mg/kg IV
  - Repeat dose: at 0.5 to 0.75 mg/kg every 2 to 10 minutes
  - Total dose: 3 mg/kg
  - Continuous infusion: 2 to 4 mg/min or 30 to 50 mg/kg per minute

COMMENTS
- Notice that there are four features to remember about dosing lidocaine: *bolus* dose, *repeat* dose, *total* dose, and continuous *drip rate*. How do you select among these dosing ranges? *Go with higher doses* if the clinical situation is urgent. *Go with lower doses and longer intervals* for those patients who will not metabolize lidocaine well and who may end up with toxic effects. These include patients who fall into the following categories:

- Elderly (greater than 70 years old)
- Liver failure
- Heart failure
- Smaller body size
- Bradycardias
- Conduction disturbances

WATCH OUT!

- You need to observe carefully for the signs of lidocaine intoxication. Remember that lidocaine is one of those drugs that forces you to walk a narrow path between giving enough to be effective and giving so much you make the patient toxic. Clinical signs of lidocaine intoxication are related to the nervous system and include the following:

- Paresthesias
- Dizziness
- Slurred speech
- Drowsiness
- Altered consciousness
- Decreased hearing
- Muscle twitching
- Seizures
- Respiratory arrest

- COMMENT: You recognize that the preceding signs are listed in order of increasing severity and that the last two are extremely severe complications. The occurrence of these symptoms reflects rising blood levels of lidocaine.

Franklin Grover McNeily

CASE 2 Continued

The medical student who is rotating on an "elective" through the Emergency Department asks whether you want to administer magnesium sulfate, stating that in an earlier rotation through the CCU all the rule-out AMI admissions received 2 g of magnesium sulfate routinely.

How would you respond?

COMMENTS

- Magnesium is an interesting agent that has attracted much attention related to the care of AMI patients. All ACLS providers should understand its current role in early hours of managing patients with a possible AMI.

Magnesium sulfate used in AMI

WHY?

- Magnesium deficiency is associated with arrhythmias and sudden death.
- Magnesium is a mild antiarrhythmic.
- Magnesium provides electrical stability in myocardium.
- Magnesium appears to possess some unknown "cardioprotective" effects.

COMMENTS

- Some observers have applied the term "temporary fad" to the use of magnesium for AMI patients. By 1993 there was increased interest in the benefits of magnesium in AMI. Several large, multicenter, randomized trials suggested an overall reduction in mortality of up to 60%. No one understood the exact mechanism of benefit.
- In the trials patients who did *not* receive magnesium sulfate died of cardiogenic shock and pulseless electrical activity (PEA). This suggested some unknown "protective" effect on the myocardium and that the benefits of magnesium came from some mechanism other than arrhythmia suppression.
- The most important study supporting the use of magnesium was the LIMIT-2 trial published in 1992. This study enrolled more than 2000 patients. In the fall of 1993, some of the same researchers presented their much larger study (LIMITS-4) of magnesium given to AMI patients. The researchers observed no benefit. These results were widely publicized, and many clinicians immediately stopped using routine magnesium for patients being admitted to rule out AMI.
- Other "magnesium defenders" have observed certain subgroups of patients who clearly appear to benefit from empirical use of magnesium, namely, known hypomagnesemic patients, such as patients with malnutrition, dietary compromise, chronic illnesses, or chronic debilitation. In the Limits-4 study low doses of magnesium were given hours after the AMI and often after thrombolytics. Needless to say, magnesium is still being studied; this is a story that "will be continued."

WHEN?

- Magnesium is the drug of choice for torsades de pointes (Class I).
- Use magnesium for cardiac arrest with known or suspected magnesium deficiency (Class I).
- Use magnesium to treat known or suspected magnesium deficiency in patients with AMI (Class I).
- Magnesium is acceptable as a prophylactic antiarrhythmic in AMI (Class IIa).

COMMENTS

- Magnesium is definitely helpful and should be given (Class I) for the first three indications. Suspected magnesium deficiency includes patients with nutritional problems (use of diuretics, alcoholism, chronic diseases, or poor dietary intake and habits). If you are treating patients who fit in these categories, be ready to use magnesium.
- Remember that serum magnesium levels do not always reflect total body stores; thus you may want to administer magnesium if the clinical picture is suggestive, even though serum levels are normal.
- The AHA does not recommend routine use of prophylactic magnesium for all AMI patients. Magnesium, however, should be considered acceptable (Class II) on the basis of current studies, but whether it is Class IIa (probably helpful) or IIb (possibly helpful) is the subject of ongoing discussion.
- The key word to remember in the AMI Algorithm is "consider": do not forget to think about magnesium administration when patients are admitted to rule out AMI.

HOW?

- Cardiac arrest: 1 to 2 g (2 to 4 mL of 50% $MgSO_4$) IV push
- Torsades de pointes: 1 to 2 g (2 to 4 mL of 50% $MgSO_4$) over 1 to 2 minutes. (Even higher doses, up to 5 to 10 g, may be needed to control the torsades de pointes.)
- AMI prophylaxis: 1 to 2 g (2 to 4 mL of 50% $MgSO_4$) diluted in 100 mL of normal saline over 5 to 60 minutes, followed with 0.5 to 2.0 g/hour up to 24 hours

COMMENTS

- Magnesium has a high margin of safety and can be given quickly and in large amounts. The safety of magnesium has been demonstrated in obstetrics for many decades: preeclamptic women often get massive amounts without serious side effects.

WATCH OUT!

- Patients with renal failure (Adjust later doses.)

- Hypotension

- Hyporeflexia

- Diaphoresis and drowsiness

- COMMENT: The kidneys excrete magnesium; therefore in patients with renal failure magnesium intoxication could develop. You can still administer the first bolus dose in the recommended amount, but later doses must be adjusted downward, particularly with more prolonged infusions (24 to 48 hours).

Franklin Grover McNeily

CASE 2 Continued

Two members of the Medical Center "cath team" enter the Emergency Department having heard "through the hospital grapevine" that a "hot" AMI was in the Emergency Department and was going to be admitted. They are interested in whether the patient will need to go to the "cath lab" for possible acute percutaneous transluminal coronary angioplasty (PTCA). What would be your response? What are the "Why? When? How? and Watch Out!" for PTCA?

Percutaneous Transluminal Coronary Angioplasty

WHY?

- With PTCA you have a method for mechanical reperfusion of the infarct-related artery.

- Mechanical reperfusion deals with the patient's core problem (a chronically narrowed artery) more directly than thrombolytics do (an acutely narrowed artery from a clot).

- Often patients who are "acutely infarcting" and need thrombolytic therapy have contraindications to thrombolytic therapy. That is when PTCA should be considered.

- PTCA provides the most effective therapy for AMI patients with cardiogenic shock or pump failure.

- PTCA provides the most effective therapy for AMI patients with occluded vein grafts from coronary artery bypass surgery.

COMMENTS

- PTCA must be considered early in AMI patients. Routinely ask, "Does this patient have indications for PTCA?" Centers that possess PTCA capabilities emphasize early decision-making about early PTCA.

- Learn whether the health center where you work has PTCA capabilities. Learn how to get in touch with the cardiology team responsible for PTCA in your institution (usually the "cardiac cath" team).

- If your professional setting lacks PTCA capacity, learn how to refer to centers that do.

WHEN?[*]

- Consider PTCA when treating the following:

  - Patients who, for more than 6 hours, have had signs and symptoms of a large, AMI, and yet for some reason thrombolytic therapy is contraindicated (Class I)

  - Patients with a "stuttering" infarction plus ECG changes but no clear indication for thrombolytic therapy (Class IIa)

  - Patients with AMI who have cardiogenic shock or pump failure within 18 hours (Class IIa)

  - Patients with a previous coronary artery bypass graft and who appear to have possible recent occlusion of a vein graft (Class IIa)

  - Patients with a possible AMI in the hospital, that is, an observed AMI with rapid access to catheterization facility (Class IIb)

  - Patients with all the indications for thrombolytic therapy but who fail to reperfuse after thrombolytic therapy

- COMMENT: The most common indications you will encounter will be the following:

  - Patients with AMI and yet contraindications to thrombolytic agents

  - Patients with AMI plus cardiogenic shock

  - Patients with previous coronary artery bypass graft and suspected new occlusion of vein graft

  - Patients who receive thrombolytic therapy for appropriate reasons but who fail to have reperfusion

HOW?

- Primary PTCA is possible only in centers with the following:

  - Personnel who are able to perform expeditious angioplasty (Recommended standard is completion within 1 hour.)

  - Immediately available catheterization laboratory

PRECAUTIONS

- The following are situations in which PTCA would be Class III (possibly harmful):

  - Attempting to dilate a more distal occluded artery in a patient with severe left main coronary artery disease

  - A patient with involvement of only a small area of myocardium

  - Attempting to dilate vessels other than the infarct-related artery during early hours of AMI

[*] ACC/AHA Guidelines for the Early Management of Patients with Acute Myocardial Infarction. *Circulation,* 82:664-707, 1990; ACC/AHA Guidelines for PTCA. *J Am Coll Cardiol* 12:529-545, 1988.

Franklin Grover McNeily

CASE 2 Continued

Mr. McNeily has now been in the Emergency Department for 35 minutes. You have performed an initial assessment, including 12-lead ECG, which displays large ST-segment elevations in leads V_2 to V_5. The nurses have started oxygen and an IV line, and he is on the monitor. They gave him a chewable aspirin, sublingual nitroglycerin, and morphine 2 mg every 5 minutes, times four doses. The thrombolytic is infusing. While you are introducing yourself to the patient's wife, the nurse says, "Please check the monitor. I think he's starting to have a tachycardia."

What are the most common arrhythmias during AMI? And what are the most important points to remember about treating AMI arrhythmias?

- There are many arrhythmias that can occur during an AMI. You should always consider these arrhythmias coming from a heart that is experiencing either **infarction** or **ischemia.** Therefore you must focus treatment on the ischemia and infarction rather than on the arrhythmia alone.

- Often the best treatment of AMI arrhythmias is aggressive treatment of the AMI itself: oxygen (check oxygen saturation level to verify good oxygenation), pain control, nitroglycerin, beta blockers, and thrombolytic agents.

- The first thing to do for all arrhythmias is to **look at the patient.** The first question to ask is "**stable or unstable?**"

- Remember: Treat the patient, not the monitor!

- Think in terms of the entire following list of arrhythmias that are possible in AMI.

LETHAL

- VF/pulseless VT
- PEA (for example, profound cardiogenic shock)

TOO SLOW

- First-degree heart block
- Second-degree heart block (types I and II)
- Third-degree (complete) heart block

TOO FAST

- VT with a pulse
- PVCs in series
- Sinus tachycardia
- Atrial flutter or atrial fibrillation
- PSVT

Important points to remember about treating the AMI arrhythmias

TOO SLOW

- Slow rates may reduce coronary flow. However, this may increase ischemia and increase the development of ventricular escape arrhythmias.

- Slow rates protect against ischemia-induced arrhythmias because faster rates put more demands on the ischemic myocardium.

- Therefore, leaving symptomatic patients (pain is the most common symptom) in a slow rate can be bad.

- However, speeding up the heart rate of patients with AMI can be *very* bad. This is because faster rates induce strain, which leads to more ischemia, which leads to more ischemic damage, more irritability, and possibly lethal arrhythmias.

- The critical rule: *Do not treat bradycardias in AMI unless forced by the symptoms.*

FIRST-DEGREE HEART BLOCK

- No treatment is needed unless there is symptomatic bradycardia.

- Monitor for progression to other blocks or arrhythmias.

SECOND-DEGREE HEART BLOCK, TYPE I

- This block is high in the conduction system and occurs at the AV node.

- This block is more likely to indicate increased vagal stimulation.

- This block seldom indicates ischemic disease of the conduction system.

- No specific treatment is indicated unless the patient has symptoms.

- Again, you must strike a treatment balance: leave the rate slow and the ischemia may worsen or escape rhythms may occur; speed the rate up and you make the ischemia worse and induce arrhythmias.

- Careful observation is usually the most prudent course.

SECOND-DEGREE HEART BLOCK, TYPE II

- This block is lower in the conduction system, occurring below the AV node.

- The block is either at the bundle branch level (frequent) or the bundle of His (less frequent).

- Remember that this block signals ischemic disease of the conduction system.

- Type II second-degree block has a high risk of progression to complete heart block.

- Complete block increases patient mortality.

- Critical point to remember: These patients have a severe injury to the conduction system at the infranodal region.

- Prepare for pacing (transcutaneous and transvenous).

This means do the following:

- Alert the person who will be responsible for insertion of transvenous pacemaker (TCP).

- Attach TCP prophylactically.

- Always give a brief trial of transcutaneous pacing to ensure that it will capture (cause mechanical beats of the heart) and that the patient can tolerate it.

- Pain may be a major problem with transcutaneous pacing; therefore, be ready to be generous with IV analgesics, muscle relaxants, and anxiolytics.

THIRD-DEGREE HEART BLOCK OCCURRING AT THE LEVEL OF THE AV NODE

- This rhythm has the following features:

  - A normal-looking QRS complex

  - A rate between 40 and 60 beats per minute

- A normal-looking QRS complex indicates that a stable junctional escape pacemaker has taken over.

- This rhythm may be transient and usually has a good prognosis.

- Watchful waiting is usually the best course; however, you should still anticipate the possible need for transcutaneous and transvenous pacing.

- Prepare for pacing (transcutaneous and transvenous) as noted earlier: notify an appropriate consultant that you have a patient who may need emergency transvenous pacing.

THIRD-DEGREE ATRIOVENTRICULAR BLOCK OCCURRING AT THE LEVEL OF BUNDLE BRANCHES

- The clue here is the wide QRS complex and a slow rate, usually less than 40 beats per minute.

- This is an infranodal block; therefore the only escape mechanism is from the ventricles below the block.

- This block usually indicates that the AMI has extensively damaged the heart.

- This is *not* a stable rhythm: episodes of asystole are common.

- You should make immediate preparations for transcutaneous pacing and use of the TCP.

SINUS TACHYCARDIA

- Sinus tachycardia is a sign of something else going on. Your job is to identify and treat that "something else."

- Identify and correct the cause, as follows:

  - Pain (analgesia)

  - Hyperdynamic state (beta blockers)

  - Hypovolemia (volume replacement)

  - Extensive myocardial damage (monitor, thrombolytics medication)

  - Infection (antibiotics, antipyretics)

ATRIAL FLUTTER WITH BLOCK

- This rhythm is due to increased left atrial pressure or extensive anterior wall damage.

- This rhythm is associated with increased mortality.

- It may represent occult heart failure.

- It may represent excessive adrenergic tone.

ATRIAL FLUTTER WITH RAPID VENTRICULAR RESPONSE

- In general, the same treatment guidelines discussed in the Tachycardia Algorithm and scenarios apply in this case, as follows:

  - Administer electrical cardioversion if the patient's condition is unstable.

  - Perform vagal maneuvers.

  - Attempt pharmacologic slowing and conversion.

  - Treat the AMI appropriately.

  - Then administer electrical conversion.

VENTRICULAR TACHYCARDIA WITH A PULSE

- This is a rhythm you should have no trouble recognizing and treating.

- Apply the treatment recommendations in the Tachycardia and Electrical Cardioversion algorithms as follows:

- Cardioversion, if patient's condition unstable

- Treatment of the AMI

- Pharmacologic treatments (lidocaine, procainamide, bretylium and so forth)

Franklin Grover McNeily

CASE 2 Continued

Following the administration of the thrombolytic agent, Mr. McNeily experiences a brief moment of PVCs and even a few seconds of monomorphic VT. He has received oxygen, morphine, nitroglycerin, aspirin, beta blocker, thrombolytic agent, and heparin. In a dramatic fashion his pain completely disappears, and his appearance of stress and anxiety begins to fade away. A postthrombolytic 12-lead ECG demonstrates definite changes in the prior ST-segment elevations, decreasing to just 1- to 2-mm elevations.

What are the major elements of Mr. McNeily's management that account for this success?

COMMENTS

- The major problem with Mr. McNeily was his delay in seeking care: waiting almost 2 hours before coming to the ED and then using private transportation rather than calling 911.

- Once he arrived in the ED, however, all the elements of excellent, contemporary care of the possible AMI patient fell into place, as follows:
  - Rapid assessment and triage
  - Clinical decision-maker already established
  - Protocol-driven initial care
  - Rapid acquisition of 12-lead ECG
  - Rapid determination of indications and eligibility for thrombolytic therapy
  - Comprehensive review of the 10 interventions to consider
  - Administration of thrombolytic agent within 30 minutes of arrival in the ED

- The combined effects of the preceding elements are probably marked myocardial salvage. By having this care provided in such an effective and well organized manner, Mr. McNeily was able to benefit from the contemporary revolution that has occurred in the care of the AMI patient.

KEY POINTS

SUMMARY

Here is a list of the most common errors that care providers make when evaluating and treating people with possible acute myocardial infarction.

- **Failure to consider and evaluate rapidly and properly (ECG, monitor, history, and physical examination) a patient with acute chest pain suggestive of AMI**
- **Searching always for the stereotypical AMI presentation: middle-aged white man with severe, crushing substernal pain, sweating, and pain radiating down the left arm**
- **Failure to consider atypical presentations for an AMI in women, the elderly, and people with diabetes, renal failure, other chronic medical conditions, and altered mental states, and in people with syncope, unexplained shortness of breath, weakness, or fatigue**
- **Failure to obtain a 12-lead ECG in a timely fashion (within 5 to 10 minutes) in patients with possible AMI**
- **Failure to administer thrombolytics in a timely fashion to patients with proper indications and no contraindications (within 30 to 60 minutes)**
- **Failure to initiate oxygen and other indicated medications in a possible AMI patient**
- **Failure to control the pain in a patient with AMI**
- **Failure to recognize exclusion criteria for use of thrombolytic therapy**
- **Administration of contraindicated medications**

Hypotension, Shock, and Acute Pulmonary Edema
Pump, Tank, Electricity, and Resistance

OVERVIEW

How would you approach the following three patients?

Case 1: Martin Williamson. *Acute pulmonary edema with normal blood pressures*

- *A 65-year-old man arrives at the Emergency Department moderately short of breath. He has rales to his scapulae and mild expiratory wheezing. A stat portable chest x-ray reveals signs of pulmonary congestion and fluid. Vital signs are as follows:*

  - *Respirations = 25 breaths/min and are somewhat labored*

  - *Heart rate = 110 beats/min*

  - *Blood pressure = 110/70 mm Hg*

Case 2: Rudolph Chelminski. *Acute pulmonary edema with elevated blood pressures*

- *A 65-year-old man arrives at the Emergency Department moderately short of breath. He has rales to his scapulae and mild expiratory wheezing. A stat portable chest x-ray reveals signs of pulmonary congestion and fluid. Vital signs are as follows:*

  - *Respirations = 25 breaths/min and are somewhat labored*

  - *Heart rate = 110 beats/min*

  - *Blood pressure = 180/120 mm Hg*

Case 3: John Tompkins. *Acute pulmonary edema with low blood pressures*

- *A 65-year-old man arrives at the Emergency Department moderately short of breath. He has rales to his scapulae and mild expiratory wheezing. A stat portable chest x-ray reveals signs of pulmonary congestion and fluid. Vital signs are as follows:*

  - *Respirations = 25 breaths/min and are somewhat labored*

  - *Heart rate = 110 beats/min*

  - *Blood pressure = 75 mm Hg systolic*

COMMENTS

- *These three patients display exactly the same clinical presentations with the single exception of their blood pressures. How do you manage a patient with acute pulmonary edema when the blood pressure is as follows:*

  - *Normal?*

  - *Extremely elevated?*

  - *Extremely low?*

- *The major goal of this chapter is to provide guidelines for managing these three clinical situations. This is obviously a more limited goal than the title of this chapter or the title of the ACLS algorithm would suggest.*

- *Shock, however, is an immense subject; entire treatises are devoted to that topic alone. The learning objectives of the ACLS Provider's Course do not extend into the full range of the shock state, such as traumatic shock, septic shock, gastrointestinal bleeding, vomiting and diarrhea with dehydration, and spinal shock.*

- *Other books and courses (such as the Advanced Trauma Life Support Courses from the American College of Surgeons) address the evaluation and treatment of the shock state.*

- *The ACLS subcommittee of the AHA does consider it important for the well-trained ACLS provider to possess an understanding and an approach to several conditions that may be encountered in people "on their way to a cardiac arrest." In addition, these guidelines are for use before invasive hemodynamic monitor-*

ing. Detailed, precise management of such patients requires invasive pressure measurements. Instrumentation for these measurements, however, takes time to implement, and will not be possible during the first minutes of management. The guidelines were prepared in light of the clinical reality that ACLS providers often must make initial management decisions without invasive monitoring.

- *The 1992 AHA Guidelines included, for the first time, guidelines on the management of*

what have been referred to as "peri-cardiac arrest conditions." Consequently the ACLS subcommittee developed the algorithm and supporting text for "shock/ hypotension/acute pulmonary edema." ACLS providers can use this algorithm to provide initial guidance for exactly the patients described earlier: patients approaching acute pulmonary edema both with and without a profound alteration of blood pressure and peripheral vascular resistance.

MAJOR CONCEPTS TO MASTER

- **Understand the Algorithm Approach to Problems of Acute Pulmonary Edema, Shock, and Hypotension.**
- **Understand use of the "cardiovascular triad" as a conceptual tool.**
- **Recognize hypotension and shock.**
- **Recognize heart failure and acute pulmonary edema.**
- **Recognize tank and resistance (volume) problems as the cause of hypotension or shock.**
- **Recognize heart rate problems ("too fast" and "too slow") as the cause of hypotension or shock.**

Critical actions

- Always apply the Five Quadrads, as follows:
  - Primary ABCD Survey
  - Secondary ABCD Survey
  - Oxygen/IV/Monitor/Fluids
  - Temperature/Blood Pressure/Heart Rate/Respirations
  - Tank (Volume)/Resistance/Pump/Rate
- Apply these quadrads within the first 5 minutes of evaluating a critically ill patient.

Skills to learn

- No specific psychomotor skills are required for these cases.

Rhythms to learn

- No specific rhythms are required; however, review the bradycardia and tachycardia cases, as these make up the "rate" portion of the cardiovascular triad of Volume/Pump/Rate.

Medications to learn

- Learn the "Why?" "When?" "How?" and "Watch Out!" for the following medications:
  - Norepinephrine
  - Dopamine
  - Dobutamine
  - Nitroglycerin
  - Nitroprusside
  - Furosemide
  - Morphine
  - Nitroglycerin
  - Amrinone

Martin Williamson

CASE 1

You are working as an "internal medicine R2" rotating for 6 weeks in the Emergency Department. Your patient is Mr. Martin Williamson, a 65-year-old retired security guard who arrives at the Emergency Department moderately short of breath. He has been triaged and taken back to Room 3A, where the nurse is just completing his assessment. As you walk up, you notice that Mr. Williamson is sitting upright on the side of the stretcher. His arms are propping him up against his knees while he leans over, working hard to breathe.

Since this is quickly appearing to be a cardiopulmonary emergency, how would you begin your evaluation and treatment of Mr. Williamson?

- Since the Primary-Secondary Survey is the unifying approach for all cardiopulmonary emergencies, you should start there. For conscious, alert patients, the Five Quadrads offer an easy-to-remember, efficient way to review 20 clinical items

- **Primary Survey**: Initial review reveals that he is conscious and breathing, with a pulse; defibrillation is unnecessary.

- **Secondary Survey**

  - *Airway:* Respirations = 25 breaths/min; air is moving in and out with each breath.

  - *Breathing:* There is obvious respiratory difficulty with intercostal and supraclavicular retractions; auscultation reveals bilateral rales to his scapulae and mild expiratory wheezing.

  - *Circulation:* Heart rate = 110 beats/min; blood pressure = 110/70 mm Hg.

  - *Differential diagnosis:* Already you are thinking of the diagnostic possibilities for a process that produces symptoms of shortness of breath and the signs of rales, wheezing, and labored breathing. To gather more information about these diagnostic possibilities, you now order a stat portable chest x-ray, arterial blood gas studies, and a 12-lead ECG and perform a more complete physical examination.

- **Oxygen/IV/Monitor/Fluids**: This quadrad should be like one word: "Oxygen-IV-Monitor-Fluids." In most Emer-gency Departments the nurses, as your co-professionals, will have already initiated these.

- **Temperature/Blood Pressure/Heart Rate/Respirations**: You have already reviewed these in the initial surveys, but often it is useful to explicitly review them again.

- **Tank (Volume)/Resistance/Pump/Rate**: What is the nature of the problem? This quadrad contains the elements of the cardiovascular triad (Volume/Pump/Rate), a conceptual tool to help understand and treat hypotension and shock during the first 30 to 60 minutes of emergency evaluations. Note that the cardiovascular triad applies in the absence of invasive hemodynamic monitoring. (See the box on p. 182 for a more in-depth discussion, and see the cases that follow.)

  - *Is there a tank problem?* Yes. The intravascular volume is increased relative to the ability of the pump to move the volume effectively. Therapy will address this volume problem.

  - *Is there a pump problem?* Yes. The heart is in congestive failure and is not pumping the blood effectively. Pulmonary congestion ensues, producing the clinical picture of acute pulmonary edema. Therapy will address this pump problem.

  - *Is there a rate problem?* No. The rate of 110 beats/min is appropriate for the clinical emergency and reflects the distress of the patient.

Martin Williamson

CASE 1 Continued

On the physical examination you note jugular venous distention and 2-plus pitting pretibial edema; the portable chest x-ray reveals signs of pulmonary congestion and fluid. The arterial blood gas levels are PO_2 = 98; Pco_2 = 28; and pH = 7.4. His 12-lead ECG displays sinus tachycardia of 110 beats/min and absence of anterior forces in the precordial leads (old anterior myocardial infarction [MI]) but without acute changes of ischemia or injury. Mr. Williamson has a history of two previous MIs.

You decide Mr. Williamson meets diagnostic criteria for acute pulmonary edema, probably caused by congestive heart failure, which in turn is due to chronic damage from his coronary artery disease. You are not sure what precipitated this episode, but you decide that therapeutic intervention for the pulmonary edema is needed immediately.

How would you now proceed?

- Look carefully at the Algorithm Approach to Problems of Acute Pulmonary Edema, Shock, and Hypotension (Fig. 10-1). It is critical to understand where Mr. Williamson stands in relation to this algorithm: he has acute pulmonary edema with a reasonable blood pressure.

- Note on the algorithm the boxes for first-line, second-line, and third-line treatments. Because he has normal blood pressure, you can start the first-line treatments and continue with the second-line and third-line treatments if he does not respond or his condition deteriorates.

FIRST-LINE TREATMENTS

- **Furosemide** (Lasix) IV 0.5 to 1.0 mg/kg
- **Morphine** IV 1 to 3 mg
- **Nitroglycerin** sublingual (SL)
- **Oxygen**/intubate as needed (prn)

- The following is a special memory aid to help you remember the four first-line agents to use for acute pulmonary edema with a normal blood pressure:

  - Remember the four letters "L-M-N-O" (alphabetical sequence) as standing for "Lasix-Morphine-Nitroglycerin-Oxygen."

FIGURE 10-1

Algorithm Approach to Problems of Acute Pulmonary Edema, Shock, and Hypotension

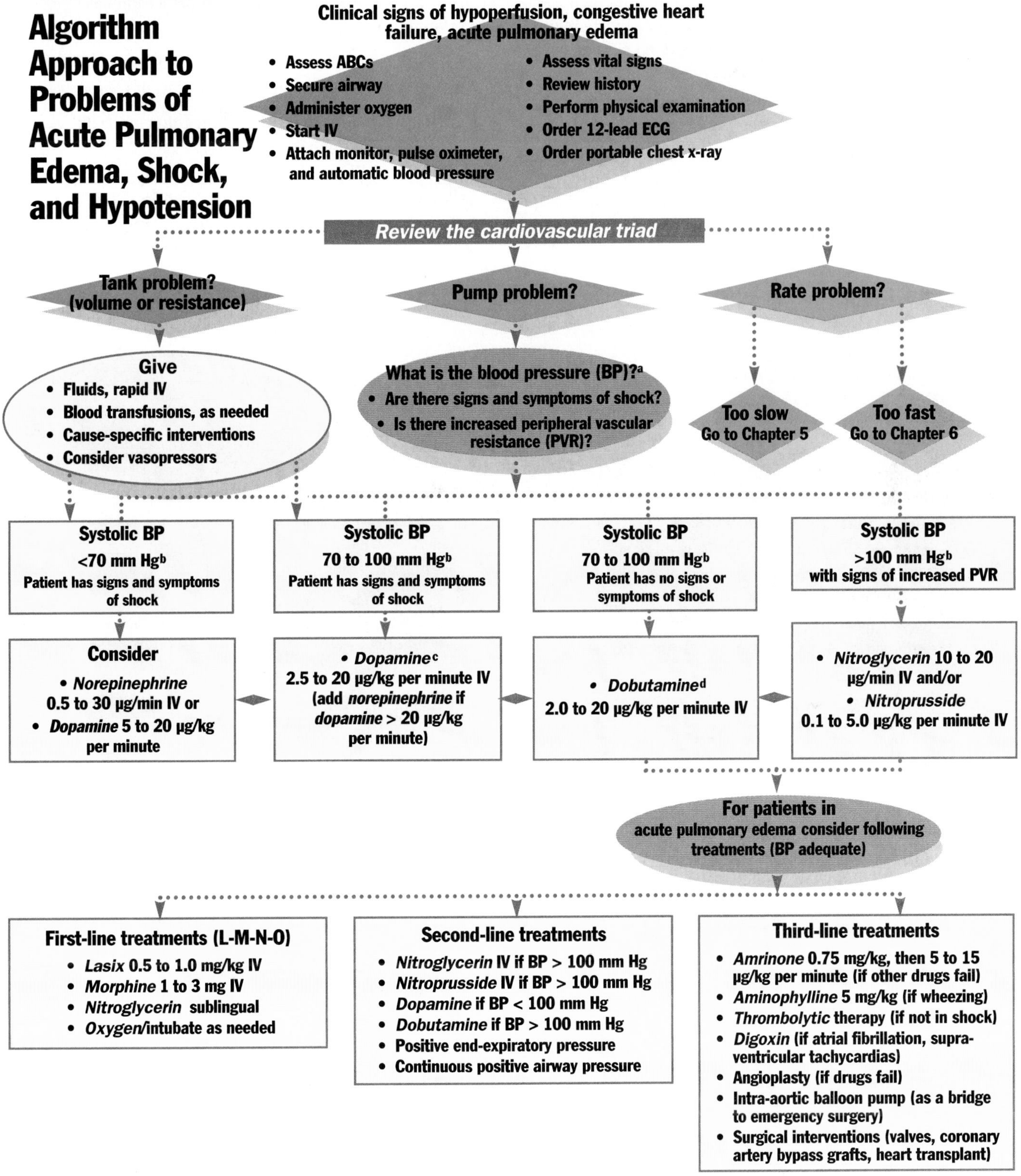

Clinical signs of hypoperfusion, congestive heart failure, acute pulmonary edema

- Assess ABCs
- Secure airway
- Administer oxygen
- Start IV
- Attach monitor, pulse oximeter, and automatic blood pressure

- Assess vital signs
- Review history
- Perform physical examination
- Order 12-lead ECG
- Order portable chest x-ray

Review the cardiovascular triad

Tank problem? (volume or resistance)

Pump problem?

Rate problem?

Give
- Fluids, rapid IV
- Blood transfusions, as needed
- Cause-specific interventions
- Consider vasopressors

What is the blood pressure (BP)?[a]
- Are there signs and symptoms of shock?
- Is there increased peripheral vascular resistance (PVR)?

Too slow Go to Chapter 5

Too fast Go to Chapter 6

Systolic BP <70 mm Hg[b]
Patient has signs and symptoms of shock

Systolic BP 70 to 100 mm Hg[b]
Patient has signs and symptoms of shock

Systolic BP 70 to 100 mm Hg[b]
Patient has no signs or symptoms of shock

Systolic BP >100 mm Hg[b]
with signs of increased PVR

Consider
- *Norepinephrine* 0.5 to 30 µg/min IV or
- *Dopamine* 5 to 20 µg/kg per minute

- *Dopamine*[c] 2.5 to 20 µg/kg per minute IV (add *norepinephrine* if *dopamine* > 20 µg/kg per minute)

- *Dobutamine*[d] 2.0 to 20 µg/kg per minute IV

- *Nitroglycerin* 10 to 20 µg/min IV and/or
- *Nitroprusside* 0.1 to 5.0 µg/kg per minute IV

For patients in acute pulmonary edema consider following treatments (BP adequate)

First-line treatments (L-M-N-O)
- *Lasix* 0.5 to 1.0 mg/kg IV
- *Morphine* 1 to 3 mg IV
- *Nitroglycerin* sublingual
- *Oxygen*/intubate as needed

Second-line treatments
- *Nitroglycerin* IV if BP > 100 mm Hg
- *Nitroprusside* IV if BP > 100 mm Hg
- *Dopamine* if BP < 100 mm Hg
- *Dobutamine* if BP > 100 mm Hg
- Positive end-expiratory pressure
- Continuous positive airway pressure

Third-line treatments
- *Amrinone* 0.75 mg/kg, then 5 to 15 µg/kg per minute (if other drugs fail)
- *Aminophylline* 5 mg/kg (if wheezing)
- *Thrombolytic* therapy (if not in shock)
- *Digoxin* (if atrial fibrillation, supra-ventricular tachycardias)
- Angioplasty (if drugs fail)
- Intra-aortic balloon pump (as a bridge to emergency surgery)
- Surgical interventions (valves, coronary artery bypass grafts, heart transplant)

(a) Guide treatment after this point by invasive hemodynamic monitoring if possible. Guidelines presume clinical signs of hypoperfusion.

(b) Rapid fluid bolus of at least 250 to 500 mL normal saline should be tried. If clinical response is inadequate, consider sympathomimetics.

(c) Start dopamine and stop norepinephrine when profoundly low BP improves. Dobutamine is preferred over dopamine when there is a hypotension with no signs and symptoms of shock.

(d) If moderate hypotension treated with dobutamine does not respond, add dopamine and reduce or eliminate dobutamine.

Adapted with permission, Journal of the American Medical Association, 1992, Volume 268, *Guidelines for Cardiopulmonary Resuscitation and Emergency Cardiac Care*, p. 2227, copyright © 1992, American Medical Association.

- In addition, you should place the patient in a sitting position, with the legs dependent. This increases lung volume and vital capacity, diminishes the work of respiration, and decreases the venous return to the heart.
- Clinical evaluations have demonstrated that the outdated approach of rotating tourniquets provides no positive benefit.

Oxygenation

- Proper oxygenation is critical for acute pulmonary edema, so pay particular attention to ensuring that oxygenation (Po_2 and oxygen saturation) and ventilation (Pco_2) are acceptable.

- Start with oxygen administration via nasal cannula at 4 to 6 L/min.
- Use oxygen saturation levels to "titrate" oxygen administration.
- Check that the oxygen saturation exceeds 97% to 98%.
- Switch to Venturi mask if oxygen saturation level still remains low. Use high-flow oxygen at a rate of 4 to 8 L/min.
- Switch to partial or nonrebreather mask if Venturi mask does not achieve 97% to 98% oxygen saturation. Nonrebreather masks can yield a concentration of 90% to 100% with reservoir bags.

Understanding and Using the Cardiovascular Triad As a Conceptual Tool *

- *The cardiovascular triad is a useful conceptual tool to use when faced with problems of hypotension, shock, and acute pulmonary edema.*

- *The starting point for Fig. 10-1 is "clinical signs of hypoperfusion, congestive heart failure, acute pulmonary edema." Just below that box is the question, "What is the nature of the problem?" This question asks the clinician to try and classify the patient's condition as a volume (tank) problem, pump problem, or rate problem.*

- *When you approach patients with hypotension or shock, always use the Five Quadrads. Note that part of the fifth quadrad in this memory aid is the cardiovascular triad, which asks the following:*

  - *Is there a volume problem (includes vascular resistance)?*

  - *Is there a pump problem?*

  - *Is there a rate problem?*

- *In this chapter we interchange the term "tank" for "volume" to better convey several of these concepts. The "tank" refers to the following parts of the vascular system:*

  - *Tank size: determined by vasomotor tone (or vascular resistance)*

  - *Tank volume: the volume inside the tank (fluid status)*

- *The cardiovascular triad holds that there are just three determinants of cardiac output, as follows:*

  - *Heart rate (the electrical system)*

  - *Pump performance (contractility)*

  - *Tank, which includes (1) tank size (vascular tone, resistance) and (2) tank volume (contents)*

- *Therefore patients with hypotension, shock, or acute pulmonary edema can be considered to have one (or a combination of two or more) of the following:*

- *Rate problems*

- *Pump problems*

- *Tank problems*

- *In addition, we can subclassify these three types of problems as follows:*

  - *Rate problems: too slow or too fast*

  - *Pump problems: primary or secondary*

  - *Tank problems: (1) absolute (volume loss: bleeding or fluid loss) and (2) relative (vasodilation, vasoconstriction, or redistribution)*

- *The value of identifying the nature of the problem is that we then can select the best therapy for that problem. In addition, when there are multiple or overlapping problems, we know the sequence of problems to treat, as follows:*

  1. *First, correct rate problems if present.*

  2. *Second, correct tank problems if present, with fluid and sometimes pressors.*

  3. *Third, treat pump problems with pressors or inotropes, or both.*

- *Each patient is different, and treatment must be individualized. The following rules, however, will help us to avoid major errors:*

- *Use fluids or pressors when the hypotension is caused by tachycardia or bradycardia (e.g., ventricular tachycardia).*

- *Use pressors instead of volume when the hypotension is caused by tank problems (e.g., shock that is due to gastrointestinal bleeding).*

- *Use fluids when the tank is already too full and the problem is due to the pump (e.g., acute pulmonary edema due to acute myocardial infarction).*

---

* Steve Miller, MD, of Boston Medical Education Group, Inc., conceptualized and developed the "cardiovascular triad." ACLS providers everywhere are indebted to Dr. Miller for this useful conceptual tool.

- Positive end-expiratory pressure (PEEP) can be used to prevent alveolar collapse and improve gas exchange.
- Continuous positive airway pressure (CPAP) can be applied during spontaneous respirations with a tight-fitting mask or endotracheal tube.
- A person skilled in intubation should be available if intubation appears imminent by the following criteria:
  - If Po_2 cannot be maintained above 60 mm Hg, despite 100% oxygen delivery
  - If patient displays signs of cerebral hypoxia (increasing lethargy and obtundation)
  - If patient displays progressive increase in Pco_2 or increasing acidosis

Nitroglycerin

WHY?

- From the perspective of the cardiovascular triad, nitroglycerin helps correct "tank" problems, primarily by making the "tank" (intravascular volume) bigger.
- Most clinicians now consider nitroglycerin to be the most effective agent for acute pulmonary edema. Nitroglycerin has the following effects:
  - Increases venous dilation
  - Inhibits venous return to the heart by its effect on the venous capacitance vessels (reduces preload)
  - Decreases systemic vascular resistance and facilitates cardiac emptying (reduces afterload)
  - Decreases myocardial oxygen consumption
  - Dilates coronary arteries
  - Increases cardiac collateral flow

WHEN?

- Acute pulmonary edema (especially with elevated blood pressure)
- Congestive heart failure
- Chest pain of suspected cardiac origin
- Unstable angina
- Hypertensive crisis or urgency with chest pain
- Elevated blood pressure in setting of AMI (especially with signs of left ventricular failure)

HOW?

- IV infusion is the route of choice for emergencies. It allows precise control of dose and greater predictability of effect.
- Infuse at 10 to 20 μg/min. Titrate to effect. Increase by 5 to 10 μg/min, every 5 to 10 minutes. Use IV infusion sets provided by the manufacturer. Do not mix with other drugs.
- Sublingual nitroglycerin tablets or isosorbide oral spray

permits the initiation of nitrate therapy earlier than personnel can start an IV line.
- Spray inhaler: Repeat every 5 minutes.
- Sublingual: Two standard 0.4-mg tablets can be given every 5 to 10 minutes as long as the systolic blood pressure is greater than 90 to 100 mm Hg. Sublingual nitroglycerin is preferred over nitroglycerin paste or oral isosorbide dinitrate because peripheral vasoconstriction leads to inconsistent skin and gastrointestinal absorption.
- Paste: Apply 1 to 2 inches with backing pad (less preferable).

WATCH OUT!

- Nitroglycerin lowers the blood pressure; therefore use with caution in patients with systolic blood pressures less than 100 mm Hg.
- Avoid dropping the blood pressure below 90 mm Hg.
- If the patient is hypertensive, limit the blood pressure drop to 30% of original levels.
- If the patient is normotensive, limit the blood pressure drop to 10% of original levels.
- Watch for headache, excessive drop in blood pressure, syncope, and tachycardia.
- Instruct the patient to sit or lie down.

Furosemide (Lasix)

WHY?

- Intravenous **furosemide** has long been a mainstay in the treatment of acute pulmonary edema because it reduces the pre-load on the heart through the following actions:
  - First, it causes an immediate decrease in venous tone and thus an increase in venous capacitance. This leads to a fall in left ventricular filling pressure and improves the clinical symptoms. This effect occurs within 5 minutes.
  - Second, it produces a marked diuresis several minutes later, which reaches a peak in 30 to 60 minutes. This diuresis, which does not need to be massive to be effective, also reduces the intravascular volume and thus the left ventricular filling pressures.
  - From the perspective of the cardiovascular triad, furosemide helps correct "tank" problems, primarily by making the "tank" (intravascular volume) bigger with the increase in venous capacitance, and then making the volume in the tank smaller (with the diuresis).

WHEN?

- For adjunctive therapy of acute pulmonary edema in patients with systolic blood pressures greater than 90 to 100 mm Hg
- Hypertensive emergencies or urgencies

HOW?

- Give IV push: 0.5 to 1.0 mg/kg over 1 to 2 minutes.

- If no response in 10 to 15 minutes, double the dose to 2 mg/kg and give slowly over 1 to 2 minutes.

- If the patient is already taking oral furosemide, the clinical rule of thumb is to administer an initial dose that is twice the daily oral dose.

- If no effect occurs within 20 minutes, double the initial dose.

- Use higher doses if the patient has massive fluid retention or renal insufficiency, or both.

WATCH OUT!

- Dehydration

- Hypotension

- Electrolyte imbalance

Morphine sulfate

WHY?

- From the perspective of the cardiovascular triad, morphine sulfate helps correct "tank" problems, primarily by making the "tank" (intravascular volume) bigger and resistance lower. Morphine sulfate has the following effects:

  - Dilates the capacitance vessels of the peripheral venous bed

  - Reduces venous return to the central circulation

  - Diminishes the preload of the heart

  - Decreases the afterload on the heart by mild arterial vasodilation

  - Reduces pain of ischemia

  - Reduces anxiety

WHEN?

- Evidence of vascular congestion (acute pulmonary edema)

- Continuing chest pain

- Blood pressure greater than 90 mm Hg systolic

- No hypovolemia

HOW?

- Give 2 to 5 mg slow IV (over 1 to 5 minutes) at frequent intervals (as often as every 5 minutes).

- Administer slowly and titrate to effect.

WATCH OUT!

- Avoid in volume-depleted patients.

- Morphine sulfate may cause severe drop in blood pressure.

- Avoid in patients with systolic blood pressure less than 90 to 100 mm Hg.

- Morphine sulfate may compromise respiration; therefore use with caution in patients with acute pulmonary edema, since they already have respiratory compromise.

- Reverse respiratory depression with naloxone (0.4 to 2 mg IV).

- Some experts are placing less emphasis on morphine as a major agent to use in acute pulmonary edema (Class IIb, possibly helpful). They question the rationale for giving a strong respiratory depressant to people who have clinical symptoms of drowning.

- NOTE: Because there are now superior vasodilators and more effective inotropes (dobutamine and amrinone), morphine administration in acute pulmonary edema will probably fade from use.

Martin Williamson

CASE 1 Continued

Over the next 30 minutes you treat Mr. Williamson aggressively and simultaneously with the four agents of the first-line treatments. You give oxygen per Venturi mask at 8 L/min which brings an initial oxygen saturation level from 94% to 98%. Morphine 2 mg is administered IV, followed 5 minutes later by a second dose after you notice no change in blood pressure. Two nitroglycerin tablets, 0.4 mg, are placed under Mr. Williamson's tongue as an initial treatment, and a second tablet is given 5 minutes later with the morphine. When the IV is started, you order Lasix 40 mg IV.

Remarkably, within 5 minutes of the nitroglycerin and morphine Mr. Williamson feels much better. His breathing is less labored, and his anxiety has decreased. After 40 minutes he asks for the urinal and produces 500 mL of clear urine. His heart rate decreases to 80 beats/min; his blood pressure drops to 90/60 mm Hg for a brief period and then returns to 100/65 mm Hg.

Does Mr. Williamson need to be admitted? Were there alternative approaches that could have been used? What if he had not improved so quickly?

- The classic, first-line "L-M-N-O" approach to acute pulmonary edema in Case 1 is usually so effective that clinicians fail to realize how ill patients in acute pulmonary edema actually are. Often the patients feel so much better that they want to go home.

- As a general rule, admit patients who come to medical attention in pulmonary edema, even if they "turn around" remarkably well.

- The clinician faces the obligation to determine why the patient's cardiac function suddenly deteriorated to such a degree that the lungs began to fill up with fluid. Occult or silent MI, even with a normal ECG, has to be considered and is a frequent cause of new-onset pulmonary edema.

- Some patients, however, become "frequent fliers" to an Emergency Department with recurrent episodes of cardiac decompensation. They can be quickly and easily "bailed out." Discharge home after consultation with their regular physician is acceptable.

- Most clinicians would have been less aggressive with Mr. Williamson, starting the first-line agents in sequence, waiting to see the response to one agent before moving to the next. Their rationale would be that Mr. Williamson was not so desperately ill that he needed multiple agents all at once. Each one could have "bottomed out" his pressure. Certainly, you should carefully watch the blood pressure when giving nitroglycerin and morphine simultaneously, as was done in Case 1.

- If Mr. Williamson had not improved so quickly you would have had to move to the second-line treatments, which are discussed later in this chapter.

Rudolph Chelminski

CASE 2

ACUTE PULMONARY EDEMA WITH ELEVATED BLOOD PRESSURE
You are working as an "emergency medicine R3" rotating for 6 weeks in the Emergency Department. Mr. Rudolph Chelminski is a 65-year-old Russian immigrant who cannot speak English. The interpreter tells you that Mr. Chelminski just arrived in the United States following a difficult 4-day immigration. He has severe hypertension for which he has taken unknown Russian medications for years. During the confusion of his departure, Mr. Chelminski lost his medications and has been without any treatment for 4 days.

Mr. Chelminski has been triaged and taken back to Room 3A, where the nurse is just completing the patient's assessment. As you walk up, you notice that Mr. Chelminski is sitting upright on the side of the stretcher. His arms are propping him up against his knees while he leans over, working hard to breathe.

How would you begin your evaluation and treatment of this anxious, lonely, and quite ill person?

- Approach Mr. Chelminski exactly as you did Mr. Williamson, using the Five Quadrads, as follows:

  - Primary ABCD Survey
  - Secondary ABCD Survey
  - Oxygen/IV/Monitor/Fluids
  - Temperature/Blood Pressure/Heart Rate/Respirations: 36.8° C, 180/130 mm Hg, 110 beats/min, and 15 breaths/min, respectively
  - Tank (Volume)/Resistance/Pump/Rate
  - Analyze the cardiovascular triad (Volume/Pump/Rate). What is the nature of the problem?
  - *Is there a tank problem?* Yes. The tank is too full. The intravascular volume is increased relative to the ability of the pump to move the volume effectively. Therapy must address this volume problem.
  - *Is there a pump problem?* Yes. Mr. Chelminsky is in congestive failure, and his heart is not pumping the blood effectively. The severe hypertension produces a dramatic increase in the afterload on the myocardium

and increases the failure. These dynamics produce the clinical picture of acute pulmonary edema. Therapy must address this pump problem.

  - *Is there a rate problem?* No. The rate of 110 beats/min is appropriate for the distress of the patient.

- To evaluate D (Differential Diagnosis of the Secondary Survey) you obtain chest x-ray, 12-lead ECG, arterial blood gas studies, and oxygen saturation levels.

- Mr. Chelminski's chest x-ray, pulmonary rales, wheezing and history of severe hypertension (now untreated) lead you to a diagnosis of acute pulmonary edema precipitated by untreated hypertension. In fact, this presentation meets the definition of *hypertensive emergency:* diastolic blood pressure elevations to 130 mm Hg or above *plus* a related systemic complication. In this case the systemic complication is the acute pulmonary edema.

- Turning to the algorithm in Fig. 10-1, we note the first-line treatments to take for acute pulmonary edema: "L-M-N-O" (Lasix-Morphine-Nitroglycerin-Oxygen). However, Mr. Chelminski presents the additional dimension of the severe blood pressure elevation, which must be treated.

- Here is a key rule to remember about the treatment of acute pulmonary edema:

  - **If the blood pressure is too high, you have to lower it.**

  - **If the blood pressure is too low, you have to raise it.**

- Three of the four first-line agents lower the blood pressure, so all three of those agents are immediately appropriate in Mr. Chelminski. (In Case 3 what to do when the blood pressure is too low is discussed.)

- We have classified Mr. Chelminski as having a primary pump problem. Therefore we can follow the arrows in Fig. 10-1 to the box where "Systolic BP" is noted to be >100 mm Hg. Two agents to help lower the elevated blood pressure are listed as follows:

  - **Nitroglycerin** 10 to 20 µg/min IV and/or

  - **Nitroprusside** 0.1 to 5.0 µg/kg per minute IV

Rudolph Chelminski

CASE 2 Continued

You initiate emergency treatment of Mr. Chelminski with all four agents listed in the first-line treatments. You start oxygen per Venturi mask at 8 L/min, carefully watching the oxygen saturation level, which rises from 92% to 96%. Morphine 4 mg is administered IV, followed 5 minutes later by a second 4 mg dose. Nitroglycerin spray (sprayed under tongue for half a second) is given as an initial treatment. You also order Lasix 80 mg IV.

You comment that "we're going to also have to add IV nitroglycerin or nitroprusside to get the blood pressure down quickly." The nurse administering the medications asks, "Well, Doctor, I sure hope you choose nitroglycerin."

What is your decision here? And why?

COMMENTS

- Both nitroglycerin and nitroprusside are effective in lowering the blood pressure in the clinical setting in Case 2.

- The main difference between the two drugs in this case is that nitroprusside may increase myocardial ischemia in patients with coronary artery disease (unclear in this patient).

- Also, nitroprusside is more difficult to use, requiring the drug reservoir to be wrapped in aluminum foil (it is light sensitive), an infusion pump, and preferably intraarterial-pressure catheters and Swan-Ganz catheters.

- See the following comments on the "Why? When? How? and Watch Out!" for nitroglycerin and nitroprusside.

Nitroglycerin

WHY? (Actions)

- Increases venous dilation
- Decreases venous blood return to heart (preload)
- Decreases cardiac afterload
- Decreases myocardial oxygen consumption
- Dilates coronary arteries
- Increases cardiac collateral flow

WHEN? (Indications)

- Acute pulmonary edema (if blood pressure is greater than 100 mm Hg systolic)
- Elevated blood pressure in setting of AMI (especially with signs of left ventricular failure)
- Hypertensive crisis

- Congestive heart failure
- Continued suspected ischemic chest pain
- Unstable angina (change in angina pattern)

HOW? (Dosing)

- IV Infusion: 10 to 20 µg/min; increase by 5 to 10 µg/min every 5 to 10 minutes.
- Use the IV sets provided by the manufacturers. Titrate to effect.
- Do not mix with other drugs.

WATCH OUT! (Precautions)

- Use with extreme caution if systolic blood pressure is less than 90 mm Hg.
- In patients with evidence of AMI, limit systolic blood pressure drop to 10% of original level if patient is normotensive (e.g., 120 to 110 mm Hg, systolic) and to 30% if patient is initially hypertensive (e.g., 180 to 120 mm Hg, systolic).
- Watch for headache, excessive drop in blood pressure, syncope, and tachycardia.
- Instruct patient to sit or lie down.

Nitroprusside

WHY?

- Potent peripheral vasodilator
- Reduces blood pressure by reducing arterial resistance
- Reduces blood pressure by increasing venous capacitance
- In heart failure, increases cardiac output by increasing stroke volume and reducing arterial resistance

- Relief of pulmonary congestion
- Decreases myocardial oxygen consumption

WHEN?

- To treat hypertensive emergencies
- To reduce afterload in heart failure and acute pulmonary edema
- To reduce afterload in acute mitral or aortic regurgitation
- Is drug of second choice in treating congestive heart failure and acute pulmonary edema in patients with coronary artery disease (Nitroglycerin is drug of first choice because of improved coronary blood flow.)

HOW?

- Begin at 0.1 μg/kg per minute and titrate upward every 3 to 5 minutes to desired effect (up to 5 μg/kg per minute).

- Solution and tubing must be wrapped in opaque material.
- Use an infusion pump.
- Action occurs within 1 to 2 minutes.

WATCH OUT!

- Can lower the blood pressure severely, causing stroke, infarction, and cardiac ischemia
- Must be used with hemodynamic monitoring for optimal safety
- Reduces coronary artery perfusion to ischemic myocardium; therefore do not use when patients with acute pulmonary edema also have coronary artery disease and myocardial ischemia

---

Rudolph Chelminski

CASE 2 Continued

Within 30 minutes of his arrival in the Emergency Department you have initiated comprehensive therapy for Mr. Chelminski. You quickly started all four agents of the first-line acute pulmonary edema protocol because the extreme elevation in blood pressure gave you "room to work." Lasix, morphine, and sublingual nitroglycerin each will lower the blood pressure, which is desired.

You thought you needed to concentrate on getting the high blood pressure down, so you added IV nitroprusside 0.1 μg/kg per minute and increased it every 3 minutes to a dose of 2 μg/kg per minute. You selected nitroprusside because it can be stopped immediately if the pressure drops too much. You were worried about "overshooting" on lowering the pressure because of the morphine, Lasix, and nitroglycerin already administered. The nurses were uncomfortable with giving the nitroprusside without invasive hemodynamic monitoring, but you promised them you would stay right with the patient until he leaves for the intensive care unit (ICU).

His blood pressure begins to steadily decrease, and by 30 minutes it measures 160/90 mm Hg. His labored breathing has become much more comfortable, and he is indicating that he needs to urinate. You begin to make arrangements for his transfer to the ICU.

COMMENTS

- Mr Chelminski demonstrates how remarkably sick patients with acute pulmonary edema and hypertensive crisis can be, and yet how dramatically they improve with effective therapy.

- Case 2 also illustrates the key role of the blood pressure in guiding the initial management of patients with acute pulmonary edema: *If the blood pressure is low you must raise it; if the blood pressure is high you must lower it.*

John Tompkins

CASE 3

ACUTE PULMONARY EDEMA WITH LOW BLOOD PRESSURE
You are working in a locum tenens position in a rural Emergency Department on the southwestern coast of Alaska. Mr. John Tompkins, a retired deep-sea-fish processor, is brought in by his anxious wife. The triage nurse became concerned at Mr. Tompkins' severe shortness of breath, his pale color, and sweaty skin. "He almost passed out before I could get him in the wheelchair."

You help the nurses get Mr. Tompkins out of the wheelchair and onto the bed. The effort totally exhausts him, and he lies back gasping for breath, with audible wheezing. His wife says he was complaining of vague chest pain several hours ago and profound weakness.

How would you begin your evaluation of this quietly suffering and extremely ill-appearing man?

COMMENTS

- Once again, use the Five Quadrads to guide your initial evaluation and treatment as follows:
  - Primary ABCD Survey
  - Secondary ABCD Survey: Reveals rales, expiratory wheezing, distended neck veins, peripheral vasoconstriction with cold and clammy skin, and delayed capillary refill on his nail beds
  - Oxygen/IV/Monitor/Fluids
  - Temperature/Blood Pressure/Heart Rate/Respirations: 37.2° C, 75 mm Hg systolic, 110 beats/min, and 25 breaths/min and labored, respectively
  - Tank (Volume)/Resistance/Pump/Rate
- Analyze the cardiovascular triad (Volume/Pump/Rate). What is the nature of the problem?
  - *Is there a tank problem?* Probably. But remember, there are two components to the tank: the size (volume) of the tank and the amount in the tank. With respect to the lungs the patient is fluid overloaded: he is in pulmonary edema. The pulmonary part of the tank is too full. The shock state, however, has produced profound vasoconstriction, which will reduce the size

of the tank. Accurate diagnosis requires invasive hemodynamic monitoring with pulmonary artery (Swan-Ganz) catheter. Such monitoring, however, will not be available to you for some time. This will be a difficult case to manage. Therapy must address both components of this volume problem.
  - *Is there a pump problem?* Yes. Mr. Tompkins is severely ill. He appears to be in congestive heart failure with acute pulmonary edema. More alarming is the severe hypotension: he appears to be in shock. Therapeutic actions must address this pump problem.
  - *Is there a rate problem?* No. The rate of 110 beats/min is appropriate for the distress of the patient.
- To evaluate D (Differential Diagnosis of the Secondary Survey) you obtain chest x-ray, 12-lead ECG, arterial blood gas studies, and oxygen saturation levels.
- Mr. Tompkins' chest x-ray, pulmonary rales, wheezing, low blood pressure, and signs and symptoms of shock lead you to the diagnosis of acute pulmonary edema with cardiogenic shock. Although the 12-lead ECG reveals only nonspecific changes, you suspect that chronic coronary artery disease and possibly an occult AMI lie at the root of Mr. Tompkins' presentation.

John Tompkins

CASE 3 Continued

You quickly complete the patient's history and physical examination. His story is one of steadily progressive shortness of breath and weakness over several hours. There is nothing to suggest occult gastrointestinal bleeding (the stool guaiac test was negative), dehydration from vomiting or diarrhea, or other significant medical illnesses.

You send for a stat finger-stick hematocrit and electrolyte and arterial blood gas studies and instruct the nurse to insert a urinary catheter to measure urine output every 15 minutes. You request a bed for admission to the Critical Care Unit. The oxygen saturation level cannot be obtained because of the profound vasoconstriction.

The nurse wants to know how fast to run the IV infusion of normal saline and whether there are any medications you want to give. What would be your response?

COMMENTS

- In a profoundly hypotensive patient like Mr. Tompkins you must be certain that the ventricular filling pressures are adequate. Since he is in acute pulmonary edema, unnecessary volume expansion could make his condition worse. Without invasive hemodynamic measures you cannot decide whether the filling pressures are adequate. You decide to just run the fluids at a keep-open rate.

- If the pulmonary edema was not present, it would be appropriate to administer **a fluid bolus of 250 to 500 mL of normal saline.** (See footnote b in Fig. 10-1.) If the patient shows some improvement, use repeat fluid boluses. If there is no response, go to pressor agents.

- Review Fig. 10-1. This algorithm contains important guidelines for the use of pressor agents and inotropic agents in patients with hypotension.

- Note that Mr. Tompkins falls under the category in the box for "Systolic BP 70 to 100 mm Hg" with "signs and symptoms of shock." Mr. Tompkins has the indications for starting dopamine 2.5 to 20 μg/kg per minute IV. You should go immediately to the high-dose "vasopressor doses" (10 to 20 μg/kg per minute).

- If dopamine at the higher dose range does not produce clinical improvement, *add* **norepinephrine 0.5 to 1.0 mg/min and tirate up to 30 μg/min IV.**

- Note that Fig.10-1 guides us regarding what drug to select if Mr. Tompkins were in acute pulmonary edema but *without* signs and symptoms of shock. In such a case, start **dobutamine** infusion at 2.0 to 20 μg/kg per minute.

- For patients so severely ill you must continue to follow the Secondary Survey D (Differential Diagnosis). Consider the possible causes of the pump failure, in particular, reversible causes. (See Table 10-1.)

TABLE 10-1

Causes of Problems With the Cardiovascular Triad: Volume/Pump/Rate

Rate Problems	Pump Problems	Tank Problems (Volume)
Too Slow • Sinus bradycardia • Types I and II second-degree heart block • Third-degree heart block • Pacemaker failures	**Primary** • Myocardial infarction • Cardiomyopathies • Myocarditis • Ruptured chordae • Acute papillary muscle dysfunction • Acute aortic insufficiency • Prosthetic valve dysfunction • Ruptured intraventricular septum	**Absolute** • Tank is empty; volume moves out of tank. 　• Hemorrhage 　• Gastrointestinal tract loss 　• Renal losses 　• Insensible losses 　• Adrenal insufficiency (aldosterone)
Too Fast • Sinus tachycardia • Atrial flutter • Atrial fibrillation • Paroxysmal supraventricular tachycardia • Ventricular tachycardia	**Secondary** • Drugs that alter function • Cardiac tamponade • Pulmonary embolus • Atrial myxomata • Superior vena cava syndrome	**Relative** • Tank changes size; therefore volume is no longer adequate; vasodilatation has occurred. 　• Central nervous system injury 　• Spinal injury 　• Third-space loss 　• Adrenal insufficiency (cortisol) 　• Sepsis 　• Drugs that alter tone

(Based upon Table 3. 1994 AHA Textbook of ACLS, pp. 1-40.)

John Tompkins

CASE 3 Continued

You start **dopamine** 10 µg/kg per minute IV, increasing it by 5 µg every 5 minutes until you get to 20 µg/kg per minute. After 15 minutes he begins to look better. His blood pressure is now 100/70; his heart rate has dropped to 96 beats/min, and respirations are still 20 per minute. However, he continues to have jugular venous distention, rales, and an S^3 gallop, and he remains short of breath. He coughs up some pink, frothy sputum. His extremities are not as cool, and capillary refill has improved to less than 1 second. The arterial blood gas studies with the patient receiving on 4 L/min of oxygen reveal that pH = 7.26, P_{O_2} = 60, and P_{CO_2} = 50.

What would you consider adding at this point?

COMMENTS

- Mr. Tompkins' blood pressure has improved, but he continues in pulmonary edema. His signs of shock are better.

- At this point you could add **dobutamine 2 to 20 µg/kg per minute IV**. Note that Figure 10-1 on p. 181 shows how, with increasing blood pressures and decreasing signs of shock, it is acceptable to try a more pure inotrope such as **dobutamine.** The combination of dopamine and dobutamine for cardiogenic shock has been used with success.

- The critical point is you have not yet begun to definitively alter the tank problems producing the acute pulmonary edema. Fig. 10-1 demonstrates that as you get the blood pressures up and signs of shock decrease, you can provide vasodilators (**nitroglycerin 10 to 20 µg/min or nitroprusside 0.1 to 5.0 µg/kg per minute or both**) to treat the acute pulmonary edema.

- Since dobutamine has vasodilation effects, you can give a trial of just dopamine and dobutamine for some minutes to see whether Mr. Tompkins improves.

- The arterial blood gas studies indicate that you need to improve the ventilation; switch to a nonrebreather mask at 12 L/min, or consider bag-valve-mask ventilations. Endotracheal intubation will be needed soon, if he does not significantly improve.

- You could also give low doses of **IV nitroglycerin** for preload reduction and also to decrease myocardial ischemia. Consider low doses of **Lasix.**

- Fig. 10-1 provides a useful listing of the second-line and third-line treatments that can be used in refractory acute pulmonary edema.

John Tompkins

CASE 3 Continued

You have been treating Mr. Tompkins for 55 minutes, and he is looking better. His blood pressure has remained stable (95 to 105 mm Hg systolic) on dopamine 15 µg/kg per minute IV (down from 20) and dobutamine 5 µg/kg per minute. You started a slow nitroglycerin infusion at 10 µg/min IV, and the blood pressure did not drop. Lasix 20 mg IV bolus has resulted in a diuresis of 400 mL of urine. The signs of peripheral vasoconstriction have abated, and the peripheral mottling has disappeared.

His most recent blood gas levels were as follows: Po_2 = 110; Pco_2 = 45, and pH = 7.3 on 100% oxygen via nonrebreathing mask. His rales have decreased, and his labored respiration is much less pronounced. You are beginning to think he can be transferred to the ICU; the on-call cardiologist has arrived and has instructed the nurses in the ICU to make preparations for insertion of an arterial pressure line and a Swan-Ganz catheter.

What if Mr. Tompkins had remained in acute pulmonary edema and either worsened or did not improve? What approaches could you have taken?

COMMENTS

SECOND-LINE TREATMENTS

- **Nitroglycerin** IV if blood pressure is greater than 100 mm Hg

- **Nitroprusside** IV if blood pressure is greater than 100 mm Hg

- **Dopamine** if blood pressure is less than 100 mm Hg

- **Dobutamine** if blood pressure is greater than 100 mm Hg

- **Positive end-expiratory pressure**

- **Continuous positive airway pressure**

- Notice that Mr. Tompkins actually received three of these four medications as part of his acute treatment. Remember the rule: In treating acute pulmonary edema, if the blood pressure is too low, you must first raise it. This is because the first-line agents all lower the blood pressure and are relatively contraindicated.

- The dopamine was used as the critical pressor-inotrope to provide arterial vasoconstriction and improve the pumping effectiveness of the heart. Thus dopamine works on both the "Tank (Volume)" and the "Pump" of the cardiovascular triad.

- Dobutamine is another potent inotrope that stimulates β_1 = adrenergic and α_1 = adrenergic receptors in the heart. Because it has vasodilatory effects that could lower the blood pressure, it becomes indicated only when the systolic blood pressure is not in the severely depressed range (70 to 100 mm Hg in Fig. 10-1).

- As a potent vasodilator, nitroglycerin is the mainstay of treatment. **Nitroglycerin** was administered to Mr.

Tompkins as soon as the dopamine and dobutamine raised the blood pressure enough to tolerate nitroglycerin's hypotensive effects. A major advantage of nitroglycerin is the ability to accurately titrate the amount of IV nitroglycerin while monitoring closely the hemodynamic effects.

- Use the other second-line vasoactive agents according to the hemodynamic subsets (Fig. 10-1), as follows:

  - **Nitroprusside** (pressure needs to come down)

  - **Dopamine** (pressure needs to come up)

  - **Dobutamine** (normotensive pump failure)

- The third-line treatments are reserved for patients with pump failure and acute pulmonary edema who resist the first-line and second-line treatments, or who have specific complications.

THIRD-LINE TREATMENTS

- **Amrinone** 0.75 mg/kg; then 5 to 15 µg/kg per minute IV (if other drugs fail) if blood pressure is greater than 100 mm Hg

- **Aminophylline** 5 mg/kg (if wheezing)

- **Thrombolytic** therapy (if not in shock)

- **Digoxin** (if atrial fibrillation, supraventricular tachycardias)

- **Angioplasty** (if drugs fail)

- Intraaortic balloon pump (bridge to surgery)

- Surgical interventions (valves, coronary artery bypass grafts, heart transplant)

- Most of the third-line treatments require invasive hemodynamic monitoring in an ICU, or specialized tertiary care facilities, but they are mentioned here for completeness.

The ACLS provider should be aware of these treatments, however, and recognize patients with the indications for such treatments as thrombolytic therapy or acute angioplasty, as follows:

- **Amrinone** (loading dose of 0.75 mg/kg over 2 to 3 minutes, followed by 5 to 15 µg/kg per minute) produces inotropic and vasodilatory effects similar to those with dobutamine.

- **Aminophylline** (loading dose of 5 mg/kg given over 10 to 20 minutes, followed by 0.5 to 0.7 mg/kg per hour) helps patients with acute bronchospasm ("cardiac asthma"), although it is used only for severe bronchospasm. Avoid aminophylline in patients with arrhythmias associated with ischemic heart disease.

- **Thrombolytics** have a limited role in patients with the combination of AMI and cardiogenic shock. Cardiogenic shock in the setting of an AMI is a classic indication for emergency angioplasty and intraaortic balloon pumping.

- **Angioplasty** has become the treatment of choice in AMI patients with presentation as cardiogenic shock.

- Table 10-1 presents several surgically correctable conditions that produce either primary or secondary pump problems. If diagnosed early some of these conditions will result in patients being candidates for acute surgical treatment, as follows:
  - Coronary artery bypass grafts
  - Repair of mitral valve insufficiency caused by ruptured chordae or papillary muscles
  - Repair of acute aortic valve insufficiency
  - Repair of prosthetic valve dysfunction
  - Repair of ruptured intraventricular septum
  - Cardiac transplantation
  - Intraaortic balloon counter-pulsation
  - Total artificial hearts, which can successfully "bridge" these patients until their operation or until a nonsurgical recovery

---

Robert Allen, MD

CASE 4

PURE VOLUME PROBLEM: OCCULT GASTROINTESTINAL TRACT BLEEDING FROM CHRONIC NONSTEROIDAL ANTIINFLAMMATORY AGENT INGESTION
You are the "attending" in the Emergency Department and have just signed out to Robert Allen, MD, your 46-year-old fellow faculty member. While sitting in the write-up area reviewing charts, one of the department secretaries comes running up shouting, "Somebody come help me. Dr. Allen has collapsed in the nurses' lounge!"

You arrive to find your pale, ashen-looking colleague being lifted from the sofa to a stretcher. Thirty minutes before, he had appeared normal and offered no complaints. He is drenched with sweat and seems confused and slightly dazed. "Does he have a pulse?" you ask. Someone replies that the pulse was 130 and weak.

As you walk quickly with the gurney to one of the examination rooms, you consider Dr. Allen's history of previous hypertension, for which you knew he refused to take medications. "Takes the fire out of my belly," he used to say.

How would you approach the initial evaluation and treatment of your colleague?

COMMENTS

For potential cardiovascular emergencies always start with the Five Quadrads, as follows:

- Primary ABCD Survey: The patient is not in cardiac arrest.
  - Secondary ABCD Survey reveals peripheral vasoconstriction with cold, clammy skin and delayed capillary refill on his nail beds. The lungs are clear without rales or congestion. Abdomen and cardiac examination are normal. You learn that Dr. Allen has been taking piroxicam 60 mg twice a day for several months for chronic low back pain. Rectal examination reveals gross melanotic stool. For the D of the Secondary Survey (Differential Diagnosis) you order chest x-rays, 12-lead ECG, electrolyte studies, white blood cell count, and hematocrit.
  - Temperature/Blood Pressure/Heart Rate/Respirations: 36.8° C, 80 mm Hg systolic, 130 beats/min, and 12 breaths/min, respectively.
  - Oxygen/IV/Monitor/Fluids: He is in sinus tachycardia.

- Analyze the cardiovascular triad (Volume/Pump/Rate). What is the nature of the problem?
  - *Is there a rate problem?* No. The rate of 130 beats/min is an appropriate response to the hypotension.
  - *Is there a pump problem?* Not clear at this time. The initial 12-lead ECG displays signs of left ventricular hypertrophy with inverted T waves in the precordial leads. He has marked hypotension: he appears to be in borderline shock.
  - *Is there a tank problem?* Probably. The tachycardia appears compensatory for the low blood pressure. The blood in the stool suggests a gastrointestinal bleeding episode that may have been induced by the chronic use of a potent nonsteroidal antiinflammatory medication.

- You decide to push a bolus of normal saline and order 500 mL of normal saline to run in "wide open."

Robert Allen, MD

CASE 4 Continued

While the fluid is running in, you complete your examination and notice that Dr. Allen is alert and oriented, although weak. His skin, initially pale and moist, rapidly begins to "pink up." Capillary refill time is less than 1 second. The weakness and dizziness begin to resolve. Within 20 minutes his blood pressure is 110/70 and his heart rate is 90 beats/min. You order a nasogastric tube placed, and during the placement Dr. Allen gags and vomits several times. The emesis is almost pure, dark blood. The initial hematocrit returns: 28%.

Dr. Allen reports that he had been feeling "like I had the flu all day," getting light-headed when suddenly standing or walking quickly. When he came to work he kept taking his temperature, thinking it should be up (it was 36.5° C), and found he had to carry a washcloth in his coat pocket to wipe his sweat-covered face before going in to see patients. He had gone to the Emergency Department restroom with cramping abdominal pain and found grossly melanotic stool in the toilet. He briefly passed out on the floor of the bathroom but recovered enough to get to the nurses' lounge before passing out again.

Does Dr. Allen have hypovolemic shock from a severe gastrointestinal bleed?

COMMENTS

- A key point to understand: You do not diagnose "shock" based on the blood pressure alone. The "shock state" refers to a condition that is taking place at the tissue level: oxygen and metabolic substrates are not being delivered to the tissues effectively enough to meet the metabolic demands. Therefore the signs of "shock" are signs of inadequate organ and tissue perfusion.

- The major signs and symptoms of shock are as follows:

  - Compensatory mechanisms: Increased heart rate, increased cardiac output and diversion of blood flow from the skin and from the mesenteric and renal circulation

  - Poor tissue perfusion: Acidosis; cyanosis; cool, mottled skin; and poor capillary refill

  - Poor organ perfusion: Mental status changes, or decreased urine output, weakness, and nausea

- "Shock" can occur with normal, increased, or decreased blood pressure. "Compensated shock" occurs when the blood pressure is slightly decreased or actually normal. "Decompensated shock" occurs with hypotension, low cardiac output, and inadequate tissue perfusion.

- A critical point in the management of shock: Identify the shock state and correct it before the tissues and organs of the patient deteriorate irreversibly. In children, especially, a key goal is recognize the subtlety of "compensated shock" and initiate therapy before the patient "decompensates" toward irreversible shock and even cardiac arrest.

- Based on the preceding definitions, Dr. Allen had "compensated hypovolemia" for several hours before his collapse in the bathroom. He could no longer maintain that compensation, suffered decreased blood flow to his brain and "passed out" twice. The ease of his fluid resuscitation suggests that he had only minimal compromise of organ and tissue perfusion.

Charlene Bradley

CASE 5

PURE VOLUME PROBLEM

You are the Emergency Department attending physician in a suburban community hospital at 8 AM. The nurse tells you that the next patient for you to see is 22-year-old Charlene Bradley, who "looks pretty sick." She was seen by the nurse practitioner the previous day for "the flu" and was given Compazine suppositories for a syndrome of nausea, vomiting, myalgias, and weakness. Her boyfriend brings her in this morning because "she's just getting worse and now she ain't talking sense."

When you enter Room 3B, it is obvious that Ms. Bradley is extremely ill. Her temperature is 38.9° C; she is flushed and warm and somewhat confused, resisting the nurse's efforts to start an IV line.

How would you approach Ms. Bradley?

- Always start with the Five Quadrads.

- The Five Quadrads can be a great help with patients like Ms. Bradley, when you are not going to be able to depend on the patient for a useful history. You can fall back on the 20 items of the Five Quadrads to make sure your evaluation is complete and to make sure you identify the most life-threatening problems, as follows:

  - Primary ABCD Survey

  - Secondary ABCD Survey reveals extremely warm, flushed skin, with an almost confluent rash across her trunk. Hands and feet are not moist; there is no clamminess. She has a bounding pulse, clear lungs, and rapid heart beat with no murmurs or abnormal sounds.

  - Oxygen/IV/Monitor/Fluids

  - Temperature/Blood Pressure/Heart Rate/Respirations: 38.9° C, 70 mm Hg systolic, 130 beats/min, and 20 breaths/min and labored, respectively.

- Analyze the cardiovascular triad (Volume/Pump/Rate). What is the nature of the problem?

  - *Is there a tank problem?* Yes! The blood pressure is low, and the tachycardia does not compensate for the relative volume problem. This is a classic clinical presentation for "warm shock" in which extreme vasodilation occurs. This is opposite from the "cool shock" of marked peripheral vasoconstriction with cold, clammy extremities. Think in terms of the two components to the tank: the size (volume) of the tank and the amount in the tank. Ms. Bradley appears to be abnormal in both components: she has relative hypovolemia because of the peripheral vasodilation (makes the tank bigger) and because of probable redistribution of fluids to third spaces (makes the volume smaller).

  - *Is there a pump problem?* No. Remember that pump problems refer to either contractility or valve problems. In this young, previously healthy woman without murmurs or rales a pump problem is unlikely.

  - *Is there a rate problem?* No. The rate of 130 beats/min is appropriate for the fever and in response to the low blood pressure.

- The Primary-Secondary Survey Approach teaches us to initiate therapy whenever we identify an urgent problem. Since you identified the profound hypotension, temperature elevation, and tachycardia on the Secondary Survey, you order a second large-bore IV catheter started and request a liter of normal saline to run wide open in each arm.

Charlene Bradley

CASE 5 Continued

As the nurses are starting the 16-gauge catheters in each antecubital space, you begin to consider the differential diagnosis. This is certainly "warm shock" in which vasodilation is most often caused by bacterial sepsis. Anaphylactic shock would also produce the decrease in systemic vascular resistance and redistribution of fluid that you are seeing here. You review the recent history with the boyfriend, who states that Ms. Bradley is taking no regular medications and that the only thing new was the Compazine suppository she took yesterday. The high temperature makes you think of urosepsis or pyelonephritis, but she has had no recent urinary tract complaints. You send off a stat "cath urine" analysis and the nurse doing the catheterization points out that there is a tampon string protruding from Ms. Bradley's vagina.

After 20 minutes of "wide-open" IVs, the automated blood pressure cuff shows a blood pressure of 70 mm Hg systolic and the heart rate remains elevated at 120 beats per minute.

How would you proceed at this point?

- Suddenly the picture becomes more clear. The discovery of the tampon and the information that Ms. Bradley's recent "flu like" illness occurred during her menstrual period makes "toxic shock syndrome" highly likely. The clinical presentation you are dealing with—fever, early erythematous rash, flushed skin, warm shock, and altered mentation—is consistent with that diagnosis.

- In addition, the working diagnosis of toxic shock syndrome has major therapeutic implications, since it gives you a greater sense of the urgency of the situation. Knowledge of the probable diagnosis tells you that therapy must be rapid and aggressive, because shock from vasodilation and fluid redistribution often requires massive amounts of fluids and vasopressors.

- NOTE: Ms. Bradley has not improved with rapid volume replacement, even though the nature of her problem is a tank problem. You must now consider **vasopressors.** Volume problems are treated (see Fig. 10-1) with either fluid (to "fill the tank") or vasopressors (to increase vasoconstriction and therefore decrease the size of the tank).

- **A key point:** Volume replacement is the treatment of choice for hemorrhagic and hypovolemic shock. *Do not treat hypovolemia with vasopressors without also giving aggressive volume replacement.* Only use vasopressors simultaneously with volume replacement or when circulating blood volume is adequate.

- Fig. 10-1 provides guidance on which vasopressors to use: **norepinephrine 0.5 to 30 µg/min IV or dopamine 5 to 20 µg/kg per minute.**

Charlene Bradley

CASE 5 Continued

You order a dopamine drip at 15 µg/kg per minute along with continued wide-open fluids in each arm. In 5 minutes you increase the dopamine to 20 µg/kg per minute and find that the blood pressure has increased to 90 mm Hg systolic. You have given a total of 4 L of normal saline and are starting to worry about fluid overload. Clearly, the "tank" needs to get smaller, so you decide to add an additional vasopressor of norepinephrine at 10 µg/min IV.

The addition of norepinephrine seems to work. The blood pressure increases to 110/70 mm Hg systolic and remains at 100 to 110 over the next hour. You drop the fluids to normal saline at 500 mL/hour and call the admitting physician covering the ICU.

Are there other "tank" problems that require volume plus specific vasoactive agents?

COMMENTS

- ACLS courses often cannot cover the richness of many resuscitation situations. The ACLS course teaches standardized approaches to common problems. The difficulty is that common problems rarely occur in a predictable manner. There are always "wrinkles" to every cardiopulmonary emergency. Therefore ACLS providers need to learn the details and "special features" of different types of emergencies.

- Toxic shock and anaphylactic shock are two examples of the preceding problem—rescuers must adjust their routine resuscitation protocols to give their patients the best chance of survival. A person collapsed in the radiology suite from a pseudoallergic reaction to contrast media may go into VF. Rigidly following the VF protocol, however, may not succeed in saving this patient because the rescuer does not realize that something else is needed. This "something else" includes very aggressive fluid replacement, IV corticosteroids, and confident use of multiple vasopressors, as were required in Case 5.

- Other "tank" problems in which simply refilling the tank may not succeed include the following; these patients need specific vasoactive agents and interventions:

  - **Septic shock**: Dopamine, norepinephrine, dobutamine, and phenylephrine

  - **Anaphylactic shock**: Epinephrine, dopamine, norepinephrine, and phenylephrine

  - **Spinal shock**: Dopamine and phenylephrine

  - **Beta blocker overdose**: Epinephrine, atropine, glucagon, dopamine, and isoproterenol

  - **Alpha blocker overdose**: Epinephrine and norepinephrine

SUMMARY

- The ACLS provider needs a systematic approach to patients with acute pulmonary edema, hypotension, and shock. These complicated clinical states challenge even the most experienced caregiver.

- We think Fig. 10-1, the algorithm for acute pulmonary edema and alterations in perfusion and blood pressure, offers a great deal of guidance in dealing with these states. The algorithm asks the clinician to determine the nature of the clinical problems by using the cardiovascular triad.

- With this tool you ask whether the problem is one or more of the following:

  - A tank problem (includes both tank size and tank contents)

  - A pump problem

  - A rate problem

- By asking these questions you not only diagnose the problem, but also receive information on treatment priorities: treat rate problems first, then volume problems, and then pump problems.

- We have incorporated the cardiovascular triad into the Five Quadrads. This list of 20 clinical items that is used to review and initiate treatment guides the ACLS provider through the initial evaluation and treatment of all cardiopulmonary emergencies. By using these conceptual tools you can help your patients in a calm, effective manner, no matter how sick they are.

Toxicologic and Electrolyte Abnormalities

OVERVIEW

ACLS providers must always consider the cause of any cardiopulmonary emergency. Identification of the cause of the cardiac arrest, however, only has value if it changes therapy. The D portion of the Secondary ABCD Survey focuses the attention of the ACLS provider, in particular, the team leader, on these two questions: Why did the person have the arrest and Are there reversible causes? Note that the algorithms for Pulseless Electrical Activity (PEA) (Fig. 5-1) and Asystole (Fig. 6-1) explicitly list "Consider Possible Causes" before the administration of medications. Often the only possibility for successful resuscitation lies with identification and treatment of reversible causes of cardiac arrest.

This chapter presents cardiac arrest cases that have specific causes and specific therapies. These causes are **toxicologic** *and* **electrolyte abnormalities**. *The "core" ACLS course does not present such cases separately, other than toxicologic and electrolyte abnormalities that lead to the four "lethal" rhythms of ventricular fibrillation (VF), pulseless ventricular tachycardia (VT), PEA, and asystole.*

We think it important, however, to present cases involving toxicologic and electrolyte problems. We recommend starting "at the top"—when things are beginning to go bad—rather than "at the bottom," after the arrest has occurred. Sometimes (but not always) ACLS providers will follow different protocols when the arrest is due to drug overdoses or metabolic or electrolyte abnormalities. On most occasions, however, once an arrest occurs, the primary approach to resuscitation remains the same, as follows:

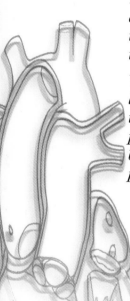

- *Airway maintenance*

- *Breathing and ventilation*

- *Circulation of blood*

- *Defibrillation when indicated*

- *Pharmacologic interventions (pressors, isotropes, rate control, and antiarrhythmics) when indicated.*

Different Emphases in Toxicologic and Electrolyte Abnormalities

You should recognize, however, the following different emphases in toxicologic and electrolyte emergencies:

- *Focus on early diagnosis—when the person is "on his or her way to a cardiac arrest."*

- *Learn specific antidotes for specific overdoses or metabolic abnormalities (when they exist).*

- *Know to adjust the ACLS protocols for specific abnormalities.*

- *Learn when to initiate novel interventions such as transcutaneous pacing, dialysis, and extracorporeal bypass.*

- *Be aware of the need to persist for longer periods of CPR and ACLS while awaiting metabolism or dissipation of the offending agent. (For example, people have survived tricyclic overdoses by being sustained for 6 to 8 hours with basic CPR chest compressions.)*

MAJOR CONCEPTS TO MASTER

- **Apply the Five Quadrads to the initial management of cardiac arrest resulting from toxicologic and electrolyte abnormalities.**
- **Know the actions to help reverse toxicologic and electrolyte abnormalities.**
- **Initiate appropriate treatment on discovery of toxicologic and electrolyte abnormalities.**
- **Apply the D=(Differential Diagnosis) of the Secondary Survey in the hunt for reversible causes of toxicologic and electrolyte abnormalities.**

Critical actions

The critical actions in treating patients with toxicologic and electrolyte abnormalities are the following:

- Perform the steps of the Primary-Secondary ABCD Survey, and the Universal, PEA, and Asystole Algorithms.
- Perform CPR when indicated.
- Properly attach and operate defibrillator/monitor.
- Recognize arrhythmias and ECG abnormalities that are due to toxicologic and electrolyte abnormalities (Tables 11-1 to 11-4).
- Recognize the need for and successful performance of endotracheal intubation.
- Establish IV access.
- Know specific treatment approaches for the major electrolyte abnormalities (Tables 11-2 to 11-4).
- Consider the differential diagnoses.

Rhythms and ECG findings to learn

Tables 11-1 to 11-4 summarize typical ECG findings with electrolyte and toxicology problems. Learn ECG findings associated with the following:

- Hyperkalemia and hypokalemia
- Hypercalcemia and hypocalcemia
- Hypermagnesemia and hypomagnesemia
- Cyclic antidepressant overdose
- Neuroleptic overdose
- Cocaine intoxication
- Beta blocker overdose
- Calcium channel blocker overdose
- Digitalis intoxication
- Narcotic overdose
- Benzodiazepine overdose

Additional medications to learn

Know the "How? When? Why? and Watch Out!" for the following:

- Glucagon

Review of the Five Quadrads Approach

PRIMARY ABCD SURVEY	SECONDARY ABCD SURVEY		
AIRWAY	**AIRWAY**	• *Ensure that chest wall moves with each ventilation.*	*rhythm and vital signs.*
• *Open the airway.*	• *Determine the effectiveness of the original ventilation and airway techniques.*	• *Listen for bilateral breath sounds.*	**DIFFERENTIAL DIAGNOSES**
BREATHING		**CIRCULATION**	• *Consider the possible causes of the cardiac emergency.*
• *Provide positive-pressure ventilation.*	• *Perform endotracheal intubation if indicated.*	• *Continue chest compressions.*	
CIRCULATION	**BREATHING**	• *Obtain IV access.*	**OXYGEN/IV/MONITOR/ FLUIDS**
• *Perform chest compressions.*	• *Determine that endotracheal tube is patent and properly placed.*	• *Attach monitor leads.*	**TEMPERATURE/BLOOD PRESSURE/HEART RATE/ RESPIRATIONS**
DEFIBRILLATION		• *Identify rhythm and rate.*	
• *Identify and shock VF/pulseless VT.*	• *Provide positive-pressure ventilations through endotracheal tube.*	• *Measure blood pressures.*	**TANK (VOLUME)/ RESISTANCE/PUMP/RATE**
		• *Administer medications appropriate for the*	

- Fab antibodies
- Flumazenil

The electrolyte disorders cases

The cases in this chapter introduce particular electrolyte and toxicologic problems. We will not present the detailed man-agement of each case because the systematic and routine approaches will be very similar: the Five Quadrads approach featuring the Primary-Secondary Survey (see box on p. 197). We do present, however, those points in diagnosis and treat-ment that are different from the routine Primary-Secondary ABCD Survey Approach.

Shannon Patterson

CASE 1

HYPERKALEMIA PLUS ACIDOSIS

You are a second-year medicine resident on duty in the Emergency Department. You are caring for a 27-year-old woman who has end-stage renal disease as a result of insulin-dependent diabetes. Recent emotional problems have led her to miss her last two scheduled dialyses, and she comes in pro-foundly weak, fatigued, and short of breath.

Your initial evaluation, following the Five Quadrads, identifies the following:

- *Decreased sensorium, slight confusion, looks ill and weak, mild rales on pulmonary auscultation*
- *Diagnostic evaluation: Finger-stick glucose level is 260; other lab tests sent for include elec-trolyte, blood urea nitrogen (BUN), creatinine, and arterial blood gas studies, portable chest x-ray, and 12-lead ECG*
- *Oxygen, nasal cannula at 6 L/min; IV, 16-gauge in left antecubital vein; monitor, Fig. 11-1; flu-ids, normal saline, keep veins open.*
- *Temperature = 36.8°, blood pressure = 130/90 mm Hg; heart rate = 98 beats/min; Respirations = 18 breaths/min and somewhat distressed.*

With this information alone you should be worried about hyperkalemia and acidosis. How would you approach this woman? What changes do you look for on the ECG to indicate an elevated serum potassium (K) level?

COMMENTS

- What you see on the rhythm strips are the following:
- Prolonged PR interval (first-degree heart block)
- Flattened P waves
- Tall, peaked (tenting) T waves
- ST segment depression, S and T wave merging
- Widened QRS complex
- You should combine the history, the physical examin-ation, and the ECG to make a tentative diagnosis of severe hyperkalemia. The known oliguric renal failure, the missed dialyses, and the weakness all support a diagnosis of hyperkalemia.
- You should consider treatment at once, even before you receive the report of the serum potassium levels.
- The serum potassium levels and the ECG generally corre-late, as displayed in Fig. 11-2 and Table 11-1.

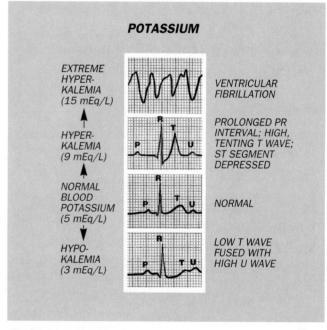

Fig. 11-1:
Potassium effects on the ECG: hypokalemia to hyperkalemia.

TABLE 11-1 Correlations Between Serum Potassium Levels and ECG

Serum Potassium Level	ECG Findings
5.6 to 6.0 mEq/L	*Tall, peaked T waves, best seen in the precordial leads; due to accelerated repolarization*
6.0 to 6.5 mEq/L	*Prolonged PR intervals; prolonged QT intervals; due to decreased impulse conduction*
6.5 to 7.0 mEq/L	*Diminished P waves, ST-segment depression (occasional elevation can be seen)*
7.0 to 7.5 mEq/L	*Delayed conduction in atrioventricular node leads to idioventricular rhythms and possibly to bundle branch blocks*
7.5 to 8.0 mEq/L	*P waves disappear; QRS complex widens; S and T wave merging; may display hyperkalemic sine wave; irregular ventricular rhythms*
8 to 12 mEq/L	*Classic hyperkalemia sine wave is seen*
> 15 mEq/L	*Frequently ventricular fibrillation deteriorating to asystole*

Shannon Patterson

CASE 1 Continued

Your first thought is to give Lasix 40 mg IV bolus, especially since Shannon's pulmonary examination indicates she is fluid overloaded; but since Shannon's renal function is so poor, that approach will not be very successful.

Just as the laboratory results come back indicating severe acidosis with hyperkalemia (K = 8.2 mEq/L; pH = 6.9), Shannon goes into a wide-complex tachycardia (Fig. 11-2).

What are the major approaches to treatment of severe hyperkalemia, and how would you treat Shannon?

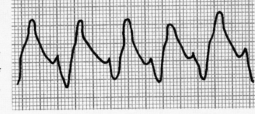

Fig. 11-2: Shannon Patterson's wide-complex tachycardia due to high potassium level.

COMMENTS

- Conceptually, it is important to understand that you can attack emergency hyperkalemia on the following fronts:

  - **Mild hyperkalemia** (5.0 to 6.0 mEq/L): Remove the potassium from the body (*diuretics, cation exchange resin, peritoneal dialysis,* or *hemodialysis*).

  - **Moderate elevations** (6.0 to 7.0 mEq/L): Also shift or redistribute the potassium from outside the cells to inside the cells (use *insulin plus glucose*).

  - **Severe elevations** (>7.0 mEq/L with toxic ECG changes): *Also* antagonize the toxic effects of high levels of potassium in the myocardium, lowering the membrane potential and reducing risks of a ventricular arrhythmia (*calcium gluconate* or *calcium chloride*).

- Table 11-2 presents the actions you can take to treat severe hyperkalemia.

- You could use all three approaches for Shannon's severe hyperkalemia with the alarming wide-complex tachycardia. She is just moments away from a lethal sine wave, idioventricular rhythm, or ventricular fibrillation (VF).

Shannon Patterson

CASE 1 Continued

You order sodium bicarbonate, one ampule (50 mEq); plus calcium chloride 10 mL of a 10% solution; plus 10 units of regular insulin; plus 50% dextrose in water, one ampule. The QRS complexes begin to narrow within 2 minutes, and the rhythm is much more regular and stable.

You call the renal dialysis team on 5-South and make arrangements to admit Shannon for further treatment. The hemodialysis team, however, will take at least 1 to 2 hours to set up. Are there any additional actions you would take?

TABLE 11-2 Emergency Treatment of Hyperkalemia

Therapy	Dose	Mechanism of Effect	Onset of Effect	Duration of Effect
Sodium bicarbonate	1 mEq/kg IV bolus	Shifts	5 to 10 min	1 to 2 hours
Calcium chloride	5 to 10 mL IV of 10% solution (50 to 100 mg)	Antagonizes	1 to 3 min	30 to 60 min
Insulin and glucose (use 1 unit insulin/5 g glucose)	Regular insulin 10 units IV; plus 1 ampule (50 g) glucose	Shifts	30 min	4 to 6 hours plus
Diuresis with furosemide	40 to 80 mg IV bolus	Removes	When diuresis starts	When diuresis ends
Cation exchange resin	Kayexelate 15 to 50 g by mouth or rectum plus sorbitol	Removes	1 to 2 hours	4 to 6 hours
Peritoneal dialysis or hemodialysis	Per institution	Removes	As soon as started	Until dialysis completed

COMMENTS

- You decide to order Kayexelate 25 g by mouth, plus sorbitol, to remove potassium entirely from the body.

- NOTE: Calcium chloride has the quickest onset of action and should have a high priority in severe emergencies. Be cautious when giving calcium to patients receiving digitalis compounds, as it may contribute to digitalis intoxication. Modify the preceding regimen by adding the calcium to 100 mL of 5% dextrose in water (D_5W), and instead of giving a calcium chloride bolus, you infuse the calcium IV over 30 minutes.

- In summary, you rapidly treated this emergency with bicarbonate, calcium, insulin plus glucose, and Kayexelate. You have arranged for renal dialysis in a few hours, which will be the most definitive treatment for this woman. While Ms. Patterson may not have had a full cardiac arrest even without such aggressive therapy, there is also the chance that you caught someone "on her way" to a cardiac arrest and prevented it.

- These actions demonstrate ACLS at its finest—preventing cardiac arrests before they happen.

Mitch Michaels

CASE 2

HYPOKALEMIA

Mr. Mitch Michaels is a 38-year-old insulin-dependent diabetic who has been experiencing one of his frequent episodes of diabetic ketoacidosis (DKA). He has been having almost intractable nausea and vomiting for 12 hours, and comes in with a supine heart rate of 110 beats/min, a blood pressure of 110/70 mm Hg, a standing heart rate of 130 beats/min, and blood pressure of 90/75 mm Hg. (He almost passed out.)

His initial blood sugar level was 550, his potassium level was 3.7, the serum bicarbonate level was 11, and his arterial pH was 7.10. His urine sugar level and ketones were 4+. The resident taking care of Mr. Michaels made a presumptive diagnosis of diabetic ketoacidosis and started treatment with rapid rehydration of normal saline at 1000 mL per hour for 2 hours, 10 units of regular insulin IV push, followed by 0.1 unit/kg per hour. Because of the low serum bicarbonate level, he gave one ampule (50 mEq) of sodium bicarbonate.

Mr. Michaels comments that he started to feel better with the normal saline, and he has begun to urinate; however, he has since developed a profound muscular weakness, almost like he is paralyzed all over his body. On the monitor screen the rhythm looks abnormal and has changed significantly since his initial rhythm on admission to the Emergency Department.

As the new attending coming on duty at 3 PM, you become quite alarmed as you hear the resident describe the treatment regimen and you see the rhythm strip (Fig. 11-3).

What do you see abnormal in the rhythm strip? And what in the treatment of this DKA raised your concerns?

COMMENTS

- The ECG displays the classic findings of hypokalemia. As serum potassium decreases, the ECG displays the following sequence of changes:
  - U waves become more prominent.
  - T waves flatten.
  - ST segment becomes depressed.
  - QT interval becomes more prolonged.
  - QRS complex widens.
  - Wide-complex tachycardias, ventricular tachycardia, or VF develops.

- The resident in his initial treatment correctly instituted rapid volume replacement and has started insulin replacement. The choice of bicarbonate therapy for the acidosis, however, simplistically assumed that since the patient had DKA, he needed sodium bicarbonate.

- This choice fails to take into account the following:
  - The serum potassium level of 3.7 mEq/L is falsely elevated because of the overall acidosis.
  - With this degree of acidosis the serum potassium level should be much higher.
  - Total body potassium losses have been severe because of the vomiting and the osmotic diuresis of the hyperglycemia.
  - Correction of diabetes and ketoacidosis should always include supplemental potassium; however, the potas-

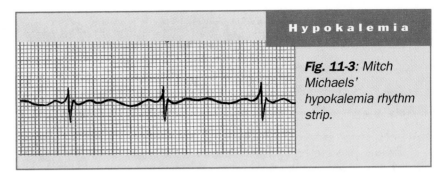

Hypokalemia

Fig. 11-3: Mitch Michaels' hypokalemia rhythm strip.

sium should be administered via a separate container (or the like) run into the volume replacement line. Do not put the potassium in the volume replacement fluid because it will be difficult to regulate the rate of potassium infusion.

- Treatment of the DKA, especially with the 50 mEq ampule of bicarbonate, will drastically lower the serum potassium level. Administration of bicarbonate will increase the serum pH even more. As the serum pH rises, potassium will move into the cells and out of the serum.

- Insulin increases the cellular uptake of glucose, and potassium follows glucose into the cells.

- The diuresis with volume replacement will also cause more loss of potassium in the urine.

- You know that severe hypokalemia can lead to profound muscle weakness (as exists here), as well as lethal ventricular arrhythmias.

Mitch Michaels

CASE 2 Continued

The initial potassium level was 3.7 mEq/L but a repeat level drawn by the nurse when the rhythm changed and the weakness increased was 2.0 mEq/L. You recognize the need for rapid potassium replacement, but you know that IV potassium itself can be lethal.

How can you estimate the amount of potassium that needs to be given? What are the best methods to guard against giving the potassium too fast and to avoid complications?

COMMENTS

- As a general rule, when serum potassium levels are in the range of 3.0 to 3.5 mEq/L, the patient will need approximately 100 mEq potassium replacement. If the serum potassium is in the range of 2.5 to 3.0 mEq/L, up to 200 mEq potassium replacement will be needed.

- In the treatment of DKA these are only rough guidelines; the total body deficits may be much greater. The key is to frequently check the serum potassium level during treatment and replacement.

- Chronic total body potassium deficits can be much larger and require much more replacement.

- Treat by infusing 10 to 40 mEq/hour. Inadvertent rapid infusions of potassium chloride can be fatal. Therefore many experts recommend never putting more than 40 to 80 mEq in a liter infusion container and recommend a maximum infusion rate of 40 mEq/hour.

- However, a patient with severe DKA may require infusion rates up to 60 mEq/hour. Thus it will take 3 to 4 hours to correct Mr. Michaels' deficits. Monitor ECG closely during rapid infusion of potassium.

Mitch Michaels	What if Mr. Michaels had a hypokalemic arrhythmia that deteriorated to a pulseless state of cardiac arrest? Would your treatment have been any different?
CASE 2 Continued	

COMMENTS

• Most experts would recommend administration rates of potassium up to 1 to 2 mEq/min during an actual cardiac arrest. This is, however, the maximal rate at which you can give potassium and still have a positive outcome.

• In addition, many experts would use magnesium 1 to 2 g IV in the setting of hypokalemic-induced cardiac arrest. Magnesium is thought to improve the electrical instability of the hypokalemic heart.

Sarah Lynch	*HYPERCALCEMIA*
CASE 3	*Mrs. Lynch is a 68-year-old, well-respected matron who has played a prominent role in community charity organizations for many years. She recently received a diagnosis of metastatic breast cancer and started*

treatment with estrogen about 2 weeks ago.

She comes into the Emergency Department because of increasing weakness, lethargy, depression, and now mental confusion over the past 24 hours. Her concerned husband reports severe hip and pelvis pain that keeps her from sleeping at night. Her serum calcium study returns a level of 13.5 mg/dL (normal = 8.5 to 10.5 mg/dL)

Several questions arise, including the following:

* *What is there about this history to suggest calcium problems?*
* *What would you expect the ECG to show (Fig. 11-4)?*
* *What treatment would you give?*
* *How would you treat her if she were to suddenly have a cardiac arrest?*

COMMENTS

The following elements in the history in Case 3 suggest a calcium problem:

• Mrs. Lynch has metastatic breast cancer, which is one of the malignancies most notorious for causing elevated calcium levels.

• Estrogen treatment of breast cancer with bone metastases can cause large elevations in calcium levels as the cancer responds.

• Weakness, fatigue, confusion, and altered mental status are common findings in severe hypercalcemia states.

• ECG shows the following changes as the serum calcium level increases:

  • Key: QT intervals are markedly shortened.
  • ST segments are shortened and depressed.
  • T waves widen.
  • Conduction slows.
  • Automaticity decreases.
  • Bradycardias are common.
  • Bundle branch blocks may occur.

• Second-degree heart block may progress to complete heart block and cardiac arrest (usually with levels above 20 mg/dL).

• **Immediate emergency treatment includes the following**:

  • Saline bolus to restore extracellular fluids and induce a diuresis.

  • Furosemide 40 to 100 mg IV (1 mg/kg every 2 to 4 hours).

  • Watch for and replace associated hypokalemia and hypomagnesemia.

  • Other treatments are more long-term and include calcitonin, mithramycin, hydrocortisone, diphosphonates (etidronate), and indomethacin.

• Treatment if a cardiac arrest occurs with known hypercalcemia includes the following:

  • Standard ACLS medications
  • Magnesium 1 to 2 g IV
  • Potassium 1 to 2 mEg/min
  • Saline bolus
  • Diuretics

Willie Burton

CASE 4

HYPOCALCEMIA

Willie Burton is a 57-year-old chronic alcoholic with a history of many previous visits to the Emergency Department where you are working. He has displayed a large variety of alcohol-related problems such as gastritis, dehydration, falls and fractures, and both acute and chronic pancreatitis. Tonight he arrives with recurrence of his severe midepigastric abdominal pain related to a recent weekend of imbibing with his street companions. The nurse reports that several things "seem different about Willie tonight," as follows:

- *His friend reports that he had a seizure during all the pain and he had never done that before.*
- *His hand curled up in spasms while the nurse was taking his blood pressure.*
- *His heart beat was irregular.*
- *Somebody started Willie on cimetidine (Tagamet) for his abdominal pain: "Don't they know he's just got alcoholic gastritis, not an ulcer?"*

You order routine "labs" on Willie, including calcium, amylase, and bilirubin studies and a 12-lead ECG. The amylase is 240 mg/dL. The ionized calcium returns as 1.8 mg/dL (normal = 4.2 to 4.8 mg/dL). (See hypocalcemia segment of Fig. 11-4.)

Several questions arise, including the following:

- *What is there about this history to suggest calcium problems?*
- *What would you expect the ECG to show?*
- *What treatment would you give to Willie?*
- *How would you treat Willie if he were to suddenly have a cardiac arrest?*

COMMENTS

- Think of **hypocalcemia.**
- Willie's risk factors for hypocalcemia include the following:
  - He is an alcoholic and presumably malnourished. This leads to hypomagnesemia, which in turn can lead to hypocalcemia.
  - He displayed a positive Trousseau's sign (carpal spasm when blood pressure cuff is applied—usually for 3 or more minutes).
  - He is on a regimen of cimetidine, which can decrease the synthesis of parathyroid hormone and lower serum calcium levels.
  - He is having a severe episode of acute pancreatitis. Pancreatic lipase breaks down fat into fatty acids, which combine with calcium to form insoluble calcium soaps. This "pancreatitis soap formation" lowers the serum calcium level dramatically.
- ECG findings: The prolonged QT interval on the ECG is the most characteristic finding in low calcium level. The

prolongation is not due to T wave lengthening but due to prolonged ST segment. The most common lethal arrhythmia that people with prolonged QT interval have is the

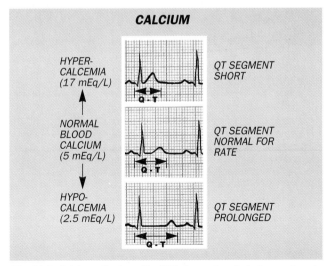

CALCIUM

HYPER-CALCEMIA (17 mEq/L)

NORMAL BLOOD CALCIUM (5 mEq/L)

HYPO-CALCEMIA (2.5 mEq/L)

QT SEGMENT SHORT

QT SEGMENT NORMAL FOR RATE

QT SEGMENT PROLONGED

Fig. 11-4: Calcium effects on the ECG: hypocalcemia to hypercalcemia.

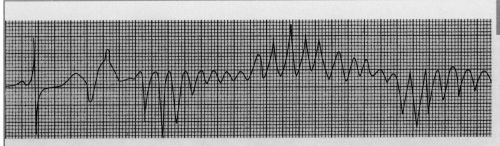

Hypocalcemia

Fig. 11-5: Hypocalcemia with long QT interval (QT interval = 0.7 seconds; RR interval; QT/RR ratio = 63%). Followed by torsades de pointes.

QRS and QT Intervals in ECG Interpretation

Electrolyte abnormalities and toxic effects of drugs frequently affect the QRS width and the QT interval on the ECG. It is easy to see why: the QRS width represents the period of ventricular depolarization; the QT intervals represent the period of ventricular depolarization plus repolarization. Many electrolytes and drugs exert their effects by prolonging (or sometimes shortening) these two periods. It is important to understand the terminology and how to measure these intervals.

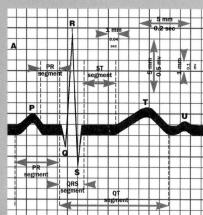

Fig. 11-6:
Electrocardiographic waves, intervals, and segments. This figure displays the normal definitions and the start-end points for measuring intervals and segments.

Fig. 11-8: *Upper limits of normal QT intervals at various heart rates (male and female).*

Data for computing heart rate, with maximum QT intervals at various rates			
HEART RATE	CYCLE TIME (0.04-second intervals)	MAXIMUM QT (seconds) MALE	FEMALE
300	5	.19	.20
250	6	.20	.22
214	7	.21	.23
187	8	.23	.25
166	9	.24	.26
150	10	.25	.28
136	11	.26	.29
125	12	.28	.30
115	13	.29	.32
107	14	.30	.33
100	15	.31	.34
93	16	.32	.35
88	17	.33	.36
78	18	.35	.38
75	20	.36	.39
71	21	.37	.40
68	22	.38	.41
65	23	.38	.42
62	24	.39	.43
60	25	.40	.44
57	26	.41	.45
52	27	.42	.47
50	30	.44	.48
46	32	.45	.50
43	34	.47	.51
41	36	.48	.53
39	38	.49	.54
37	40	.51	.56
35	42	.52	.57
34	44	.53	.58
32	46	.54	.60
30	50	.57	.62

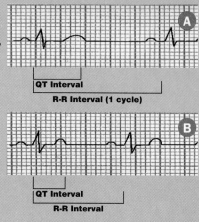

Fig. 11-7: *Relationship between QT interval and RR interval. The QT interval comprises about 40% of each cardiac cycle (the cardiac cycle = a RR interval). Greater than 40% represents abnormal QT prolongation. The QT interval, however, must always be measured in relationship to the rate. The faster the heart rate, the shorter the normal QT interval. In Fig. 11-7, B, the heart rate is much faster than the rate in Fig. 11-7, A, and the QT interval is therefore much shorter. However, the ratio of the QT intervals to the RR interval remains about 0.37.*

QT-Interval Abnormalities

Fig.11-9: *Examples of rhythms with QT-interval abnormalities.*

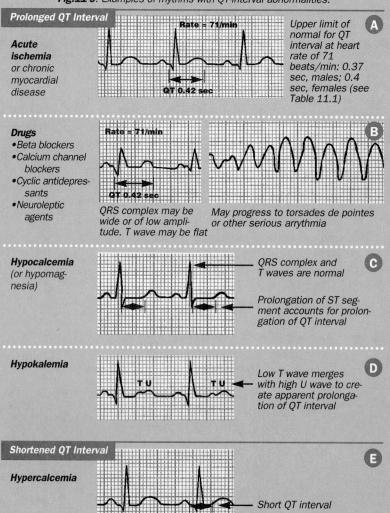

Prolonged QT Interval

Acute ischemia or chronic myocardial disease

A — *Upper limit of normal for QT interval at heart rate of 71 beats/min: 0.37 sec, males; 0.4 sec, females (see Table 11.1)*

Drugs
• Beta blockers
• Calcium channel blockers
• Cyclic antidepressants
• Neuroleptic agents

QRS complex may be wide or of low amplitude. T wave may be flat

B — *May progress to torsades de pointes or other serious arrythmia*

Hypocalcemia (or hypomagnesia)

C — *QRS complex and T waves are normal / Prolongation of ST segment accounts for prolongation of QT interval*

Hypokalemia

D — *Low T wave merges with high U wave to create apparent prolongation of QT interval*

Shortened QT Interval

Hypercalcemia

E — *Short QT interval*

form of VT known as torsades de pointes. (See Fig. 11-5 to 11-9 and Table 11-1 QRS and QT intervals in ECG interpertation.)

- Treatment is indicated in this case because Willie is symptomatic, displays an abnormal ECG with cardiac irregularity, and probably is going to get worse before he gets better.
- **Treatment:** Calcium chloride 10% solution (1 g in 10 mL = 272 mg calcium). Give 100 mg in 100 mL of D₅W over

10 to 20 minutes. Over the next 6 to 12 hours give a total of 1 g by continuous IV drip.

- Cardiac arrest (particularly if bradyasystolic arrest or PEA and particularly in patients with chronic renal failure: Give full ampule of calcium chloride (1 g in 10 mL of a 10% solution). If a cardiac arrest occurs, consider multiple electrolyte abnormalities such as associated hypomagnesemia and hyperkalemia. (See later in this chapter for additional treatment for those problems.)

Lamar MacDonald

CASE 5

HYPOMAGNESEMIA

You are the cardiologist on call for your group practice when you receive word that Lamar MacDonald has begun to have seizures. You admitted Mr. MacDonald several hours before for acute diarrhea and dehydration, chronic alcoholism, chronic pancreatitis, and diabetes secondary to pancreatic destruction. He was admitted to the coronary care unit with frequent premature ventricular contractions (PVCs) and mild ST-segment depression and to rule out myocardial infarction (MI). His potassium level is 3.7 mEq/L; ionized calcium level is 3.8 mg/dL; amylase level is 88 mg/dL; other laboratory values were all "one end or the other of the normal range," but none were markedly deranged.

Several questions arise, including the following:
- *What is there about this history to suggest a magnesium problem?*
- *What would you expect the ECG to show?*
- *What immediate treatment would you give to Lamar?*
- *How would you treat Lamar if he were to suddenly have a cardiac arrest?*

COMMENTS

- The new onset of seizures in Mr. MacDonald, given the other elements in his history, should make you think of hypomagnesemia *(normal serum magnesium level = 1.5 to 2.0 mEq/L; hypomagnesemia is a level less than 1.4 mEq/L; severe deficiency is a level less than 0.5 mEq/L).* These elements are as follows:
- Chronic malnutrition that is due to the chronic alcoholism. Poor nutrition is the most common cause of decreased total body magnesium.
- The low potassium and low calcium levels support the probability of chronic malnutrition, as follows:
  - Chronic pancreatitis and acute diarrhea can both lead to gastrointestinal tract magnesium losses.
  - Insulin dependency is associated with decreased magnesium.
  - The seizures may be a sign of hypomagnesemia.
  - The arrhythmias, PVCs, and ST-segment depression are signs of hypomagnesemia.
- The ECG in hypomagnesemia shows the following (note the overlap with low potassium and low calcium levels):

- Prolongation of the PR and QT intervals
- Wide QRS complexes
- ST-segment depression
- Broad, flat T waves with precordial T wave inversion
- Emergency treatment of hypomagnesemia is indicated because of the seizures and the arrhythmias as follows:
  - Magnesium sulfate 1 to 2 g IV over 5 to 10 minutes. (Rapid administration is acceptable when significant adverse effects from the hypomagnesemia exist.)
  - Follow initial 1 to 2 g with 4 to 6 g over next 24 hours.
  - NOTE: Initiate additional interventions for the seizures and the arrhythmias.
- Treatment of cardiac arrest in association with low magnesium levels is as follows:
  - Magnesium sulfate 1 to 2 g IV push.
  - Follow routine ACLS Guidelines.
  - Hypokalemia, hypocalcemia, and hypophosphatemia may also be present and may necessitate concomitant therapy if arrest remains refractory.

The toxicologic cases
Cyclic antidepressant and neuroleptic overdose

- Case 5 covers two large groups of medications people often ingest in suicide attempts. ACLS providers should learn the basic principles of treatment that apply to all of these agents, rather than learn many details that apply to just a few of these agents.

- We present these two medication types together (each containing many specific agents) for the following reasons:

  - Often patients take both types of agents in their desperate states of depression and disturbance.

  - The agents provide similar clinical consequences, with only minor differences in their effects on the ECG.

  - The immediate treatment of these patients is similar.

- The ACLS response to patients who have taken these medications and who have had cardiac arrest is largely the same.

- The major agents include those listed next.

  - **Cyclic antidepressants**
    - Tricyclic antidepressants
    - Monocyclic and bicyclic antidepressants
    - Trazadone (Desyrel)
    - Fluoxetine (Prozac)

  - **Major tranquilizers: Five classes of neuroleptics**
    - Phenothiazines (Compazine, Thorazine)
    - Thioxanthenes (thiothixene)
    - Dibenzoxazepines (loxapine)
    - Butyrophenone (Haldol)
    - Dihydroindolone (molindone)

Janelle Ratcliffe

CASE 6

CYCLIC ANTIDEPRESSANT DRUG OVERDOSE
You are a resident physician on duty in the Emergency Department. Suddenly a cluster of college students arrives at the doors half-carrying a young woman with her arms draped over their shoulders. She appears unconscious, and her legs are buckling and not bearing any of her weight. The friends shout out that they found her "passed out" in one of the nearby college dorms with two empty pill bottles nearby. She has a history of depression and was under professional care from both the student health center and a local private psychiatrist. She had written an incoherent letter with themes of low self-esteem, parental conflict, unsatisfactory personal relationships, and overwhelming feelings of despair.

You help place Janelle onto a nearby stretcher and roll her into the first treatment room. During that transfer you checked her level of consciousness (reduced, but responsive to deep pain stimulation), her carotid pulse (present and slow), her breathing (deep, slow respirations) and her gag reflex (markedly reduced). You ask one of the friends whether he brought the empty pill bottles to the Emergency Department, but he had not. "I'll go get them right now. They are back in the room!"

How would you approach the immediate care of Janelle?

COMMENTS

- The Five Quadrads approach provides a good guide to the things to quickly review and institute.

- **Primary ABCD Survey** reveals the following:

  - Reduced consciousness
  - *A:* Open airway but absent gag reflex
  - *B:* Spontaneous breathing
  - *C:* Pulse present
  - *D:* Not in VF

- **Secondary ABCD Survey**

- *Airway and Breathing:* You recognize at once that Janelle will need endotracheal intubation because of her reduced

level of consciousness, the need to protect her airway (minimal gag reflex) in general, and the need to protect her airway during the performance of gastric lavage. You tell the charge nurse to prepare for an "urgent" intubation, which you will perform.

- *Circulation:* Start large-gauge IV lines in both arms, attach monitor leads, examine rhythm strip, and order 12-lead ECG.

- *Differential Diagnosis:* Cover many items here as you begin to think about Janelle's problem including the following:

  - Send the friends back for the empty pill bottles. One bottle had 50 amitriptyline 50-mg tablets dated a week previously (she should have taken 21 pills per her prescription, leaving 29 for the overdose); one bottle contained 50 trazodone 50-mg tablets dated 2 days ago (she should have taken 6, leaving 44 for the overdose). The drugs were prescribed by different physicians and were obtained from different pharmacies, suggesting an element of planned deception by Janelle.

- This is a severe overdose; cyclic antidepressants are the major cause of subsequent overdose death in patients who reach the hospital alive.
- Order chest x-ray.
- Order electrolyte, calcium, magnesium, BUN, glucose, and creatinine studies.
- Order arterial blood gas studies.
- Order gastric lavage, but start with activated charcoal 50 g down the tube first, before starting the lavage; then proceed with several liters of saline (until clear).

Follow lavage with instillation of an additional 50 g of activated charcoal with sorbitol.

- *Oxygen/IV/Monitor/Fluids:* Already started, with fluid of choice being normal saline at 1000 mL/hour.
- *Vital signs:* Respirations = 12 breaths/min; blood pressure = 90/60 mm Hg heart rate = 120 beats/min; temperature = 38.2° C.
- *Tank/Resistance/Pump/Rate:*
  - **Is there a tank problem causing the hypotension?** Yes. Cyclic antidepressants in excessive amounts act as vasodilators, causing "enlargement of the tank."
  - **Is there a pump problem?** Yes. Cyclic antidepressants reduce myocardial contractility and pumping effectiveness.
  - **Is there a rate problem?** Yes. One of the early signs of cyclic antidepressant overdose is sinus tachycardia.

Janelle Ratcliffe

CASE 6 Continued

Your secondary, more detailed examination reveals that Janelle is having severe cyclic antidepressant intoxication. This manifests itself as an anticholinergic overdose. She has confusion and mental status changes and appears delirious (mad as a hatter). Her pupils are dilated (blind as a bat); her skin is flushed and erythematous (red as a beet). Just as the clinic assistant completes the 12-lead ECG, Janelle has a complete grand mal seizure.

What do you expect to see on the ECG in tricyclic antidepressant (TCA) overdoses? What would be your immediate treatment for the seizures?

COMMENTS

The major ECG signs in cyclic antidepressant intoxication are the following:

- ST-segment and T-wave changes.
- QRS complex is prolonged.
- QT interval is prolonged.
- Right-axis deviation of the QRS complex.
- Bundle branch blocks.
- Atrioventricular (AV) conduction blocks with aberrant conduction.
- Ominously broad, slurred QRS sine waves (if pulseless, PEA).
- Ventricular arrhythmias

- Intraventricular conduction blocks (showing up as widened QRS complexes and QT intervals) are an early and sensitive indicator of TCA overdose.

- Although cyclic antidepressant overdoses can cause lethal ventricular arrhythmias, these are not their primary mechanism of death. The cyclic antidepressants profoundly depress myocardial contractility. Most TCA deaths occur

from hypotension and interventricular conduction abnormalities, rather than from ventricular arrhythmias.

SEIZURE TREATMENT

- The seizures that occur with cyclic antidepressant intoxication are usually brief and short-lived and do not necessitate immediate treatment other than respiratory support, hyperventilation to a pH of 7.5, and alkalinization. (See later comments.) Treat recurring seizures aggressively, however, because they can lead to the development of greater acidosis, which increases the toxic effects of TCAs.

- Most toxicologists would now recommend immediate treatment with a benzodiazepine if TCA-induced seizures persist. Phenobarbital is the agent of second choice.

- In the past, Dilantin was widely used in cyclic antidepressant overdose to treat the seizures and to treat the cardiac conduction defects. Evidence would suggest that Dilantin has little documented effectiveness and at best should be classified as Class IIb (acceptable, possibly effective) for this indication.

- Physostigmine has been used with anecdotal success but is generally *not* recommended. Most toxicologists now think there is no use for this agent in TCA overdoses.

Janelle Ratcliffe	*You have now been pushing normal saline at 1000 mL/hour and have ordered Ativan 2 mg IV. The seizures have not recurred. Janelle has worsening hypotension. The cardiac monitor displays a variety of PVCs, steadily widening QRS complexes (duration now >100 ms) and*
CASE 6 Continued	

a prolonged QT interval. The blood pressure has dropped to 80 mm Hg systolic.

What sequence of interventions should you now initiate, given this steadily worsening condition?

COMMENTS

- **Alkalinization** to a pH of at least 7.5 has become the mainstay of treatment for the cardiovascular toxic effects of cyclic antidepressants. Alkalinization decreases the binding of cyclic antidepressants to the myocardial membrane. This helps overcome the action-potential blockade that tricyclics produce. The hypertonic effects of sodium bicarbonate, when it is given as a bolus, can affect the myocardial action potential and decrease arrhythmias.

- Use alkalinization whenever patients have QRS duration greater than 100 ms; ventricular arrhythmias, or hypotension that does not respond to the initial 500 mL normal saline bolus.

- Alkalinization is accomplished as follows:

  - Hyperventilation is safe, reversible, and instantly available; use first. Some experts disagree on the use of hyperventilation to achieve alkalinization. Hyperventilation, by decreasing cerebral perfusion, can increase the risk of seizures. Cyclic antidepressant overdose patients are already at an increased risk for seizures.

- Follow with bolus sodium bicarbonate: 1 to 5 mEq/kg over 1 to 2 minutes.

- Follow with continuous infusion sodium bicarbonate: 50 to 100 mEq (two ampules in 0.25 normal saline) at 150 to 200 mL/hour. (Some experts recommend intermittent bolus infusions to achieve the antiarrhythmic effects of the hypertonicity.)

- Goal pH is 7.45 to 7.55; blood pressure normalizes; QRS duration narrows to less than 100 ms.

- If more prolongation of the QT interval or torsades de pointes develops, use **magnesium** sulfate 1 to 2 g. Give IV bolus if condition is unstable or over 1 to 5 minutes in more stable conditions; up to 5 to 10 g may be used.

- If hypotension does not respond to the sodium bicarbonate and the normal saline, use pressor agents with predominately an alpha-adrenergic effect as follows:

  - Norepinephrine (considered the pressor of choice by many experts because cyclic antidepressants cause depletion of endogenous norepinephrine stores)

  - Epinephrine

  - High-dose ("pressor dose") dopamine

Janelle Ratcliffe	*The next 60 minutes are very much touch-and-go with Janelle. She gradually begins to respond in terms of her hypotension, tachycardia and bradycardia, the ventricular irregularities, the broadening QRS complex, and lengthening QT intervals. You hyperventilated Janelle 's*
CASE 6 Continued	

lungs after the lavage to a pH of 7.6.

You have administered the following:

- *Normal saline, 1 L*
- *Sodium bicarbonate 3 mEq/kg over 1 to 2 minutes*
- *Sodium bicarbonate 100 mEq (two ampules) in the "quater normal saline" to run at the rate of 200 mL/hour.*
- *Magnesium 2 g IV bolus over 5 minutes*
- *Norepinephrine infusion to run at 20 µg/min, dropping back when the blood pressure reached 110 mm Hg systolic*

You monitored the serum pH and dropped back on the sodium bicarbonate rate when pH = 7.6.

You admit Janelle to the intensive care unit (ICU). She gets a catheter for invasive hemodynamic monitoring. Her critical care "attending" notifies the "pump team" that they may have a patient who needs hemoperfusion with activated charcoal or resin. You know that this will remove only a few milligrams of the drugs because they are bound so tightly to the body tissues. Nevertheless, no one wants to neglect a chance to perhaps save her life.

What would you have done if Janelle had not responded as described here and instead had a full cardiac arrest?

- The former recommendations to use physostigmine are Class III (harmful), but some would accept its use if patient is clearly in extremis and not responding to any other actions.

COMMENTS

- Certainly the standard ACLS protocols would be followed, including defibrillation and careful attention to the airway. The specific things to make sure to get done (assuming asystolic or PEA arrest) are the following:

  - **Hyperventilation**
  - **Sodium bicarbonate** in large doses (up to 5 mEq/kg IV push)
  - **Defibrillation** for VF
  - **Epinephrine,** using high doses (0.1 mg/kg)
  - **Magnesium sulfate** 1 to 2 g IV
  - **Norepinephrine**
  - NOTE: Avoid procainamide in TCA overdose because it has tricyclic-like properties.

- More controversial agents that have been used during cardiac arrest (especially during the "peri-cardiac arrest period" before the pulse vanishes) include the following:

  - Dilantin (rarely used now)
  - Digitalis (rarely used now)
  - Physostigmine (almost never used now)
  - Charcoal hemoperfusion
  - Cardiopulmonary bypass

- Perhaps most important, *do not give up on patients with cyclic antidepressant overdose too soon.* These drugs appear to be powerful poisons that resist all interventions. You can see the patient deteriorate, despite all your efforts. However, the effects of these agents do not continue indefinitely. If the patient can be maintained until the drug effects dissipate, you may save a life. Think in terms of the possible need for prolonged periods of basic CPR. The "world records" for basic CPR survival have been set with TCA overdose patients. There are case reports of survival after 3,4, and even 6 hours of CPR.

Janelle Ratcliffe

CASE 6 Continued

If Janelle had consumed an overdose of neuroleptic agents (for example, large amounts of Haldol or Thorazine) how would this management have been different?

COMMENTS

- In fact, the management is surprisingly similar, although few textbooks discuss the management in combination.

- ECG changes: The QT interval becomes quite prolonged and the QRS complexes become widened, just as with cyclic antidepressant overdose. Ventricular arrhythmias, including torsades de pointes and AV dissociation, occur and are managed in the same way.

- The other approaches mentioned for cyclic antidepressant

overdose apply to neuroleptic overdose as well, including the following:

- Aggressive alkalinization
- Benzodiazepines for seizures
- Magnesium sulfate
- Norepinephrine for hypotension and shock
- Charcoal decontamination and hemoperfusion
- Prolonged CPR and resuscitation efforts

Douglas Walker Newcome

CASE 7

COCAINE INTOXICATION

As an Emergency Department physician, you are evaluating Mr. Douglas Walker Newcome, a well-known 42-year-old product litigation attorney. Mr. Newcome arrives at the Emergency Department with complaints of crushing chest pain, shortness of breath, a severe headache, and pounding pulse. His condition is managed as a possible AMI with rapid triage and evaluation to Room 1, where his initial vital signs are as follows: temperature, 36.8° C; heart rate, 120 beats/min; blood pressure, 120/180 mm Hg; and respirations, 18 breaths/min.

According to the Emergency Department routine for chest pain patients he receives 12-lead ECG, Oxygen/IV/Monitor, one-half aspirin (160 mg), two sublingual nitroglycerin tablets, and morphine sulfate 2 mg IV (see Chapter 9). The 12-lead ECG reveals sinus tachycardia, occasional PVCs, and 2-mm ST-segment elevation in the precordial leads (V_4 to V_6).

As you are looking at the 12-lead ECG, Mr. Newcome begins to cry, sobbing, "I knew I should have stopped using that crap! Look what it has done." As you follow up on these statements you learn that Mr. Newcome has been "snorting nose candy"— relatively pure powdered cocaine— for

CONTINUED

Douglas Walker Newcome

CASE 7 Continued

the past 6 months. He had increased the frequency from recreational use on weekends to additional use during the week, particularly during recent professional pressures. He admits to "snorting two big lines" just before his chest pain began, about an hour ago.

How will this information change your approach to Mr. Newcome's care? What are the major complications you are going to look for?

COMMENTS

- The first issue to sort out is the ST-segment elevations on the 12-lead ECG. He clearly appears to be having a **cocaine-induced MI** (since the full ECG criteria are met). Current controversy exists over the mechanism of infarction in cocaine users. Some studies have observed 50% of the AMIs to be due to acute coronary artery spasm and 50% due to coronary artery thrombosis.

- Administration of thrombolytics always poses a risk of cerebral hemorrhage. This risk, however, is increased in cocaine users because they have had previous bouts of severe hypertension with their drug use. If the AMI was due only to spasm, thrombolytic therapy would be ineffective and would expose the patient to an unnecessary risk of a severe, disabling stroke.

- Therefore for cocaine-induced MI, some experts recommend delaying the administration of thrombolytics until you obtain additional indications of acute thrombosis such as cardiac enzyme studies, echocardiography, or, most definitively, acute coronary angiography.

- The ischemia should be treated aggressively, combining the usual AMI protocols with the following special adjustments for the cocaine intoxication:

  - Aspirin

  - Oxygen

  - Nitroglycerin (Use IV route here to lower the elevated blood pressures and dilate coronary arteries.)

  - Morphine is appropriate.

  - Benzodiazepines are particularly useful in cocaine intoxication and can bring down the blood pressure and slow the tachycardia as well.

  - Magnesium sulfate is acceptable and has some beneficial effects in terms of prophylaxis against cocaine-induced arrhythmias.

  - Avoid beta blockers because full, unopposed, cocaine-induced alpha vascular effects may increase coronary artery spasm.

- Since Mr. Newcome appears to be having several other side effects of the cocaine use, it is important to the acute management of two complications of cocaine: severe hypertension and PVCs.

SEVERE HYPERTENSION

- Cocaine produces what is, in effect, an overdose of norepinephrine, epinephrine, dopamine, and serotonin. Cocaine first stimulates the release of these agents and then blocks their reuptake.

- Treat with a **benzodiazepine** ("such as" diazepam 5 to 20 mg IV) first.

- Vasodilators like **nitroglycerin** 10 to 20 µg/min IV would be an ideal method of lowering the blood pressure in this setting because nitroglycerin is already a major agent to use for AMI.

- Avoid betablockers like propranolol or esmolol for treating hypertension only, because a beta blocker will leave the alpha effects of cocaine relatively unopposed and can induce severe excess of alpha effects (even more severe hypertension). This is a deviation from usual AMI management in which persistent tachycardia and blood pressure elevation are powerful indications for the use of beta blockade.

- **Nitroprusside** 0.1 to 5.0 µg/kg/per minute IV can be used for severe hypertension.

- Consider **phentolamine,** a pure alpha blocker (use 1 to 10 mg titrated as a dilute solution over 2 to 3 minutes) to lower blood pressure.

- **Labetalol** (5 to 20 mg IV) may be an exception to the prohibition against beta blockers for cocaine-induced hypertension. Since labetalol has both alpha-blocking and beta-blocking effects, it will oppose the alpha effects of cocaine. This remains an area of disagreement among toxicologists.

PREMATURE VENTRICULAR TACHYCARDIAS

- Treat with diazepam 5 to 20 mg IV over 5 to 20 minutes.

- Use lidocaine with caution. See the next section.

Douglas Walker Newcome

CASE 7 Continued

You initiate the following therapy for Mr. Newcome:
- *Oxygen, aspirin per AMI routine*
- *Diazepam 5 mg IV, repeat every 15 minutes if persistent elevations of blood pressure and heart rate.*
- *Morphine 2 mg IV, every 5 minutes for persistent ischemic pain*
- *Nitroglycerin 10 µg/min IV and titrated up to control blood pressure*
- *Magnesium sulfate 2 g, IV infused over 20 minutes*

With the preceding regimen you notice a marked improvement in his symptoms of pain, tachycardia, and hypertension. The decision, after rapid consultation with the cardiology service on call, is to withhold thrombolytic therapy at this time and take Mr. Newcome directly to the cardiac "cath lab."

In the cath lab, Mr. Newcome is noted to have open coronary arteries without significant narrowing and to have no thrombosis. However, during the dye infusions, Mr. Newcome begins to have brief runs of VT, that degenerates into VF over a 30-second period.

How would you adjust the standard ACLS protocols now that you are dealing with an acute cocaine-associated VT/VF cardiac arrest?

COMMENTS

- The ACLS Pulseless VF/VT Algorithm (see Fig.4-1) should be applied to cocaine-associated cardiac arrest in the standard guideline approach with the following exceptions:

  - **Lidocaine** (1 to 1.5 mg/kg) should be used much more cautiously, especially for VT with a pulse, because both lidocaine and cocaine lower the seizure threshold. The combination of these two agents markedly increases the risk of severe seizures, even *status epilepticus*.

  - Space out the **epinephrine** dose to every 5 to 10 minutes. Avoid completely the use of higher doses of epinephrine that are acceptable in refractory VF/VT arrest.

  - **Propranolol** (3 to 5 mg IV every 5 minutes) for refractory VF/VT is acceptable though not confirmed in multiple studies.

  - Consider **labetalol** (5 to 20 mg) if the VF/VT arrest persists after use of the agents just listed.

- NOTE: Mr. Newcome survived the "cath lab" arrest after two shocks and a bolus of lidocaine 1 mg/kg. He did well in the coronary care unit, ruling out an AMI, and swearing "on my word as a lawyer" that he would never use cocaine again.

Kristin Hendricksen

CASE 8

BETA-BLOCKER OVERDOSE

Kristin Hendricksen is a 24-year-old Norwegian exchange student who has been living with her aunt and uncle in Ballard, Washington. She had become acutely despondent after receiving a telephone call from Bergen informing her that her mother and brother had been killed in an automobile accident. She went to her uncle's bathroom medicine cabinet and took approximately 20 propranolol (Inderal) 40-mg tablets over a 15-minute period. She gradually became confused and semidelirious and, when discovered by her aunt 45 minutes later, was weak and unable to walk.

The medics have started an IV, started oxygen, and placed her on a monitor. She has profound sinus bradycardia of 35 beats/min with a marked first-degree block of 0.28 seconds and a blood pressure of 75/50 mm Hg. The medics are asking for advice on initial field treatment.

Several questions arise, including the following:
- *What would you expect the 12-lead ECG to show?*
- *What treatment would you advise the medics to give?*
- *What will be your therapeutic approach when she arrives at the Emergency Department?*
- *How would you treat her if she were to suddenly have a cardiac arrest?*

- Case 8 is a potentially lethal dose of a common beta blocker. The beta blockers have powerful negative inotropic, chronotropic, and vasodilatory effects. The condition of victims may decline very rapidly and may include the following:
  - Altered mental status
  - Hypotension
  - Sinus bradycardia
  - Seizures
  - Pulseless electrical activity (PEA)
  - Profound heart block
  - Hypoglycemia
- The 12-lead ECG will show the following profound, direct cardiovascular effects on conduction through the myocardium:
  - Bradycardia
  - AV block
  - Widening of the QRS complex
  - Peaked T-wave changes
  - ST-segment changes
- On clinical examination there will be evidence of suppression of myocardial contractility, as following:
  - Cardiac output falls, hypotension ensues.
  - Myocardial perfusion falls.

- The fall in myocardial perfusion leads to further cardiac deterioration, including PEA and cardiac arrest.
- Immediate therapy (give this order to the paramedics) includes the following:
  - **Saline bolus** of 500 to 1000 mL
  - **Atropine** 0.5 to 1.0 mg IV for the bradycardia (though rarely effective in bradycardias and heart blocks caused by beta blockers)
  - **Epinephrine** 2 to 100 µg/min for the hypotension
- Further immediate therapy in the Emergency Department (this is listed in the recommended sequence) is as follows:
  - Continue the epinephrine infusions.
  - **Glucagon** 1 to 5 mg IV (over 1 min). Glucagon enhances myocardial contractility, heart rate, and AV conduction by acting at a receptor site distinct from the beta receptors. Many experts consider it the drug of choice in the management of beta blocker overdose. (Be alert for glucagon-induced vomiting.)
  - **Dopamine** infusion at 10 to 20 µg/kg/min.
  - **Calcium chloride** 5 to 20 mL IV.
  - **Pacing:** Either transcutaneous or transvenous.
  - Additional pressor agents to try if insufficient response to the above interventions include **dobutamine, norepinephrine,** and **isoproterenol.**
- In special situations consider cardiopulmonary bypass and intraaortic balloon pump.

Kristin Hendricksen

CASE 8 Continued

Since Kristin had taken a lethal dose of a beta blocker, all the following interventions were used: saline bolus, epinephrine infusion plus dopamine infusion at 20 µg/kg per minute, calcium chloride, and glucagon.

She briefly lost her pulse, and CPR compressions were started. The major interventions for PEA and profound shock were instituted (endotracheal intubation, higher doses of epinephrine, atropine, and the addition of norepinephrine), and a pulse returned after 8 minutes. Transcutaneous pacing was started at 120 milliamperes (mA) at 80 beats/min with excellent results for about 1 hour.

She gradually became unresponsive to the pacing stimulus, and preparations were begun for cardiopulmonary bypass. Isoproterenol was added to the dopamine and epinephrine plus additional doses of glucagon and calcium chloride. With this regimen she was able to maintain a blood pressure of 90/60 mm Hg for another 2 hours. At this point she began to displays signs of dissipation of the overdose.

The ICU nurses were able to gradually wean her off the pressors, and after 8 hours it became clear that she was going to recover. Within 24 hours she was sitting up talking, and she eventually made a complete recovery.

What important lesson did this experience teach?

- A major lesson in Case 8, especially true for young patients with a good heart before the overdose, is "Do not give up." Beta blockers, like calcium channel blockers, present another form of toxic overdose that is completely reversible within hours if you can manage to keep the patient alive while waiting for the drug effects to wear off.

- The patients often have a perfectly normal heart that is just temporarily suppressed by the overdose of the medication. Do not fail to give these patients every possible chance, including prolonged efforts at pacing and CPR, and even cardiopulmonary bypass and intraaortic balloon pump.

Henrietta Cipa

CASE 9

CALCIUM CHANNEL BLOCKER OVERDOSE

Mrs. Cipa is a 77-year-old Russian immigrant being treated for a variety of medical problems, including severe hypertension, chronic congestive heart failure, cardiopulmonary disease, and coronary artery disease.

Her alarmed children bring her into the Emergency Department at 11 PM stating that they fear Mrs. Cipa had consumed far too many of her nifedipine 20-mg-tablets. They found 20 pills missing from a recently filled bottle of 60 tablets. The bottle date suggested that only four pills should be gone. Since Mrs. Cipa often became confused at night when she took her medications, this "accidental overdose" is a distinct possibility.

As you begin your evaluation of Mrs. Cipa, suspecting a possible calcium channel blocker overdose, you have several questions, including the following:
* *What would you expect the 12-lead ECG to show?*
* *What would be your immediate approach to treatment in the Emergency Department?*

COMMENTS

* Calcium channel blocker overdose has many of the same toxic effects as beta blocker overdose, including the following:
  * Negative inotropic effects
  * Negative chronotropic effects
  * Vasodilatory effects
* The clinical problems are almost entirely cardiac and include conduction system abnormalities and suppression of cardiac contractility, as follows:
  * Hypotension
  * Sinus bradycardia
  * Conduction abnormalities that may include QRS-complex widening and QT-interval lengthening. (PEA is the cardiac arrest finding.)
  * Heart blocks, particularly prolonged first-degree block, but also second- and third-degree blocks.
  * Central nervous system depression ranging from drowsiness to confusion and coma
  * Seizures (rarely)
  * Hyperglycemia

* Immediate therapy (follow outlined sequence if clinical condition not improving) is as follows:
  * **Saline bolus** of 500 to 1000 mL.
  * **Calcium chloride** 1 to 4 g. This is 10 to 40 mL of 10% solution. (Calcium chloride comes in 10-mL vials: 100 mg/mL equals 1 g per vial. (Goal is to elevate the serum calcium level by 1 to 2 mg/dL.)
  * **Glucagon** 1 to 5 mg IV. (This may have positive effects on myocardial contractility and AV conduction, but successes have been mostly anecdotal case reports.)
  * **Epinephrine** infusion at 2 to 100 μg/min.
  * **Dopamine** infusion at 10 to 20 μg/kg per minute.
  * Repeat **calcium chloride** 5 to 10 mL of 10% solution (after epinephrine has sensitized the myocardium).
  * **Dobutamine, norepinephrine,** and/or **isoproterenol** if still refractory.
  * **4-Aminopyridine.** (This drug is experimental in the United States but has had success in Europe, where it is more widely available.)
  * **Pacing:** Either transcutaneous or transvenous.
* **Cardiopulmonary bypass** in special situations.

Henrietta Cipa

CASE 9 Continued

Mrs. Cipa developed first-degree heart block, sinus bradycardia at 50 beats/min, hypotension at 90/60 mm Hg, and QRS widening. You treated her with saline infusion (only 250 mL/hour for 4 hours), calcium chloride, and glucagon. A dopamine drip of 15 μg/kg per minute was needed for about 90 minutes, and transcutaneous pacing adhesive electrode pads were applied prophylactically. She was observed in the coronary care unit for 48 hours and did well.

If she had unexpectedly had a full cardiac arrest, how would you have treated her?

COMMENTS

* The arrest would have had the "overlap" features of PEA and profound hypotension. Thus the algorithms you follow would combine those two algorithms as follows:

* **Epinephrine** and **atropine** for the PEA. (Atropine would probably not have been effective.)

- Normal **saline bolus** to assure a "full tank" and counteract the effects of the calcium channel blocker-induced vasodilatation.

- Immediate **transcutaneous pacing (TCP).**

- **Norepinephrine** and **dopamine** as the hypotension pressor agents.

- **Dobutamine** as the inotropic agent.

- In addition, you would want to add the agents listed above specifically for calcium channel blocker overdose:

  - **Calcium chloride**

  - **Glucagon**

Gary Adams

CASE 10

DIGITALIS INTOXICATION:

Mr. Gary Adams is a 67-year-old retired gas station owner who has been taking digitalis for many years. Recently he began taking digoxin 0.25 mg twice a day, instead of once a day as directed, because of increasing feelings of weakness and fatigue. "If one helps then two should be even better." In addition, his physician had placed him on hydrochlorothiazide 50 mg bid for some "swelling in my legs" about 3 weeks ago, but without potassium supplementation.

He presents to the Emergency Department because of some nausea, vomiting, and progressive weakness. His family members report that he has appeared more confused over the past several days and that he did not want to come to the hospital. He also feels "palpitations" and that his "heart is beating funny." You find that his BP is 110/70; heart rate is 45 with first-degree heart block and a PR interval of 0.28 seconds; rhythm is frequent PVCs, junctional escape beats, and some runs of paroxysmal atrial tachycardia. His potassium level is 3.2 mEg/L; BUN is 50; and creatinine is 2.3.

You suspect digitalis intoxication with this history and the unusual rhythms. The stat digoxin level was 4 ng/mL (therapeutic range is 0.5 to 2.0 mg/mL).

Several questions should be considered, including the following:

- *Is this acute or chronic digitalis intoxication?*
- *What is the basic therapy of digitalis intoxication?*
- *What is the therapy of the various digitalis intoxication syndromes?*
- *What will you do if cardiac arrest develops?*

COMMENTS

- There are useful distinctions to make between acute digitalis intoxication, which is usually due to accidental or intentional overdose, and chronic digitalis intoxication, which is usually unintentional and is due to gradual decline in renal function in elderly patients placed on diuretics and long-term digitalis. (See Fig. 11-10 for progressive effects of digitalis intoxication on the ECG.)

- *Acute intoxication:* is associated with more supraventricular tachyarrhythmias with AV blocks; serum potassium may be markedly elevated and indicates the level of toxicity; serum digoxin level shows marked elevation.

- *Chronic intoxication:* more ventricular arrhythmias occur than supraventricular, but almost anything can occur; serum potassium is low or normal; digoxin level shows mild elevation or may even be therapeutic.

- Two clinical issues to consider with digitalis intoxication:

  - Is the toxicity acute or chronic?

  - Are the hemodynamics stable or unstable?

- Basic therapy in chronic digitalis intoxication that will correct most arrhythmias is:

  - Volume replacement

  - Potassium replacement

  - Magnesium replacement

- **Drug-Specific Antibodies (Digibind):** Digoxin-specific fragment antibodies (Fab) are IgG fragments of sheep antidigoxin antibodies that have revolutionized the management of acute digitalis intoxication. They are also useful for chronic toxicity. Digibind is the key to treating many of the specific digitalis-induced arrhythmias.

  - Fab fragment antibodies can completely reverse toxicity within 30 minutes. One 40 mg vial of Fab binds 0.6 mg of digoxin.

  - Fab dose: the dose should be based on the patient's weight and steady-state serum digoxin level (See 1994 *ACLS Textbook*, p. 10-21). In more urgent clinical situations, a dose of 10 to 20 vials can be empirically administered.

Recommendations for specific digitalis-induced arrhythmias

DIGITALIS-INDUCED BRADYCARDIAS

- Atropine 0.5 mg IV

- Use transcutaneous or transvenous pacemaker,

if absolutely necessary. In general, however, avoid pacemakers since patients with digitalis intoxication are prone to pacemaker-induced rhythm disturbances.

- Digibind (6 to 20 vials given IV).

DIGITALIS-INDUCED VENTRICULAR ECTOPY

- Volume replacement
- Potassium replacement
- Magnesium 2 g IV over 1 to 5 minutes; then infusion of 1 to 2 g/hour
- Lidocaine 1 to 1.5 mg/kg IV
- Dilantin IV
- Digibind (6 to 20 vials IV)

DIGITALIS-INDUCED VENTRICULAR TACHYCARDIA

- **Stable VT**
  - Digibind 10 to 20 vials given IV plus the following:
  - Lidocaine bolus 1.5 mg/kg, infusion of 3 mg/min; if needed, add the following:
  - Magnesium 2 g over 1 to 2 minutes; then infusion of 1 to 2 g/hour for 30 to 60 minutes to allow for effects of Digibind
- **Unstable VT**
  - Immediate cardioversion. (Use lower energy levels of 25 to 50 J to start because of possible post-counter-

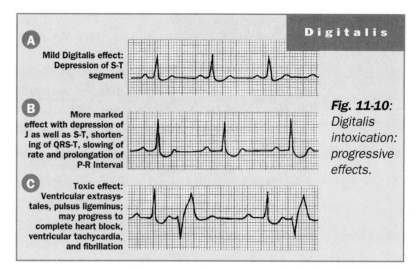

Digitalis

A Mild Digitalis effect: Depression of S-T segment

B More marked effect with depression of J as well as S-T, shortening of QRS-T, slowing of rate and prolongation of P-R Interval

C Toxic effect: Ventricular extrasystales, pulsus ligeminus; may progress to complete heart block, ventricular tachycardia, and fibrillation

Fig. 11-10: Digitalis intoxication: progressive effects.

shock rhythm deterioration in patients with digitalis intoxication.)

- Digibind (10 to 20 vials). This will take time to work, so add the following:
- Lidocaine 1 to 1.5 mg/kg
- Magnesium 2 g IV push; then up to 5 g over 2 to 5 minutes

DIGITALIS-INDUCED VENTRICULAR FIBRILLATION

- Standard ACLS: Shock, endotracheal intubation, epinephrine, lidocaine 1.5 mg/kg, Then
- Magnesium 2g IV push, PLUS the following:
- Digibind 20 vials (or as many as available up to 20)

Sum Doode

CASE 11

NARCOTIC OVERDOSE

You are on duty in the Emergency Department when a 1971 Toyota Corolla drives up to the door and three barefoot teenagers dressed only in tattered blue jeans jump from the car. They reach into the back seat and bring out another similarly dressed 18-year-old man who appears unconscious and unresponsive.

"I think he got some bad heroin," one shouts. "Take care of him!" As you and the clinic assistant transfer the young man to a nearby gurney, the three "friends" jump into their Corolla and rapidly drive off.

As you roll Mr. Doode into Room 1, you quickly check his carotid pulse and note that it is present. Upon looking for respirations, however, you observe that he is not breathing and is becoming more cyanotic and mottled.

How would you manage this respiratory emergency?

COMMENTS

- Case 11 presents a classic case of an acute narcotic overdose in which respirations have ceased (or at least have been inadequate), yet cardiac function remains. Your major effort here should be to reverse the respiratory arrest while providing respiratory support.

- Initiate the Primary-Secondary Survey as rapidly as possible. Many Emergency Departments are so familiar with this scenario that often intubation is delayed to determine whether the narcotic antagonist **naloxone** will suffice.

Bag-valve-mask ventilations are used to support the patient until the IV access is gained and naloxone is administered.

THERAPY

- Treat using standard ACLS protocols, but add the following:
- **Naloxone** 2 mg IV; repeat every 2 to 5 minutes up to 10 mg to nonresponders.
- Half-life ranges from 15 to 45 minutes, so watch for relapse into coma.
- **Naloxone infusion** 0.8 to 1.0 mg/hour is titrated to effect. (Mix 8 to 10 mg in 1000 mL of D_5W).

Sum Doode	
CASE 11 Continued	

With a rapidity that never ceases to amaze the hardened Emergency Department staff, Mr. Doode awoke within 15 seconds of the administration of naloxone 2 mg IV. He looked around, and on seeing the staff slapped his forehead and said, "Oh bummer, not again!" Virtually no other history was forthcoming. Mr. Doode had obvious needle tracks up and down both forearms. After 15 minutes' observation he displayed no change in his sensorium, continuing to curse and abuse the nursing staff.

To make his original room available for subsequent emergencies, he was moved to the hallway where he could rest but remain under observation. Twenty minutes later one of the nurses asked, "Where's Mr. Charmer?" at which point the empty stretcher was noted. A quick search revealed that Mr. Doode had vanished from the vicinity. "I bet he doesn't come back for his registration card," smiled one of the nurses.

COMMENTS

- Patients who respond well to naloxone should be observed for their respiratory response while the naloxone half-life of 15 to 45 minutes passes. Many patients with longer-acting narcotics in the bloodstream lapse back into unconsciousness or respiratory compromise.

- The naloxone infusion (0.8 to 1.0 mg/hour) can be very effective in those patients taking longer-acting narcotics.

Clive Holmberg	
CASE 12	

BENZODIAZEPINE OVERDOSE

A 27-year-old rugby player had fallen, landing hard on his right shoulder with his arm extended. He suffered an obvious anterior shoulder dislocation. He was placed in Room 3 with oxygen saturation monitor, two IVs, ECG monitor, suction device, oxygen supply, and ventilation equipment. To facilitate reduction, the orthopedic resident ordered meperidine 50 mg IV and midazolam 2 mg IV.

These agents appeared to have no effect on the vigorously complaining young man. Midazolam 2 mg IV was repeated every 5 minutes with virtually no effect. After 12 mg had been given, the resident asked the "ED attending" what to add for better sedation and analgesia. While walking back to check on the patient, the attending and resident were greeted by the nurse, who shouted, "We need some help in here. I think this guy just stopped breathing!"

How would you approach this iatrogenic respiratory emergency? What agent is now used as a specific antidote to benzodiazepine overdoses?

COMMENTS

- The young man in Case 12 has acute respiratory depression resulting from the high doses of benzodiazepine that he was given.

- The Primary-Secondary Survey must be initiated quickly; provide good ventilations and oxygenation to this patient while obtaining flumazenil (Romazicon), a benzodiazepine receptor antagonist.

- **TREATMENT**:

  - Flumazenil 0.2 mg (2 mL) administered IV over 60 seconds. In reversal of conscious sedation, 80% to 90% of patients will wake up within 60 seconds. Amnesia will be their major complaint.

  - Repeat 0.2 mg IV at 1 minute intervals until a total maximum does of 1 mg has been given.

  - For resedation (which may occur in 3% to 9% of patients), repeat doses may be given at 20-minute intervals as needed. Give at no more than 1 mg (given at 0.2 mg/min), and give no more than 3 mg in any 1 hour.

WHAT IF THIS HAD BEEN A CASE OF SUSPECTED BENZODIAZEPINE OVERDOSE? HOW WOULD YOU CHANGE THE ADMINISTRATION OF FLUMAZENIL?

For management of suspected benzodiazepine overdose you give the Romazicon more slowly, and you give more:

- Flumazenil 0.2 mg IV over 30 seconds. Wait 30 seconds. If level of consciousness is not satisfactory, give the following:

- Flumazenil 0.3 mg IV over 30 seconds. If not satisfactory, give the following:

- Flumazenil 0.5 mg IV over 30 seconds at 1-minute intervals up to a cumulative dose of 3 mg.

- If there is no response within 5 minutes of a cumulative dose of 5 mg flumazenil, benzodiazepine is unlikely to be the cause of the sedation.

KEY POINTS

SUMMARY

- The cases in this chapter attempt to expand the traditional ACLS focus on cardiac arrest rhythms and algorithms.
- Instead, we ask the questions that we emphasize throughout this book: Why did the person go into the arrest? If you saw this person 30 minutes before the arrest, would you know enough to prevent it?
- We focus on the treatment of potentially lethal electrolyte and toxicologic emergencies, which, if administered rapidly and aggressively, could actually prevent the cardiac arrest.
- In addition, we focus on how the treatment of the cardiac arrest would differ depending on what caused the arrest.
- Since many of the arrests you will treat in your career will follow electrolyte and toxicologic emergencies, we think these approaches must be learned by every professional who treats cardiac emergencies.

Effects on ECG of Electrolyte and Drug Intoxication

HYPERKALEMIA

- *Prolonged PR interval (first-degree heart block).*
- *P waves almost disappeared.*
- *Tall, peaked (tenting) T waves.*
- *ST-segment depression; S and T wave merging.*
- *Sine-wave pulseless electrical activity, wide-complex tachycardias, ventricular tachycardia, VF.*

HYPOKALEMIA

- *T waves flatten down.*
- *ST segment becomes depressed.*
- *QT interval becomes more prolonged.*
- *QRS complex widens.*
- *Wide-complex tachycardias, ventricular tachycardia, VF.*

HYPERCALCEMIA

- *Key: QT intervals markedly shortened.*
- *Automaticity is decreased.*

- *ST-segments are shortened and depressed.*
- *T waves widen.*
- *Bundle branch blocks may occur.*
- *Second-degree heart block may progress to complete heart block and cardiac arrest (usually with levels above 20 mg/dL).*

HYPOCALCEMIA

- *Prolonged QT interval.*

HYPOMAGNESEMIA

- *Note the overlap with low potassium and low calcium levels.*
- *Prolongation of the PR and QT intervals.*
- *Wide QRS complexes.*
- *ST-segment depression.*
- *Broad, flat T waves with precordial T-wave inversion.*

TOXIC EFFECTS OF CYCLIC ANTIDEPRESSANTS AND MAJOR TRANQUILIZERS (NEUROLEPTICS)

- *ST-segment and T-wave changes.*
- *QRS duration is prolonged.*
- *QT interval is prolonged.*
- *Right-axis deviations of the QRS complex.*

- *Bundle branch blocks.*
- *Atrioventricular conduction blocks, aberrant conduction.*
- *Ominously broad, slurred QRS sine waves.*
- *Ventricular arrhythmias.*
- *Pulseless electrical activity.*

BETA BLOCKER OVERDOSE

- *Bradycardia.*
- *Atrioventricular block.*
- *Widening of the QRS complex.*
- *Peaked T wave.*
- *ST-segment changes.*
- *Further cardiac deterioration leading to pulseless electrical activity, cardiac arrest.*

CALCIUM CHANNEL BLOCKER OVERDOSE

- *Sinus bradycardia.*
- *QRS-complex widening and QT-interval lengthening.*
- *Heart blocks, particularly prolonged first-degree block, but also second- and third-degree blocks.*
- *Pulseless electrical activity.*

TABLE 11-3

Toxicologic and Electrolyte Abnormalties

Clinical Problem	Typical ECG Findings	Treatment Approaches
ELECTROLYTE ABNORMALITIES		
HYPERKALEMIA *ECG changes are listed in order increasing potassium levels.*	• *Tall, peaked (tenting) T waves.* • *Prolonged PR interval (first-degree heart block).* • *Prolonged QT intervals.* • *P waves diminished.* • *ST-segment depression; S and T wave merging; node conduction problems.* • *Sine wave pulseless electrical activity (PEA).* • *Wide-complex tachycardias, ventricular tachycardia (VT), ventricular fibrillation (VF).*	• *Sodium bicarbonate 1 mEq/kg IV bolus.* • *Calcium chloride 5 to 10 mL IV, 10% solution (50 to 100 mg).* • *Regular insulin 10 units IV plus one ampule (50 g) glucose.* • *Furosemide 40 mg to 80 mg IV bolus.* • *Kayexelate 15 to 50 g by mouth or rectum, plus sorbitol.* • *Peritoneal dialysis or hemodialysis.*
HYPOKALEMIA	• *U waves become more prominent.* • *T waves flatten down.* • *ST segment becomes depressed.* • *QT interval becomes more prolonged.* • *QRS complex widens.* • *Wide-complex tachycardias, VT, VF.*	• *If serum potassium (K) level = 3.0 to 3.5 mEq/L, need ≈ 100 mEq K replacement.* • *If serum K level = 2.5 to 3.0 mEq/L, need ≈ 200 mEq K replacement.* • *Infuse 10 to 40 mEq/hour. (Never put >40 to 80 mEq in 1-L bottle.)*
HYPERCALCEMIA *Normal total calcium = 8.5 to 10.5 mg/dL.* *Normal ionized calcium = 4.2 to 4.8 mg/dL.*	• *Key: QT intervals markedly shortened.* • *Automaticity is decreased.* • *ST segments are shortened and depressed.* • *T waves widen.* • *Bundle branch blocks may occur.* • *Second-degree heart block may progress to complete heart block and cardiac arrest (usually with levels above 20 mg/dL).*	**Urgent treatment** • *Normal saline (NS) bolus: Induce diuresis.* • *Furosemide 40 to 100 mg IV (1 mg/kg every 2 to 4 hours).* • *Replace K and magnesium (Mg) as needed.* **Cardiac arrest** • *Standard ACLS plus.* • *Mg sulfate 1 to 2 g IV push.* • *Potassium 1 to 2 mEq/min.* • *NS bolus.* • *Diuretics.*

CONTINUED

HYPOCALCEMIA *Normal total calcium = 8.5 to 10.5 mg/dL.* *Normal ionized calcium = 4.2 to 4.8 mg/dL.*	• *Prolonged QT interval due to prolonged ST-segment.* • *May have VT or torsades de pointes.*	**Urgent** • *Calcium chloride 10% solution. (1 g in 10 mL = 272 mg calcium.) Give 100 mg in 100 mL D_5W in 10 to 20 minutes.* • *In the next 6 to 12 hours give a total of 1 g by continuous IV drip.* **Cardiac arrest** • *Full ampule of calcium chloride (1 g in 10 mL of a 10% solution).*
HYPOMAGNESEMIA *Normal level = 1.5 to 2.0 mEq/L.* *Severe hypomagnesemia = 1.4 mEq/L.* *Severe = <0.5 mEq/L.*	• *Prolongation of the PR and QT intervals.* • *Wide QRS complexes.* • *ST-segment depression.* • *Broad, flat T waves with precordial T-wave inversion.*	**Noncardiac arrest** • *Mg sulfate 1 to 2 g IV over 5 to 10 minutes.* • *Follow initial 1 to 2 g with 4 to 6 g in next 24 hours.* **Cardiac arrest** • *Mg sulfate 1 to 2 g IV push.*

DRUG OVERDOSES

CYCLIC ANTIDEPRESSANTS AND MAJOR TRANQUILIZERS *(NEUROLEPTICS)*	• *ST-segment and T-wave changes.* • *QRS duration is prolonged.* • *QT interval is prolonged.* • *Right-axis deviations of the QRS complex.* • *Bundle branch blocks.* • *Atrioventricular (AV) conduction blocks, aberrant conduction.* • *Ominously broad, slurred QRS sine waves.* • *Ventricular arrhythmias.* • *Pulseless electrical activity.*	• *Hyperventilation to pH = 7.5.* • **Benzodiazepine** *(first choice) or* **phenobarbitial** *(second choice) for seizures.* • **Sodium bicarbonate** *1 to 5 mEq/kg over 1 to 2 minutes.* • **Bicarbonate** *infusions 50 to 100 mEq (1 to 2 ampules in 0.25 NS) at 150 to 200 mL/hour.* • **Mg** *1 to 2 g IV bolus if unstable; over 1 to 5 minutes if stable; up to 5 to 10 grams total.* • *Pressors if needed (****norepinephrine, epinephrine, high-dose dopamine****).* • *Charcoal hemoperfusion.* • *Cardiopulmonary bypass.*

CONTINUED

| COCAINE | • *Sinus tachycardias.*
• *Supraventricular tachycardias*
• *VT/VF.*
• *Cocaine-induced acute myocardial infraction (AMI).* | **Not in cardiac arrest**
• *Consider delay of thrombolytics until enzyme levels return from laboratory.*
• **Benzodiazepines** *for increased blood pressure and heart rate.*
• **Mg sulfate** *may prevent cocaine-induced arrhythmias.*
• *For definite AMI treat per usual AMI protocols.*
• *Use* **nitroglycerin** *(10 to 20 ug/min) or nitroprusside (0.1 to 5 ug/kg/min IV) to lower blood pressure and heart rate.*
• **Phentolamine** *1 to 10 mg titrated as a dilute solution over 2 to 3 minutes to lower blood pressure.*
• **Labetalol** *(5 to 20 mg IV): Consider for severe hypertension. Both alpha blocking and beta blocking remain areas of controversy.*
For cardiac arrests
• *Use lidocaine cautiously*
• *Space out epinephrine to every 5 to 10 minutes.*
• *Consider* **propranolol** *3 to 5 mg every 5 minutes or* **labetalol** *5 to 20 mg if VF persists.* |
| BETA BLOCKERS | • *Bradycardia.*
• *AV block.*
• *Widening of the QRS complex.*
• *Peaked T waves changes.*
• *ST changes.*
• *Further cardiac deterioration leading to PEA, cardiac arrest.* | • *Saline bolus of 500 to 1000 mL.*
• *Atropine 0.5 to 1.0 mg IV if bradycardic.*
• *Epinephrine 2 to 100 ug/min, if hypotensive.*
• *Glucagon 1 to 5 mg IV (over 1 minute).*
• *Dopamine infusion at 10 to 20 ug/kg per minute.*
• *Calcium chloride 5 to 20 mL IV.*
• *Pacing: transcutaneous or transvenous.*
• *Additional pressor agents if poor response to preceding interventions: dobutamine, norepinephrine, isoproterenol.* |

CONTINUED

CALCIUM CHANNEL BLOCKERS	• Sinus bradycardia. • QRS-complex widening and QT-interval lengthening. • Heart blocks, particularly prolonged first-degree block, but also second- and third-degree blocks. • Pulseless electrical activity.	• Saline bolus of 500 to 1000 mL. • Calcium chloride 1 to 4 g (10 to 40 mL of 10% solution). Goal is to elevate serum calcium level by 1 to 2 mg/dL. • **Glucagon** 1 to 5 mg IV (positive effects on myocardial contractility and AV conduction). • **Epinephrine** infusion at 2 to 100 ug/min for low blood pressure. • **Dopamine** infusion at 10 to 20 ug/kg per minute for low blood pressure. • Repeat **calcium chloride** 5 to 10 mL of 10% solution (after epinephrine has sensitized the myocardium). • **Dobutamine, norepinephrine,** and/or **isoproterenol** if still refractory. • **4-Aminopyridine.** (experimental in United States). • **Pacing:** Either transcutaneous or transvenous. • **Cardiopulmonary** bypass in special situations.
DIGITALIS	Many arrhthymias are possible including the following: • Bradycardias. • Ventricular ectopy and VT.	**Basic therapy** • Volume replacement. • Potassium replacement. • Magnesium replacement. • Digoxin-specific antibodies (Digibind). One 40 mg vial of Fab binds 0.6 mg digoxin. • Fab dose is based on weight and digoxin level. **Urgent therapy** • Give 10 to 20 vials empirically. • Arrhythmias: Usual therapy plus generous use of magnesium and Fab fragments.

CONTINUED

| NARCOTICS | • *No specific effects on the ECG.*
• *Bradycardia and asystole follow the respiratory depression.* | • *Treat using standard ACLS protocols, but add the following:*
• **Naloxone** *2 mg IV; repeat every 2 to 5 minutes up to 10 mg to nonresponders.*
  • *Half-life ranges from 15 to 45 minutes, so watch for relapse into coma.*
• **Naloxone infusion** *0.8 to 1.0 mg/hour, titrated to effect (mix 8 to 10mg in 1000 mL of D5W).* |
| BENZODIAZEPINES | • *No specific effects on the ECG.*
• *Bradycardia and asystole follow the respiratory depression.* | • **Flumazenil** *0. 2 mg (2 mL) administered IV over 15 seconds; used to reverse sedation from benzodiazepine overdose; 80% to 90% patients wake up in 60 seconds.*
• *Repeat 0.2 mg IV at 1 minute intervals until a total maximum does of 1mg has been given.*
• *For resedation (may occur in 3% to 9% of patients) give repeat doses at 20 minute intervals as needed. Give no more than 1 mg (given at 0.2 mg/ min), and give no more than 3 mg in any 1 hour.* |

TABLE 11-4

Correlation Between ECG Abnormalities and Clinical Problems

Typical ECG Abnormalities	Clinical Problems
P waves diminished	Hyperkalemia
PR intervals prolonged	Hyperkalemia
	Hypomagnesemia
	Hypercalcemia
	Beta blockers
	Calcium channel blockers
	Cyclic antidepressants
	Neuroleptics
QRS widened	Hypomagnesemia
	Hypercalcemia
	Beta blockers
	Cyclic antidepressants
QT interval prolonged	Hyperkalemia
	Hypocalcemia
	Cyclic antidepressants
	Neuroleptics
	Calcium channel blockers
QT interval shortened	Hypercalcemia
ST-segment depression	Hyperkalemia
ST-segment shortened	Hypercalcemia
	Beta blockers
T waves tall and peaked	Hyperkalemia
	Beta blockers
T waves wider	Hypercalcemia
T waves flatter	Hypomagnesemia
U waves appear	Hypokalemia

Drowning

OVERVIEW

When treating cardiac arrest associated with drowning, be aware of important differences between treating drowning victims and treating victims of nontraumatic cardiac arrest.

The cases in this chapter bring out the unique features of treating the drowning victim and provide guidelines for how to approach these emergencies.

These major differences are as follows:

- *Drowning is a primary respiratory event, not cardiac; management must focus on the airway.*

- *Drowning represents a form of trauma; victims of drowning are also managed as victims of trauma.*

- *Drowning usually occurs in an environment that poses problems of rescuer safety; rescuer safety must not be ignored.*

- *Drowning often adds the challenge of hypothermia to the patient and the rescuers; manage drowning victims as victims of hypothermia.*

- *Drowning often represents a tragedy that could be prevented; drowning can be the end result of violations of common sense and violations of decent child care.*

MAJOR CONCEPTS TO MASTER

- Hypoxia is the major problem in drowning. Most cardiac arrests that occur in association with drowning are really secondary cardiac arrests—secondary to the damage done by the extreme hypoxia of drowning. Therefore the top three concerns in drowning become "airway, airway, airway." Rapid initiation of advanced airway management plays the major role in resuscitation from drowning. This contrasts with rapid initiation of defibrillation, which plays the major role in so many other cardiopulmonary emergencies.

- Prevention is a major theme in drowning. As in cardiac arrest that is due to trauma, our major goals should be to prevent the original trauma, plus prevent the secondary cardiac arrests that ensue. Once a person deteriorates to an unconscious, breathless, and pulseless state in the setting of trauma or drowning, the chances for a successful outcome diminish to the vanishing point.

- *Rescuer safety* should never be forgotten. A key rule in emergency medicine: Never have the rescuer become a second victim. Rescue of drowning victims occurs on or near the water, and this exposes the rescue team to the same hostile environment. Emergency personnel use many emergency techniques to rescue people from the water. Such techniques are beyond the scope of this handbook. We encourage all ACLS providers, however, to learn more about field rescue techniques. You never know when such skills will be a matter of saving a life— yours as well as the victim's.

- Drowning should be recognized as a traumatic event. You use different approaches when associated traumatic injuries are possible. In particular, the responsibility to protect and stabilize a potentially unstable spine rests with the rescuer. CPR, airway maintenance, and ventilation must be performed in light of possible associated trauma.

- **Hypothermia frequently occurs in association with drowning. Cold water emergencies add the disorder of hypothermia to the equation, increasing the trauma to the victim and increasing the danger to the rescuer.**
- **Appropriate treatment of the drowning victim requires knowledge of rewarming techniques and the treatment of hypothermia. These techniques are presented in Chapter 14.**

Critical actions

- Ensure rescuer safety.
- Learn the key principles of prehospital care: extricate-rescue-resuscitate-stabilize-transport.
- Apply the Five Quadrads to the initial management of drowning victims, as follows:

- Perform the steps of the Primary-Secondary Survey from the Universal Algorithm.
- During airway opening always provide cervical spine stabilization.
- Perform CPR when indicated.
- Hunt for ventricular fibrillation (VF); it is always a possibility.
- Oxygen/IV/Monitor/Fluids.
- Provide advanced life support when indicated.
- Consider differential diagnoses, including significant hypothermia.
- In post-resuscitation care monitor for development of respiratory complications (pneumonia, pneumonitis, adult respiratory distress syndrome [ADRS], and pulmonary edema).

Bobby Ray Presley

CASE 1

Bobby Ray Presley, a 16-year-old high school sophomore, was "horsing around" at a large family Labor Day picnic. One cousin shoved Bobby Ray particularly hard, and he fell backward into the pool, slipping as he did so and striking the water at a "head-first" angle. Only several minutes later did someone notice that Bobby Ray was no longer adding his raucous laughter and enthusiastic shoves. In fact, Bobby Ray had not resurfaced after being pushed into the pool and had remained on the bottom, unconscious and unnoticed, for at least 3 minutes. His natural buoyancy brought him floating back, face down, to the surface. Suddenly someone spotted him and screamed, "Oh my god! Something's happened to Bobby!"

Several friends quickly removed Bobby Ray from the water and brought him to the poolside, placing him on his abdomen. At first all the bystanders watched in dismay at his blue, cold, and unresponsive body. Finally, one of the adults ran up shouting, "He's drowned! Quick! Do the Heimlich maneuver! I've seen it on TV." One of the other bystanders commented, "Well, shouldn't we do CPR first? I think you only do the Heimlich maneuver for choking people who are moving around."

The man vigorously grabbed Bobby's torso and pushed him over to his back, the head rolling loosely back and forth with the turning. "No, you've got to get the water out of the lungs before we can get the air in." The man straddled the 16-year-old's body and began a series of vigorous thrusts to Bobby Ray's midsection, just below the ribcage. After several thrusts he paused to look at Bobby Ray's mouth and saw no water emerging. "Well, I better push harder," the man said, and returned to the vigorous thrusting.

This time, a large amount of stomach contents welled up from the mouth, containing a mixture of chili, baked beans, and barbecued ribs. One of the bystanders reached over and turned Bobby Ray's head to the side so that the food would drain out; however, it was too thick and remained stagnant in his mouth. "Let's start chest compressions while we wait for the ambulance." No one came forward to perform mouth-to-mouth breathing.

You are a paramedic on duty when the 911 call comes in. You hear "teenage boy drowns in his family pool" and hear nothing of the circumstances of the event. You walk quickly up to the poolside and see many people standing around. You notice that one man was doing chest compressions and another person was leaning over, holding Bobby's head in his hands.

What important features of drowning does this scene illustrate? What is the current teaching about the Heimlich maneuver for drowning? How would you care for this patient?

Case 1 presents the following important concepts to remember about drowning and near-drowning episodes:

- Drowning should always be considered and treated as a *traumatic* event. As outlined in Chapters 13, 14, and 15, cardiac arrest associated with trauma must be treated differently. You must immobilize and protect the cervical spine, and you must maintain a heightened awareness of the possibilities of other injuries. These include not only obvious falls, diving injuries, and boat capsizings, but also a wide range of minor, unseen collisions occurring underwater.

- Cervical spine injuries are always a possibility in drowning and near-drowning events, and much attention must be given to proper protection of the cervical spine. Fig. 12-1 displays the technique for shallow water rescue with neck stabilization in the water. Every swimming pool and public swimming area should have backboards and cervical collars available and should be staffed with personnel who know how to perform CPR, know how to immobilize and protect the spine, and know how to do CPR for someone who has a possible cervical spine injury. These are special skills, and the public has the right to expect these skills to be available in public swimming areas. With Bobby Ray, we have the terrible tragedy of a paralyzing cervical spine injury that will leave the young man in a wheelchair for the rest of his life.

- Death from drowning is a *respiratory* death. This means your primary interventions must focus on opening and protecting the airway and providing adequate *oxygenation* (getting oxygen in) and adequate *ventilation* (getting carbon dioxide out). Hypoxia is your major opponent in drowning and must be fought aggressively. Cardiac arrest in drowning is almost always a *secondary* event following excessively prolonged hypoxia (but there are exceptions: see Case 3). In children, in particular, a pulseless, apneic state is usually a late, preterminal state and is very ominous. Work hard to keep the patient from getting to that point.

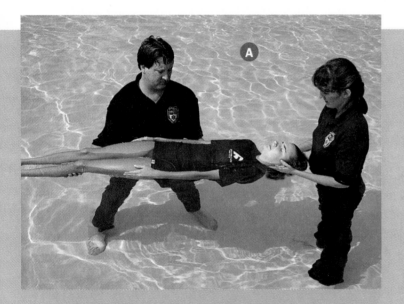

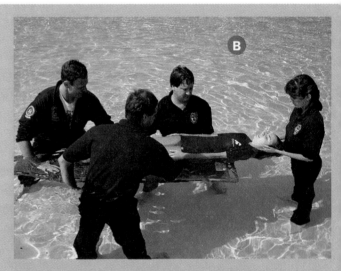

Fig. 12-1, A to G: Neck stabilization in shallow water rescue.

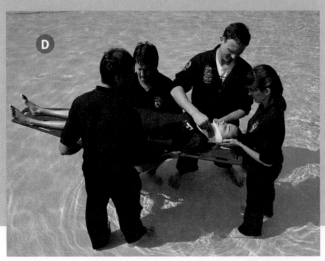

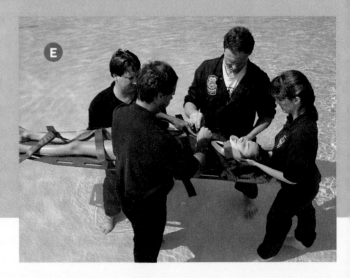

- Since drowning produces *respiratory arrests* in which hypoxia leads to *cardiac arrest,* you must provide ventilations as soon as possible. This means beginning the ABCs in the water, before you get the victim to shore. Fig. 12-2, *A* and *B,* demonstrates the performance of rescue breathing in shallow water, and Fig. 12-3 shows a technique for rescue breathing in deep water, in which a life belt provides victim buoyancy while the rescuer provides ventilations.

- The Heimlich maneuver must *not* be performed as the first intervention in drowning victims. In this scenario the rescuers, well-intentioned though they were, committed at least two dangerous errors, as follows, by their misunderstanding of the place of the Heimlich maneuver in drowning resuscitation:

  - First, by their efforts to perform the Heimlich maneuver, they may very well have contributed to the C5-6 transection of the spinal cord that left Bobby Ray permanently paralyzed. We can never know this for sure. The full, irreversible spinal injury may have occurred the moment the victim made contact with the bottom of the pool on his original fall.

- On the other hand, the final transsection of the spinal cord may have occurred later, for example, when Bobby Ray was pulled from the water without proper immobilization, during the unsupported turning and manipulations of the body, or during the inappropriate Heimlich thrusts done at the start of the resuscitation attempts.

- Furthermore, the Heimlich maneuver unquestionably produced the regurgitation of stomach contents that resulted in complete airway obstruction, aspiration of gastric contents, and a severe post-resuscitation pneumonitis that necessitated 7 days on the ventilator.

- Although the Heimlich maneuver has clearly saved lives in the situation of conscious, choking victims, there has been no scientific evidence that the maneuver should be performed at the start of a drowning resuscitation to "get the water out of the lungs." No valid data confirm the hypothesis that drowning victims' lungs are full of water or that they need to have their lungs "unplugged" from all the water sucked in during the drowning.

- Field personnel who intubate the tracheas of drowning victims report that they rarely encounter lungs and respiratory pathways "full of water" when they look down their laryngoscopes. Only minimal amounts of water are required to induce the laryngospasm that frequently occurs with drowning. As shown in Fig. 12-4, it is submersion with resultant lack of oxygen that produces the problem, not aspirating water into the lungs. When the head finally sinks below the water surface, air to breathe is no longer available. The victim does not continue efforts to breathe underwater and consequently does not suck in vast quantities of water.

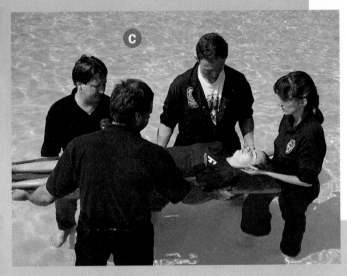

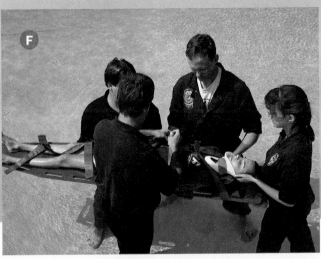

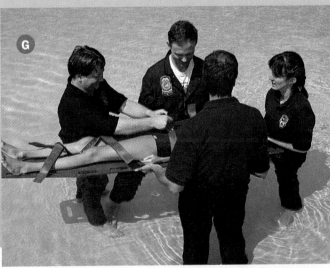

Fig. 12-1: *Continued.*

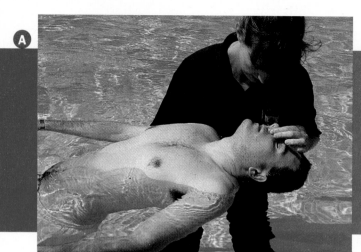
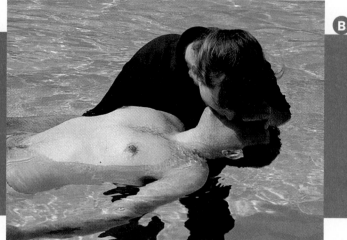

Fig. 12-2, A and B: *Rescue breathing, shallow water.*

- Both the AHA and the American Red Cross endorse the use of the Heimlich maneuver *once the rescuers establish that the airway is obstructed* (after two breaths and repositioning the airway). The following is a reasonable and straightforward approach to drowning victims:

  - Provide A—an Airway (with C-spine stabilization precautions).

  - Provide B—two breaths.

  - If the two breaths do not enter the lungs easily, reposition the airway, paying particular attention to the chin-lift maneuver.

  - If ventilation is still unsuccessful, try the Heimlich maneuver.

- The routine, systematic approach to the drowning victim should continue to follow the recommendations of the Primary-Secondary Survey and the Five Quadrads (see the box on p. 230).

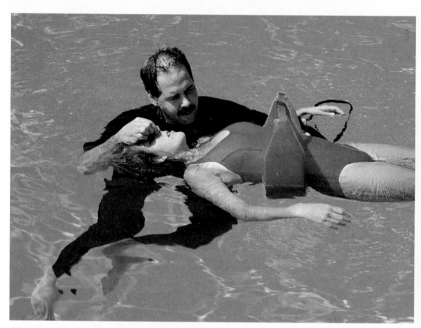

Fig. 12-3: *Rescue breathing, deep water.*

| **Bobby Ray Presley** **CASE 1 Continued** | *You realize that this is a drowning associated with a dive and fall and therefore a possible cervical spine injury. You ask one of the EMTs on the scene to return to your ambulance and get the full-length backboard and rigid cervical spine collars. You ask one of the* |

bystanders, "Please keep doing CPR until I tell you to stop."

How would you apply the Five Quadrads with the Primary-Secondary Survey to this scenario? (see box on p. 230.)

Primary Survey

AIRWAY

- You immediately direct your partner to provide in-line cervical spine immobilization (not traction), with a jaw thrust. This requires moving the neck back to the neutral position. You do this slowly and carefully without rough or sudden movements.

- The food in the mouth is immediately apparent, so you begin to clear the airway with the hand-powered, portable suction device.

BREATHING

- Once you remove most of the food, you take the oropharyngeal airway and insert it into the mouth.

- You attach the oxygen tubing to the inlet valve on the bag-valve-mask and begin hyperventilations.
- The lungs appear to be rising bilaterally and symmetrically.

CIRCULATION

- At this point, while you are "bagging," you tell the bystander doing CPR to stop the chest compressions while you check for a pulse at the carotid artery. There is no pulse, and you tell him to start chest compressions again.

DEFIBRILLATION

- The chest is dried off quickly with a towel, and a quick look with the paddles reveals that the rhythm is not VF or ventricular tachycardia (VT). The monitor screen shows slow, organized complexes of 20 to 30 per minute.

DISABILITY

- At this point you are not able to evaluate neurologic dysfunction during the cardiac arrest and resuscitation efforts. You notice, however, that Bobby Ray has a full erection, and this registers as an ominous sign in suspected spine injuries.

Secondary Survey

AIRWAY

- You turn over the bag-valve-mask to one of the EMTs. You begin preparation for endotracheal intubation. There is no delay in your steady movement to advanced airway control of this patient.

BREATHING

- Using good in-line cervical spine immobilization, you are able to intubate the trachea on the second try.
- You notice that there is considerable food debris in the hypopharynx and just above the tracheal opening. Otherwise the trachea is clear, and there is not a trace of water from the pool.
- After attaching the bag and inflating the endotracheal tube cuff, you observe good bilateral chest movements, and good breath sounds in the midaxillary regions; the end-tidal CO_2 detector also indicates that the tube is in the lungs.

CIRCULATION

- A repeat pulse check shows that Bobby Ray remains in full cardiac arrest.
- Your partner was already starting a 14-gauge IV line in the right arm, and she soon announces, "IV is in. Are you ready for epinephrine?"
- The monitor screen on the defibrillator provides a rhythm display, and you notice now that the rhythm is an organized QRS complex at 40 beats/min.
- "Yes, go ahead with epinephrine 1 mg IV bolus and follow immediately with atropine 1 mg IV. Make sure you run in some fluids after each drug and elevate the arm during the 'chaser' bolus of fluid."

DIFFERENTIAL DIAGNOSIS

- You are growing increasingly worried about the possibility of a cervical spine injury, given the history you have been hearing.
- You know that hypothermia can always be a contributing factor during a resuscitation attempt, so you direct someone to dry Bobby Ray off thoroughly, remove his clothing, and provide him with passive external rewarming (i.e., place a blanket over him). Core temperature must be followed in the post-resuscitation period.
- Your thoughts are that this was a head injury with loss of consciousness upon hitting the bottom of the pool. This probably produced a cervical spinal column fracture and spinal instability. Whether an associated spinal cord injury occurred with the original fall is unknown. The unstable spine may have led to a spinal cord injury during the unstabilized removal from the water or during efforts to perform the unnecessary Heimlich maneuvers.
- While unconscious under the water, Bobby Ray was unable to breath, and severe hypoxia ensued. This hypoxia led to a cardiac arrest. You think that good respiratory support and appropriate cardiac stimulants should restore spontaneous circulation.
- You will need to tell the emergency physicians about the large amount of food aspiration, which will require special attention in the post-resuscitation period.
- The epinephrine, atropine, and hyperventilation with 100% oxygen through the tube appears to be restoring cardiac function. After 2 minutes, your partner reports that she can feel a carotid pulse, and the subsequent blood pressure measured 100/70 mm Hg at a heart rate of 85 beats/min.

OXYGEN/IV/MONITOR/FLUIDS

- Oxygen, started; IV, started; Monitor, attached; Fluids, normal saline at keep-open rate. (Avoid excessive fluids because of the high risk of post-resuscitation pulmonary edema and pneumonitis.)

VITAL SIGNS

- Temperature, 35.8° C; heart rate, 85beats/min; blood pressure, 100/70 mm Hg, respirations, 12 breaths/min and spontaneous.

CARDIOVASCULAR QUADRAD

- **Tank:** No reason to suspect hypovolemia.
- **Resistance:** Peripheral vascular resistance is increased because of the cool water hypothermia.
- **Pump:** A major pump problem existed here. The asystolic arrest (pump failure) was secondary to hypoxia; the hypoxia was secondary to drowning. However, by restoring good airway control, reversing the hypoxia, and providing appropriate pharmacologic treatment, you managed to restore spontaneous cardiac activity.
- **Rate:** Not a problem.

The Five Quadrads Applied to Resuscitations in Drownings

Primary Survey

AIRWAY

- *Provide in-line cervical spine immobilization (not traction). May need to move the neck to the neutral position. Do this slowly and carefully without rough or sudden movements.*
- *Open the airway with jaw-thrust maneuver.*
- *Clear the airway of any visible foreign bodies.*
- *Insert oropharyngeal airway.*

BREATHING

- *Provide positive-pressure ventilations through open airway with appropriate technique (bag-valve-mask, pocket face mask, mouth-to-mask).*
- *Ensure that lungs rise bilaterally and symmetrically.*
- *If unable to ventilate lungs, reposition jaw, try other airway opening techniques (finger sweep, hand-powered or battery-powered portable suction device, Heimlich maneuver).*
- *Provide supplemental oxygen. (Attach oxygen tubing to the inlet valve on the bag-valve-mask and begin hyperventilations.)*

CIRCULATION

- *Check carotid pulse.*
- *If no pulse, provide chest compressions.*

DEFIBRILLATION

- *Assess the rhythm with automatic or conventional defibrillator.*
- *If VF/VT, deliver shocks per protocols.*

DISABILITY

- *The D for "disability" reminds the caregiver to consider the brain. In advanced trauma life support the "disability" survey looks for significant neurologic injuries such as paralysis, brain contusions, and subarachnoid and subdural hemorrhage.*

Secondary Survey

AIRWAY

- *Prepare for endotracheal intubation.*
- *Using good in-line cervical spine immobilization, perform endotracheal intubation.*
- *Suction the airway for debris, water, and other foreign materials.*

BREATHING

- *Attach ventilation bag.*
- *Provide positive-pressure ventilation; observe for bilateral and symmetric chest rise.*
- *Listen on each side for breath sounds in the mid-axillary regions and the front of the chest.*
- *Listen for the absence of ventilation sounds over the epigastric region.*
- *End tidal-CO_2 detectors, esophageal detectors, and other techniques can also be used to verify tube placement.*
- *Tube placement may also be confirmed via laryngoscope.*
- *If necessary, remove the endotracheal tube and reattempt intubation.*

CIRCULATION

- *Start large-gauge IV line in the antecubital vein.*
- *Attach cardiac rhythm monitor.*
- *Provide rhythm-appropriate cardiac medications.*

DIFFERENTIAL DIAGNOSIS

- *Consider in a systematic fashion the possible causes of the respiratory-cardiac failure.*
- *Focus on reversible and treatable causes.*
- *Consider role of hypothermia; treat appropriately.*

Oxygen/IV/Monitor/Fluids

- *Oxygen line, started; IV, started; monitor, attached; fluid, normal saline at keep-open rate. (Avoid excessive fluids because of the high risk of post-resuscitation pulmonary edema and pneumonitis.)*

Vital Signs

- *Temperature/Blood Pressure/Heart Rate/Respirations.*

Cardiovascular Quadrad

- ***Tank:*** *Suspect hypovolemia.*
- ***Resistance:*** *Abnormal peripheral vascular resistance can profoundly affect resuscitation outcomes.*
- ***Pump:*** *Major cardiac dysfunction may be reversed by restoring good airway control and reversing hypoxia, and by providing appropriate pharmacologic treatment.*
- ***Rate:*** *Consider whether it is too fast or too slow.*

Bobby Ray Presley

CASE 1 Continued

Bobby Ray's cardiac function steadily improves, and during transport to the Emergency Department, he begins to make spontaneous respiratory movements. In the Emergency Department, you tell the attending physician about the food aspiration and the fear of significant spinal cord injury. Your fears are confirmed, for the young man has indeed suffered permanent loss of neurologic function below the C5-6 level.

What lessons about drowning can we learn from these unfortunate events?

COMMENTS

The tragic scenario in Case 1 displays the following important dimensions of drowning and near-drowning episodes:

- Associated trauma (head injury and paralysis) may have led to the drowning; therefore watch for cervical spine trauma that damages the spinal cord.

- Immobilize the head, cervical spine, back.

- Pay most attention to the airway, ventilation, and oxygenation. These efforts alone may be sufficient to restore spontaneous cardiac activity, as happened in Case 1.

- The Heimlich maneuver should not be performed as the first action in the treatment of drowning events. Use it only when indicated (i.e., to treat the inability to move air effectively into the lungs).

Roy Hawkins

CASE 2

ALCOHOL, EXHAUSTION, DROWNING, HYPOTHERMIA
You are with a crew of paramedics called to Lake Stevens for a drowning victim. A 40-year-old man, fishing without a life preserver, had caught no fish. To assuage his disappointment, he had been drinking beer steadily throughout the afternoon. While standing in the bow of the boat to recycle a portion of the beer, he stumbled and fell out of the boat, striking his head during the fall. A bystander on shore could see that Mr. Hawkins tried but could not reach the gunwale of the boat to pull himself up.

He began to swim toward shore but soon became fatigued, struggled briefly while calling for help, and then drifted under the water. He remained submerged for about 10 minutes before some other fishermen who had come over to help managed to locate his body and pull him from the dark lake water. You arrive at the dock just as the rescue boat is pulling up.

What general features of drowning does this event represent? How would you approach the care of this patient?

COMMENTS

The case of Mr. Hawkins presents many elements typical of adult drownings as follows:

- He lacked adequate safety devices on his boat.
- He fell in while not wearing a life preserver.
- He was engaged in unsafe behavior near the water (the precariously balanced micturation).
- He is intoxicated from alcohol.
- He showed poor judgment in abandoning the boat and trying to swim to shore.
- He had some degree of trauma associated with the event.
- He had poor swimming skills.
- He became fatigued.

- He became submerged in dark lake water, delaying his rescue.
- Some lakes are quite cold, adding hypothermia to the equation.

- Your approach to Mr. Hawkins should again follow the Primary-Secondary Survey Approach, modified for possible trauma, and possible hypothermia, as follows:
  - Immobilize the cervical spine.
  - Administer early and aggressive advanced airway management.
  - Provide intubation with in-line cervical spine stabilization.
  - Prevent further heat loss.
  - Provide active and passive external rewarming.

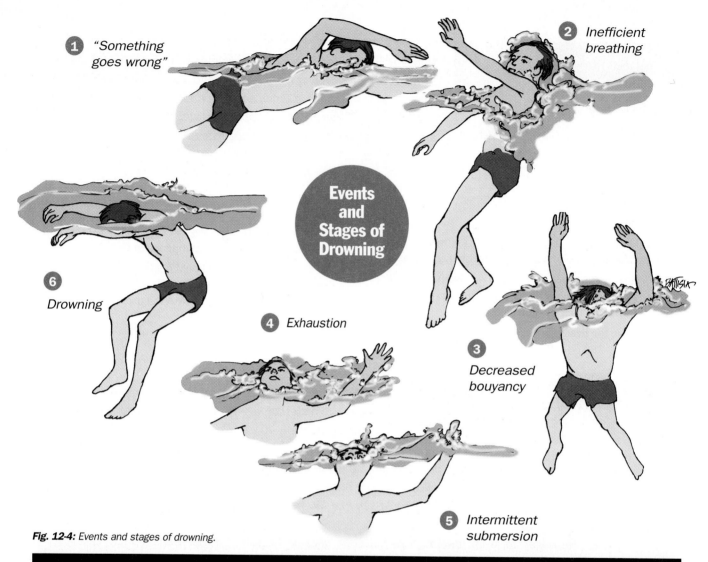

Fig. 12-4: *Events and stages of drowning.*

DETAILED LEGEND (FIG. 12-4)

1. **"Something goes wrong":** Swallowing water, fatigue, inability to cope with currents, injuries, cold weather and water, entanglement in kelp or seaweeds, loss of orientation, intoxication from alcohol or other drugs, poor swimming skills.

2. **Inefficient breathing:** Follows the increasing panic from whatever went wrong.

3. **Decreased buoyancy:** Follows the inefficient breathing (decreased residual volumes and decreased tidal volumes).

4. **Exhaustion:** Becomes more and more exhausted, fatigued, and hypoxic.

5. **Intermittent submersion:** Struggles to breathe with intermittent submersion. Victim tries to inhale air as long as possible, but decreased buoyancy and exhaustion leads to head slipping beneath the water and eventually a brief inhalation of water into the trachea. In 15% of all drownings, this induces laryngeal spasm, closing the airway and leading to death from asphyxiation.

Victims do not continue to inhale water into lungs at this point.

6. **Drowning:** Complete exhaustion and slipping under the water; complete hypoxia with loss of consciousness, convulsions, cardiac arrest, and drowning.

Note on terminology: The distinctions between "drowning" and "near-drowning" are poorly drawn. Some experts define "near-drowning" as involuntary submersion for a period of time but with spontaneous recovery once pulled from the water. "Drowning" is reserved for those people who become submerged long enough to become unconscious and to stop breathing. They do not spontaneously recover without resuscitation efforts. Some experts also distinguish between drowning with and without a pulse, claiming that loss of cardiac function during drowning implies much more severity. These ill-defined clinical states have led to much of the imprecise debate over use of the Heimlich maneuver in drowning cases.

Roy Hawkins

CASE 2 Continued

Your first steps after initiating CPR with Mr. Hawkins are to place him on a backboard and place him in a rigid cervical collar. You follow the Primary-Secondary ABCD Survey. Soon Mr. Hawkins' trachea is intubated, and his lungs hyperventilated, and he is monitored and receiving CPR.

The cardiac monitor displays narrow-complex bradycardia at 40 beats/min and no pulse. You therefore follow the Pulseless Electrical Activity (PEA) Algorithm using epinephrine and atropine.

You hope for rapid recovery of a perfusing rhythm. If this does not occur, you will need to pay close attention to other reversible problems associated with PEA, such as tension pneumothorax, cardiac tamponade, acidosis and other electrolyte disturbances, and occult hypovolemia.

Mr. Hawkins, however, begins to show signs of responding within 1 minute of intubation. He gradually recovers spontaneous cardiac function and then spontaneous respiratory function. By the time you arrive at the Emergency Department, he is fighting the endotracheal tube and beginning to open his eyes and respond.

What else should be considered in the Emergency Department? Should Mr. Hawkins be admitted?

COMMENTS

- No matter how good Mr. Hawkins looks to the emergency physicians, drowning or near-drowning victims should always be admitted to the hospital. Aspiration pneumonitis, ARDS, and pulmonary edema often develop hours after drowning and near-drowning episodes. If complications such as these are to occur, it is far better that they do so in the hospital, under observation, rather than at home.

Rev. William Ord Graves

CASE 3

VF-INDUCED DROWNING
The Suburban Senior Center has instituted a new "Aquacize" class for seniors that features dance aerobics followed by aerobic swimming. You are an EMT-D who received a 911 call for the Reverend William Ord Graves, a 70-year-old retired minister. Rev. Graves was observed to have some brief swimming difficulties while putting in his regular laps, and then to slip quietly under the water. He was recovered in less than a minute and given CPR by the lifeguards. However, when you arrive 4 minutes after the original emergency, he still has no pulse and no respirations and CPR is in progress.

You know that "definitive" drowning treatment is airway support and management. As an EMT-D, however, you are not trained to perform endotracheal intubation. Given this history, what is a major consideration? How will you approach this person?

COMMENTS

- Case 3 is a classic story for a primary cardiac event leading to drowning and, in turn, leading to a secondary respiratory event. This is an important distinction—events that look like drowning with no pulse and no breathing generally start with a respiratory problem that leads to hypoxic cardiac arrest. Here, however, you have a patient who went into exercise-associated VF, lost cerebral perfusion, became unconscious, and then became submerged beneath the water.

- By being systematic and following the Five Quadrads, you will identify the primary cause here—VF. In your system, EMT defibrillation, or first-responder defibrillation programs, have become the standard of care. With your automated external defibrillator (AED) you will be able to definitively treat Rev. Graves.

- He is defibrillated successfully by two shocks from your AED. By the time medics arrive, he is beginning to regain consciousness and has an adequate spontaneous circulation. He suffered a mild pneumonitis during his hospitalization but was discharged 7 days later with a new, automatic, implantable defibrillator.

- NOTE: in some locations the senior center would have available an AED right in the exercise facilities. Staff members would be trained in CPR and in the use of an AED. Such programs are becoming more and more common in the United States. Good ACLS providers must be familiar with these AEDs, which they may encounter in unexpected public situations.

David Perkins

CASE 4

THREE-YEAR-OLD DROWNS IN UNGATED, 3-SIDE-ENCLOSED SWIMMING POOL

You are on duty in the Emergency Department of a large academic medical center. You learn that the medics are on their way in with a 3-year-old child found floating face down in a neighbor's private swimming pool. The medics have intubated the child, noted the rhythm to be asystole, and started an intraosseous line and have administered epinephrine 0.01 mg/kg (1:10,000, 0.1 mL/kg) followed 3 minutes later by 0.1 mg/kg of 1:1000.

The Emergency Department resuscitation does not go well. The child displays no cerebral or cardiac function. After 30 minutes you decide to stop resuscitation efforts. The family members are on their way to the hospital, but the nurses tell you that the neighbors, in whose yard the drowning occurred, are very distraught and are waiting in the interview room to speak to someone.

What are some important details to learn about this drowning, particularly for the purpose of preventing such events in the future?

Darin Day

CASE 5

EIGHT-MONTH-OLD DROWNS IN BATHTUB

You are the EMT called by the 911 dispatcher for an "infant drowned in a bathtub." You arrive at the third-floor walk-up apartment in "the projects" to find a scene of chaos and tragedy. You learn that a 12-year-old older sibling had been given daily responsibility for her 8-month-old sister while the single mother worked each day. Today the 8-month-old had soiled her diaper for the third time and had been placed with some disgust in the bathtub with the water running. While filling the tub, the 12-year-old baby-sitter left briefly to answer the telephone. The caller was her boyfriend, and the conversation lingered on for several minutes. When she returned to the bathroom, she found the tub overflowing and the infant floating face down in the water.

The girl became confused and panicked, and left the child, still in the bathtub, to go get a neighbor for help. Several minutes passed before they returned and removed the child from the water and finally made a 911 call.

Your efforts are far too late. You initiate CPR and ventilations, but you know they will be futile. Paramedics arrive, intubate the infant's trachea, start an intraosseous infusion, give epinephrine, and then transport the infant to Children's Medical Center. You learn later that the resuscitation efforts were stopped within 5 minutes at the Medical Center.

What lessons does this tragic death teach us?

COMMENTS

- The drownings in Cases 4 and 5 present pediatric cases. One could argue that pediatric cases do not belong in this "adult" life support book. Drowning, however, cannot be satisfactorily discussed without addressing issues of *prevention.* It is only through prevention that we can reduce some of the terrible toll that drowning and other cardiopulmonary emergencies impose on our patients.

- The private swimming pool was a disaster waiting to happen. All private swimming pools are like magnets for small children. It seems almost a matter of time before ungated and unenclosed private swimming pools will be the scene of a tragedy like the case of David Perkins.

- The swimming pool followed the "letter of the law" regarding private pools in that it was enclosed on three sides. There was no way children could wander into the pool area from outside the house because of the high fence surrounding the yard. Regrettably, the pool owners elected to use their house as the fourth side for the pool—a decision that studies have shown to be incorrect for preventing infant and child drownings.

- It was easy for the visiting child, when briefly unobserved, to walk through the sliding doors of the den to the shining poolside where the water sparkled with such appeal. Experts tell us that if the pool had been enclosed on all four sides by independent fencing, not incorporating the house as the fourth side, this tragedy could have been prevented.

- In addition, the single gate for the pool fencing should be self-closing and self-locking, with a locking mechanism that could foil, or at least slow up, enterprising explorers like David Perkins. David's young life has been cut short by the emphasis on economy and convenience taken by his neighbors.

- The tragedy of Darin Day can also teach us lessons. One is the inappropriateness of giving such child-care responsibilities to younger siblings, particularly those who lack the maturity to provide appropriate supervision.

- Another lesson is to recognize how quickly and easily infants, when unsupervised, can drown. Studies have reported tragedies like those of Darin Day and David Perkins, where infants drown in toilets, diaper pails, wading pools, and mere inches of bathtub water. Unsupervised children have been known to hold their infant siblings under the water, to stand on the infant's head, or to sit on the infants*: All in play, of course, but in complete unawareness of the consequences.

- The lesson here is unambiguous—responsible, mature, adult supervision must be provided for all infants and children when they are near the water—even water as innocent as the bathtub and the wading pool.

*Jensen LR, Williams SD, Thurman DJ, Keller PA. Submersion injuries in children younger than 5 years in urban Utah. West J Med 1992 Dec.; 157(6):641-4. In this study **all** bathtub drownings occurred while the victim was bathing with a young sibling without adult supervision. All drownings in pools resulted from unintentional falls into ungated and unfenced pools rather than during swimming and wading activities.

KEY POINTS

SUMMARY

Drownings and near-drownings take a depressing toll on often young and vigorous lives. This toll can be reduced if all ACLS providers approach these emergencies with skill and organization, as follows:

- **Perform the steps of the Primary-Secondary ABCD Survey, and defibrillation when indicated.**

- **Stabilize the cervical spine before performing any airway maneuvers whenever there is a possibility of cervical spine injuries.**

- **Perform all steps of the Five Quadrads.**

- **Look for and treat hypothermia.**

- **Intubate the patient's trachea, and assess tube placement and the adequacy of ventilations.**

- **Continue to monitor the patient after return of spontaneous circulation.**

- **Be alert for post-resuscitation respiratory complications.**

- **Do not perform the Heimlich maneuver before attempting ventilations.**

- **Take every possible opportunity to support prevention activities, including the following:**
  - **Safe pool design**
  - **Enclosed private pools provided by responsible pool owners**
  - **Self-closing and locking gates**
  - **Trained lifeguards**
  - **Fully equipped public swim areas (including backboards, cervical collars, and even AEDs in some settings)**
  - **Swimming and lifesaving classes**
  - **Citizen CPR training**
  - **Babysitter training programs**

FILE 13. Electric Shock and Lightning Strike

OVERVIEW

Cardiac arrest due to electric shock or lightning strike, or both, requires management approaches that differ from "routine" ACLS. The following are these major differences.

- *Most electric shocks and lightning injuries, unlike nontraumatic sudden cardiac arrest, are avoidable.*

- *Resuscitations in these cases can expose the rescue team to some element of danger, either from the source of electric shocks or from subsequent lightning strikes. Therefore rescuer safety is critically important. Careless safety violations can turn the rescuer into an additional victim. The rescuers need the following additional skills:*

- *Know how to remove victim from source of electricity and know when not to do so.*

- *Have some knowledge of how to turn off electricity at the power source.*

- *Both electric shock and lightning strikes should be considered as "cardiac arrest associated with trauma" (see Chapter 15). Remember the possibility of associated trauma, particularly cervical spine trauma, entrance and exit point burns, and deep thermal burns.*

- *In these resuscitation attempts, the rescuers will have to implement "reverse triage" (treat the most severely injured victims first).*

- *Rescuers will need to continue rescue efforts longer than usual with asystolic arrest. Asystole due to electric shock and lightning strike has a better prognosis in these patients.*

- *Rescuers will need to support victims' respirations for a much longer time to allow recovery. This is because reversible respiratory arrest may persist after restoration of spontaneous circulation.*

MAJOR CONCEPTS TO MASTER

- Know how to ensure rescuer safety.
- Know how to turn off electricity at power source, or at least recognize that it needs to be done, and know how to contact responsible agencies.
- Know how to remove victim from source of electricity and when not to do so.
- Know how to manage "cardiac arrest associated with trauma" (see Chapter 15) because cardiac arrests resulting from electric shocks and lightning strike should be considered traumatic cardiac arrests.
- Know principles of "reverse triage" (treat the most severely injured victims first).
- Asystole has a better prognosis in these patients; therefore continue rescue efforts longer with their asystolic arrest.
- Since reversible respiratory arrest may persist after restoration of spontaneous circulation, know to support victims' respirations for longer than normal periods.

Critical actions

- Follow the **Five Quadrads** approach, modified in the following manner:
  - Cervical spine immobilization during all airway maneuvers
  - Treatment as trauma victims
  - More prolonged treatment for victims in asystole
  - More prolonged respiratory support for patients who have prolonged respiratory arrest

Skills to learn

- Safe maneuvers around sources of electricity.
- Safe maneuvers during lightning storms.
- Know how to remove victim from source of electricity and when not to do so.
- Know principles of "reverse triage" (treat the most severely injured victims first).

Chuck Norton

CASE 1

CONTACT WITH POWER LINES THROUGH CHERRY PICKER

Chuck Norton, a 33-year-old employee of the local power company, was walking beside the company's "cherry picker" truck. He reached his right hand up to grasp a side handrail. Moments before, his partner in the truck cab had extended the empty "cherry picker" basket upward so that the metal arm of the basket made contact with an overhead, high-voltage power line. Insulated by the rubber tires, the workman in the cab escaped electric shock. Chuck, however, was suddenly seized with tetanic contractions of his right hand and arm as the current passed from the power line, through the metal of the truck, to the handrail, down Chuck's arm, and into the ground. Witnesses stated later that they could actually see an electric current arc from Chuck's ankle (his boot soles were rubber) to the ground.

Chuck gave a sudden cry that was heard by several fellow workers. He collapsed into unconsciousness. The first bystanders ran up to find him still hanging by his contracted hand. They shouted to the workman in the cab to move the cherry picker off the power line. When contact was broken Chuck's hand opened and he fell heavily to the ground. Two of the workmen checked quickly for consciousness, breathing, and a pulse. When none were noted, they started two-person CPR.

You are a member of the first-responding paramedic unit. EMT-Ds had arrived 4 minutes after the arrest, and you arrived 4 minutes after the EMT-Ds (8 minutes since the arrest). The EMT-Ds had used an automated external defibrillator (AED) to deliver three shocks, and although a spontaneous rhythm had returned with a palpable pulse of 50 beats/min, there were no respirations. What special features of cardiac arrest following electric shock do you have to keep in mind?

COMMENTS

- Case 1 contains many features to remember about electrical shock emergencies.

- Alternating current produces tetanic contraction of the muscles, which may cause prolonged contact with the electric source. This increases the probability of more severe damage to the heart and brain from the electric energy and from deep thermal burns. Electric energy is converted to thermal energy in the muscles, and it is this conversion to heat that produces severe burns in electric shock accidents.

- Alternating current most often produces ventricular fibrillation, (VF) rather than asystole, the most common lethal rhythm produced by direct current. Cardiac damage is due to the following:

- Direct effects of the current on the myocardium

- Coronary artery spasm during the tetanic contractions

- Greater chance of hitting the vulnerable period of the cardiac cycle (R-on-T phenomenon)

- Rescuer safety should be a major concern in electric shock accidents. Shut off the power at its source. This is the safest technique. Attempts to remove Chuck from his tetanic grip on the handrail would have been unsuccessful and would have exposed the other workers as well. Nonconducting materials such as wooden poles, boards, or ropes can be used to push or pull the victim from the power supply (Fig. 13-1).

- The pathway the current takes (Fig. 13-2) can influence the degree of injury as follows:

  - Mr. Norton suffered a "vertical electric shock" (hand-to-leg), meaning the current passed vertically from his hand and down and out his lower leg.

  - "Horizontal" or transthoracic electric shock passes from one hand or arm to the other (hand to hand).

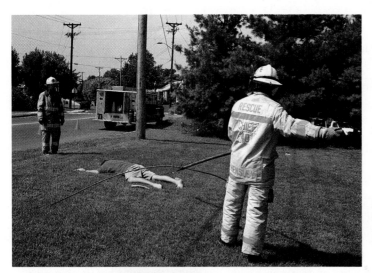

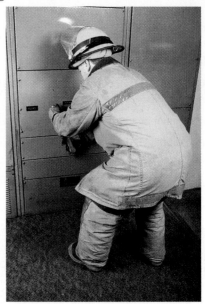

Fig. 13-1: *Ways of getting electric line from victim and shutting off power source.*

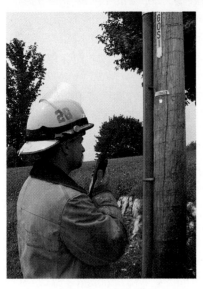

Current on this pathway passes through the heart and increases the risk of cardiac damage from current injury and by inducing VF or ventricular tachycardia (VT).

- "Straddle" shock passes from one foot to the other (foot to foot). This is the least dangerous shock because no vital organs are in the current pathway.

- Mr. Norton responded well to the early defibrillation delivered by the EMT-Ds using AEDs. This is a credit to this well-organized EMS system, which had implemented an early defibrillation program. Defibrillation at 8 minutes by the paramedics probably would have been unsuccessful.

- Notice that Chuck continues to be apneic, despite return of spontaneous circulation. This is a critical phenomenon to remember—electric shock can produce prolonged periods of respiratory paralysis through the following mechanisms:

  - Brain paralysis of respiratory centers
  - Tetany of diaphragm and chest wall musculature
  - Prolonged paralysis of respiratory muscles

- Anticipate the need to provide respiratory support much longer than with primary cardiac arrest. Often, untreated respiratory arrest in electric shock injuries leads to hypoxic cardiac arrest.

- All ACLS protocols remain the same for cardiac arrest induced by electric shock. Therefore follow the recommended indications for defibrillation, intubation, and rhythm-appropriate medications.

- You must, however, consider electric shock injuries as traumatic events. You must assume until proven otherwise that traumatic injuries are present. This is particularly true for cervical spine injuries and represents one change from standard ACLS protocols.

Chuck Norton

CASE 1 Continued

As you greet the EMT-Ds working on Mr. Norton, you notice that he has not been placed on a backboard and that the neck is not in a rigid C-collar. You ask that those be obtained and direct the EMT-Ds providing the bag-valve-mask to be careful with the neck extension. How would you approach the resuscitation attempt at this point?

COMMENTS

Always initiate the Five Quadrads approach, starting with a quick review of the Primary-Secondary ABCD Survey.

PRIMARY ABCD SURVEY

- **Airway:** Airway is maintained open with an oropharyngeal airway but without cervical spine immobilization. This is being corrected.

- **Breathing:** Bag-valve-mask ventilations appear to be producing appropriate, bilateral chest expansion.

- **Circulation:** There is a palpable pulse, but the blood pressure measures only 80/50 mm Hg.

- **Defibrillation:** The AED adhesive pads are in place, and the monitor screen shows a narrow-complex, sinus rhythm at 50 beats/min.

SECONDARY SURVEY

- **Airway:** You recognize the need for endotracheal intubation, since there is no spontaneous respiration. Despite the return of a pulse and blood pressure, electric shock injury is associated with delayed return of respiratory function, and you know the airway needs to be protected.

- **Breathing:** You successfully intubate Mr. Norton using the orotracheal route and maintaining in-line cervical spine immobilization (no traction!) while doing so. You check tube placement with an esophageal detector device and by five-point auscultation (front of chest, left and right, midaxillary line, left and right, epigastrium). The endotracheal tube appears in place.

- **Circulation:** Your partner proceeds with starting a 16-gauge intracatheter in the right antecubital vein. You order atropine 0.5 mg for the bradycardia, choosing a lower dose than you would use for cardiac arrest, since he has a palpable pulse. Because he had just been in VF that had converted with shocks, you decide to give a bolus of lidocaine 1 mg/kg to "stabilize the post-VF rhythm."

- **Differential Diagnosis:** There appears to be no mystery here as to why Mr. Norton went into cardiac arrest. You focus now on maintaining a stable rhythm and good respiratory support.

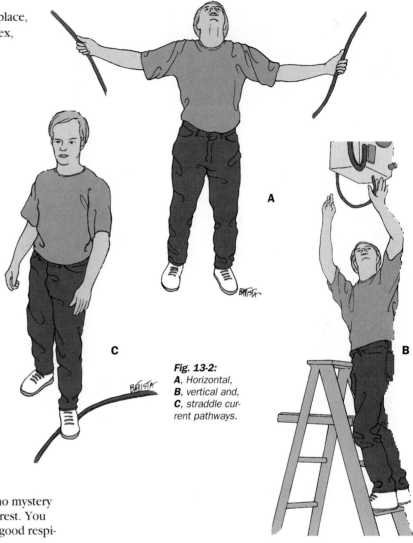

Fig. 13-2:
A, Horizontal,
B, vertical and,
C, straddle current pathways.

Chuck Norton

CASE 1 Continued

You also remember something someone told you about clothes catching on fire after electric shock, so you check for smoldering clothing, shoes, and belt buckles and find, much to your surprise, that the belt buckle is extremely hot (but not smoldering).

Chuck now appears ready for transport. What are your major tasks during transport to the Emergency Department?

COMMENTS

- Your tasks during transport are **maintenance.** You have a patient with spontaneous circulation, although he is a little hypotensive.

- You need to continue to ensure good oxygenation and ventilation, since he is not yet spontaneously breathing.

- You must continue to protect the cervical spine and to assume that other injuries may have occurred.

- You know that the early intubation was particularly appropriate because the airway may swell as a result of electric burns in the upper airway. This could have been a major mistake. Dealing with an obstructed airway resulting from soft tissue swelling during ambulance transport would present a major challenge.

Chuck Norton

CASE 1 Continued

You arrive safely at the Emergency Department and report that Chuck has begun to breathe spontaneously. His vital signs remain appropriate and stable.

What are some special considerations that the physicians in the Emergency Department will need to keep in mind for a patient surviving cardiac arrest due to electric shock?

COMMENTS

- The electric energy of the shock is converted to heat. Therefore much of the damage to people who survive cardiorespiratory arrest is burn injury with tissue destruction and hypovolemic shock.

- The two important actions that the physicians in the Emergency Department need to consider are to treat the hypovolemia and prevent renal shutdown resulting from myoglobinuria. Therefore the treatment is as follows:

  - Use *normal saline* or *lactated Ringer's solution* to keep urinary output at 1 to 1.5 mL/kg per hour (50 to 100 mL per hour).

  - Use alkalinization to keep blood pH above 7.45. Use normal saline plus one ampule of *sodium bicarbonate* and run the infusion to keep urine at 50 to 100 mL per hour.

- Induce an osmotic diuresis (*mannitol* 25 g, then 12.5 g/hour).

- After resuscitation and return of spontaneous respirations there are a number of complications that may occur following severe electric shock injury. The clinicians must be alert for the following:

  - Persistent coma
  - Severe agitation
  - Seizures
  - Hypovolemia
  - Renal shutdown from myoglobinuria
  - Metabolic acidosis from burns and tissue destruction
  - Vascular spasm and thrombosis
  - Damage from being thrown or falling from the original current
  - Deep tissue burns and injuries, which may require plastic surgery, debridement, or fasciotomies

Lamar E. Lee III and Jackson Woodrow Davis

CASE 2

STRUCK BY LIGHTNING PLAYING GOLF

You and your paramedic partner are "patrolling your zone" down by the Piggly Wiggly when you receive a call of several "men down" after being struck by lightning at the 17th hole of the Callenwolde Country Club.

The dispatcher reports that four senior golfers took shelter under a large tree during a thunderstorm. To the horror of people watching from the Club House, a bolt of lightning struck the tree, running down the tree trunk, and out the lower limb under which the men stood. All four men were knocked down, and two men were unconscious when the first bystanders arrive.

As you pull up in your rig, you notice that one of the men is sitting up talking to some bystanders, and one is lying on his back but moving his head and arms and making eye contact with people. The other two, to your dismay, appear to be receiving CPR from the bystanders. There appear to be four victims, two of whom appear to have severe cardiopulmonary emergencies.

What are some important features of cardiac arrest that result from lightning strike? What is "reverse triage?" How would you and your team members handle this call?

COMMENTS

- Lightning strikes produce 50 to 300 fatalities per year, with many more people struck but surviving. Some studies have observed only a 30% mortality rate, which is surprising, given the magnitude of energy in a bolt of lightning. One theory holds that often the lightning "flashes over" the victim, doing minimal damage. This phenomenon may have occurred in Case 2 since two of the victims appear to be reasonably well.

- Figure 13-3 displays a fascinating photograph of a 41-year-old woman struck on the right side of her neck through a necklace. The lightning produced a cutaneous "lightning print" of its pathway through the woman's neck, chest, and abdomen and out the left leg. This "lightning print" probably represents a form of "flash-over" that saved the woman's life. The woman was in her 26th week of pregnancy, and the lightning flash struck the baby's head in utero, causing its death.

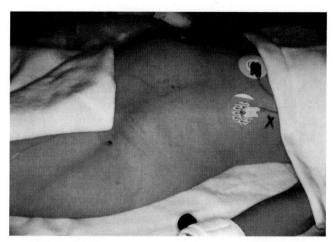

Fig. 13-3: *A 41-year old woman in her 26th week of pregnancy was struck by lightning while standing under a tree during a thunderstorm. The lightning entered her body on the right side of the neck through a necklace, went toward the ground, was deflected by the baby's head, and left the woman's body through the left leg, marking its way by a cutaneous "lighting print." The woman survived, but the baby died. (From N Engl J Med 330:1492, 1994.)*

- Some of the lightning current (200 amperes in lightning, compared with 30 to 40 amperes in typical defibrillation shock) may pass through the heart, producing cardiac arrest.

- Since lightning strikes are massive jolts of direct current, they tend to instantaneously depolarize the entire myocardium, producing asystole rather than the VF produced by the alternating current from line power. In many patients the spontaneous automaticity of the myocardium recovers, and the heart resumes beating.

- Respiratory paralysis that is due to either brain injury or respiratory muscle spasm may also occur, severely compromising oxygenation. These respiratory

sequelae of lightning strike may in turn produce hypoxic cardiac arrest.

- **Reverse triage** comes into play, as follows, when you have multiple victims of lightning strike. (It also applies to electric shock, but those accidents seldom involve multiple victims.)

  - In regular triage you place the lowest priority on patients who appear on clinical examination to be dead (i.e., the full cardiac arrest victims). Because cardiac arrest resulting from trauma has a high mortality rate no matter what therapy you employ, prompt care for the other victims should not be sacrificed on behalf of a futile effort.

  - With lightning strikes, however, victims who appear on clinical examination to be dead may have only temporary myocardial "stunning," temporary respiratory paralysis, or a reversible arrhythmia like VF.

  - You should "reverse triage" these victims and evaluate and treat them immediately (Fig. 13-4). This response may prevent progression from respiratory arrest to both respiratory and cardiac arrest.

- You approach the two victims in Case 2 exactly as you would any other cardiopulmonary emergency: you use the Five Quadrads and the Primary-Secondary Survey technique—with a few necessary modifications.

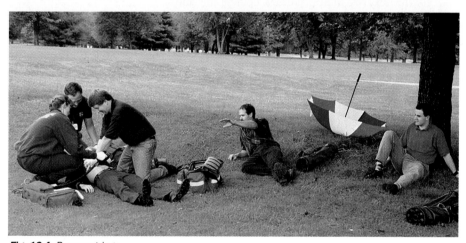

Fig. 13-4: *Reverse triage.*

Lamar E. Lee III and Jackson Woodrow Davis

CASE 2 Continued

You and your partner split up to perform rapid Primary-Secondary Survey of the two victims. You evaluate Lamar E. Lee and find that he is in full cardiac arrest, unconscious, without a pulse, and without breathing. He needs a full resuscitation effort.

Your partner shouts out that Jackson Woodrow Davis is unconscious, with a weak, thready pulse and slow, labored respirations. His inadequate respirations will lead to full cardiac arrest if he does not get respiratory support quickly. The EMT first-responder unit arrives at this time with four volunteer EMTs ready to help.

What sequence of interventions would you now direct?

For *Lamar* you direct the following sequence of interventions.

PRIMARY SURVEY

- **Airway:** Perform cervical spine immobilization with backboard and rigid cervical collar; open airway with the jaw-thrust method.

- **Breathing:** Insert oropharyngeal airway and begin bag-valve-mask ventilations with 100% oxygen at 15 L/min.

- **Circulation:** Continue CPR, since there is no pulse.

- **Defibrillation:** The EMT-Ds attach their AED and find that the rhythm is asystole and "no shock indicated" over three assessment periods.

SECONDARY SURVEY

- **Airway:** You proceed with orotracheal intubation with in-line cervical spine immobilization (no traction).

- **Breathing:** You verify tube placement and provide bag-valve-mask hyperventilations.

- **Circulation:** Whereas you would normally attempt to obtain IV access, you decide, since you are the only ACLS-trained person, to use the endotracheal route for the next two indicated drugs, epinephrine and atropine. For the epinephrine use 3 mg mixed in 10 mL of normal saline and injected down the endotracheal tube followed by hyperventilation. For the *atropine* use 2 mg diluted in 10 mL, and inject the contents down the tube as well, followed by vigorous "bagging."

  - As an alternative, you could have remained at the victim's head and moved from performing intubation to starting an internal or external jugular vein IV line.

  - You could have simply turned the "bagging" over to one of the EMT-Ds and moved down and started the antecubital line in one of the arms. With IV access you would inject epinephrine 1 mg IV bolus plus atropine 1 mg IV bolus, each drug followed by 10 mL saline flush.

  - You plan to repeat each of those medications in 3 minutes, increasing the *epinephrine* dose to 5 mg.

- **Differential diagnosis:** You recognize that prolonged asystole is expected in cardiac arrest resulting from lightning strike and that the respiratory support must be continued aggressively for long periods.

- You began this resuscitation challenged because you were the only ACLS person managing this cardiac arrest. The Primary-Secondary Survey provides you with a priority listing as to how to proceed. You should move steadily in the sequence presented by the ABCD listing: while EMT-Ds were doing CPR, you intubated the victim's trachea.

Then you moved to giving medications down the endotracheal tube or starting an IV line and then to medication administration.

- The word had gone out that a second ACLS unit is needed, and 15 minutes after the original call a second unit arrives. One member of this team is directed to take their defibrillator and monitor to Mr. Davis, who appears to be recovering well (discussed next). The other member comes to help you, and you ask him to start a peripheral IV line, and inject another round of medications (*epinephrine,* and *atropine*). Since the asystole persists in an intubated and ventilated patient, you decide to add *sodium bicarbonate* 1 mEq/kg.

- After 20 minutes of resuscitation efforts, Mr. Lee displays a wide-complex ventricular escape rhythm that produces a palpable pulse of 50 beats/min and a blood pressure of 90/60 mm Hg. You stop CPR efforts and transport him with continued ventilatory assistance to the nearest Emergency Department. You learn later that Mr. Lee was admitted to the intensive care unit, where he had a stormy and unstable course, dying in cardiogenic shock 18 hours later. He never displayed signs of return of brain function.

For *Jackson Woodrow Davis* ("Bubba" to his friends) your partner directs the following sequence of interventions.

PRIMARY SURVEY

- **Airway:** Perform cervical spine immobilization with backboard and rigid cervical collar; open airway with the jaw-thrust method.

- **Breathing:** Insert oropharyngeal airway and begin bag-valve-mask ventilations with 100% oxygen at 15 L/min.

- **Circulation:** There is a weak pulse with a systolic blood presure of 70 mm Hg, so CPR is not needed.

- **Defibrillation:** The patient is not in full cardiac arrest, so rhythm assessment to "hunt for VF" is not indicated at this time.

SECONDARY SURVEY

- **Airway:** Your partner begins preparations for orotracheal intubation with in-line cervical spine immobilization (no traction); however, he notices that bagging with 100% oxygen is making the pulse stronger and faster. He shouts, "His pulse is so much stronger I'm going to just keep bagging for a bit and see if he starts breathing again."

- **Breathing:** Ventilations with the bag-valve-mask continue for 1 minute; then your partner stops bagging and watches Bubba closely. After 15 seconds he takes a deep, gasping breath, which is followed 10 seconds later by another. Over the next minute the respirations increase in frequency and become steady, regular, and strong, and your partner decides to not perform intubation.

- **Circulation:** Your partner starts a 14-gauge catheter in the left antecubital vein. The monitor and defibrillator, which just arrived, display a sinus bradycardia of 45 beats/min. He administers *atropine* 0.5 mg IV push, followed 5 minutes later by a second 0.5 mg IV dose.

- **Differential diagnosis:** The origin of the respiratory compromise is not in question here; cardiac bradycardia and hypotension have responded well to good ventilation support.

What do you think made the difference in outcomes for these two ACLS emergencies?

COMMENTS

- Lamar Lee had a full cardiorespiratory arrest following the lightning strike, going into asystole and respiratory paralysis. His age (72 years) may have played a role here, leading to underlying cardiovascular disease that contributed to his bad outcome. The severity of his injury from the lightning may have been simply incompatible with life, despite the most optimal resuscitation efforts.

- Bubba had a better outcome because he never lost his pulse and never completely stopped breathing. By supplying early and effective ventilation and oxygenation, cardiac dysfunction and deterioration to a full cardiac arrest were prevented. He provides a good example of how proper airway management can prevent a bad outcome.

KEY POINTS

SUMMARY

The Primary-Secondary Survey, combined with the rest of the Five Quadrads, provides a systematic approach to managing electric shock and lightning strike emergencies. The only special features that have to be remembered are the following:

- **Rescuer safety must be considered, to avoid turning the rescuer into an additional victim.**

- **Consider victims to have "cardiac arrest associated with trauma."**

- **Remember the possibilities of associated trauma, particularly cervical spine trauma, entrance and exit point burns, and deep thermal burns.**

- **Know how to remove victim from source of electricity.**

- **Know principles of "reverse triage" (treat the most severely injured victims first).**

- **Continue rescue efforts longer with asystolic arrest because asystole has a better prognosis in these patients.**

- **Aggressively support victims' respirations for longer periods to allow recovery. This is because reversible respiratory arrest may persist after restoration of spontaneous circulation.**

- **Be prepared to watch for the post-resuscitation complications in all victims who manage to survive and recover: hypovolemia, burns, renal shutdown, and myoglobinuria.**

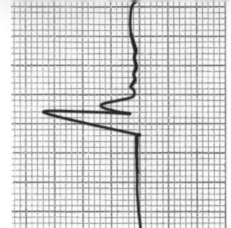

O V E R V I E W

Cardiac emergencies associated with hypothermia are managed differently from cardiac arrests of other causes. While you will continue to apply the **Five Quadrads** *and the* **Primary-Secondary Survey***, you will need to modify the approach in several respects. As with the other special resuscitation situations (drowning, electric shock, trauma, pregnancy, lightning, and drug overdoses), we find it most useful to use D (Differential Diagnosis) in the Secondary Survey as the place to consider the resuscitation modifications.*

In hypothermia the emergency care provider encounters a cold myocardium that is usually getting colder. Treatment includes not only the usual efforts at resuscitation, but also specific attempts to rewarm the patient. Both the problems encountered and the probability of success vary by how low the temperature dropped, how long the temperature remained low, and how fast and effectively the heart and blood can be rewarmed.

You must ascertain the core temperature. This is critical because core temperature determines the following:

- *Resuscitation protocols used*

- *Rewarming approaches used*

- *Resuscitation problems encountered*

The major new concepts to learn are the immediate need for stopping heat loss and starting rewarming and how the resuscitation, the clinical problems, and the rewarming method vary according to the core temperature.

MAJOR CONCEPTS TO MASTER

To maximize success in treating hypothermic patients you must learn the following:

- How to stop further heat loss.
- How to rewarm the victim. Use different rewarming approaches depending on the setting (prehospital, Emergency Department, operating room, or intensive care facility).
- How to monitor core temperature.
- Modifications of defibrillation and medication protocols for hypothermic cardiac arrest.
- Special techniques for monitoring the rhythm in the hypothermic patient.
- Indications and methods of rewarming, including the following:

- Passive external rewarming
- Active external rewarming
- Active internal rewarming

- How to recognize those victims who need rapid mobilization to facilities that can perform advanced core rewarming (for example, extracorporeal bypass rewarming and peritoneal lavage rewarming).

- The need to distinguish a cardiac arrest that started out normothermic but that occurred in a cold environment, from a cardiac arrest caused by progressive cooling of the heart. The condition of a person who has a sudden ventricular fibrillation (VF) arrest and falls down in snow is profoundly different from that of a person with a broken leg who lies

- in the snow for hours and gradually cools down to where she or he goes into cardiac arrest.
- The need to have a high index of suspicion for subtle forms of hypothermia. For example, "urban hypothermia" occurs when people are chronically exposed to cool rather than cold ambient temperatures or people may have disabilities or mental incapacitation that renders them unable to prevent or protect themselves against heat loss.
- The need to have a high index of suspicion for hypothermia anytime a thermometer registers its lowest value, even though that value may not be truly hypothermic, for example: 35° C (95.0° F).
- The need to have a high index of suspicion for hypothermia anytime a person has been submerged in water. Always consider a drowning victim to be hypothermic. This is true no matter what the ambient water temperature.
- Remember, "a person is not dead until he or she is warm and dead." This basically means the following:
  - You must give every victim, even one without signs of life, a chance to see if his or her heart and spontaneous circulation will restart when warmed to a higher temperature.

- The criteria we usually employ to indicate death cannot be used on deep hypothermic victims unless the victim displays obvious lethal damage. Raise the body temperature to at least 30° C to 32° C (86° F to 89.6° F), and establish whether there is any return of spontaneous cardiac activity, before pronouncing the victim dead.
- Full recovery may occur even if the person appears "dead and frozen" when first discovered. Tissues and organs, especially the brain, need less oxygen when hypothermic. Therefore, chances of survival and neurologic recovery after hypothermic cardiac arrest are greatly increased.
- You can precipitate VF easily in the hypothermic patient. Avoid rough movement and procedures and excessive activity.
- Always move hypothermic patients gently, in the horizontal position for the following reasons:
  - their compensatory mechanisms are not operating effectively
  - the vertical, upright position could precipitate hypotension and circulatory collapse.

Critical actions

- Do not expose the rescuer to the danger of hypothermia.
- Always stop further heat loss and preserve remaining body heat.
- Determine core temperature using proper equipment.
- Start *appropriate* rewarming. (Technique is determined by setting and core temperature.)
- Monitor the rhythm.
- Perform CPR in normal fashion.
- When indicated, always perform endotracheal intubation, even though there is some possibility of inducing VF.
- When ventilating the lungs, always provide warm, humidified oxygen.
- Limit defibrillations to the first series of shocks if the VF appears to be refractory, as follows:
  - This is especially true if you know the core temperature is below 30° C (86° F).
  - Repeat defibrillations for VF are acceptable after central rewarming has elevated core temperature to greater than 30° C (86° F).
- Give IV medications further apart than standard intervals, or withhold medications until further central rewarming has occurred. This is done because of the following:

- The hypothermic heart often does not respond to drugs.
- Hypothermic patients have reduced drug metabolism and excretion.
- Multiple doses or infusions may accumulate to dangerous or toxic levels.
- Look for, assess, and treat coexisting diseases or underlying conditions that may have precipitated or increased the risk of hypothermia. This assessment is of critical importance to the outcome in hypothermic patients. Such conditions include the following:
- Drug and alcohol intoxication
- Infectious diseases
- Metabolic or endocrine disorders
- General disability, especially in the elderly

Specific skills to master

- How to assess patients with different degrees of hypothermia
- How to use the Hypothermia Algorithm (Fig. 14-1)
- Techniques and equipment for measuring body core temperature (rectal, esophageal, and tympanic)
- Techniques and equipment for heat preservation and rewarming *in the field*

Tanya Vander Schmidt
and Jorritt Mueller

CASE 1

You are a paramedic who has volunteered to help search for two cross-country skiers. Crystal is your 2-year-old Labrador retriever search-and-rescue dog. The two skiers are Jorritt Mueller, a 23-year-old Dutch exchange student, and Tanya Vander Schmidt, his 20-year-old Austrian girl friend. The day before, they had gone out for a 15-mile round-trip ski tour carrying only a small backpack filled with lunch, water, and an extra sweater. By 8 PM they had not reported back to their friends' cottage. The friends called the ski lodge, and the search and rescue team was called out. Now, at 10 AM the next day, you, Crystal, and two other volunteers have been combing the downhill portion of what would have been the return route for the two skiers.

You notice unmistakable signs of a small avalanche on the hillside above you. You realize, by visualizing a line backward from the trail, that the avalanche must have intersected the cross-country ski trail. With mounting fear you send Crystal out on a "cast" in front of you, shouting, "Search for them!" to guide her sweeps. Suddenly, up ahead, Crystal gives the unmistakable barks and displays of a "find." She is digging in the tumbled chunks of the avalanche, barking with great excitement.

Your paramedic partner radios to the base camp that you may have a find. With Crystal barking proudly, you and the other paramedics dig down, locating first a hand, then the rest of the man, Jorritt Mueller. His limbs are stiff and immobile, arrayed in distorted positions. When he is finally removed, you observe the completely cyanotic appearance of death, with open, staring eyes, and his mouth full of snow. You reach your hand inside his ski parka and feel the cold, stiff muscles of his abdomen and chest.

Would you initiate resuscitation efforts on this unfortunate young man? If so, what would your approach be?

COMMENTS

- Case 1 poses extremely difficult decisions for the emergency rescuer. We have all heard the phrase "no person is dead until he or she is warm and dead." In addition, everyone has read dramatic newspaper accounts of people rescued from severe hypothermic cardiac arrest when their initial appearance suggested frozen death.

- You know, however, that Mr. Mueller has not suffered a cardiac arrest secondary to hypothermia. All evidence suggests that Mr. Mueller has suffocated. As his primary disaster, he was covered with snow in the avalanche and was unable to breathe. His heart stopped beating from asphyxiation. He suffered a primary respiratory arrest followed by secondary cardiac arrest.

- This victim of hypothermia represents an already dead body cooling down because it was packed in ice—and it was packed in ice hours ago. It would be a waste of resources to initiate resuscitation efforts on Mr. Mueller if the limited personnel could be used to a better advantage.

- Similar circumstances apply in hypothermia associated with cold water drownings. Again, resources are often wasted when people assume drowning in cold water is

markedly different from drowning in warm water. The primary event is not hypothermia but asphyxiation. In such events a normothermic heart stopped because it was deprived of oxygen, not because it got cold. The prognosis is dismal if resuscitation efforts are delayed more than a few minutes.

- We all are gratified when we see newspaper accounts of a small child retrieved from under the ice 30 to 45 minutes after submersion. What the newspapers fail to report, however, is the much greater number of children and adults who are never resuscitated or who recover to a life of severe neurologic compromise.

- These are not easy decisions. Emergency personnel should always have a low threshold to do everything they are trained to do. The second layer of personnel, the physicians and intensive care providers, need to be very forthright in stopping efforts sooner rather than later, especially when the chances of meaningful recovery are remote.

- Frustrated by the lack of extra personnel, you decide to leave the young man unattended in the snow and that you and Crystal and the other two paramedics will keep searching for the lost skier.

246

FIGURE 14-1

Hypothermia Treatment Algorithm

Actions for all patients suspected of hypothermia:
- Remove wet clothing
- Guard against heat loss and wind chill exposure (use blankets and insulating equipment)
- Keep patient in horizontal position (use stretchers during extrications)
- Avoid all rough or excess movements
- Assess and closely monitor core temperature
- Assess and closely monitor cardiac rhythm[a]

Perform Primary ABCD Survey:
Assess responsiveness, breathing, and pulse

If pulse and breathing present

What is core temperature?

34° C to 36° C (mild hypothermia)
- Passive rewarming (blankets)
- Active external rewarming (heating source over any of body areas)

30° C to 34° C (moderate hypothermia)
- Passive rewarming (blankets)
- Active external rewarming of truncal areas only[b,c]

< 30° C (severe hypothermia)
- Use active internal rewarming techniques (see below)

Active internal rewarming techniques[b]
- Warm IV fluids (43° C)
- Warm, humid oxygen (42° C to 46° C)
- Peritoneal lavage (KCl-free fluid)
- Extracorporeal rewarming
- Esophageal rewarming tubes[d]

Continue internal rewarming until:
- Core temperature >35° C or
- Return of spontaneous circulation or
- Resuscitative efforts cease

If pulse or breathing absent

- Start CPR
- Defibrillate ventricular fibrillation or ventricular tachycardia (VF/VT) up to a total of 3 shocks (200 J, 300 J, and 360 J)
- Intubate
- Ventilate with warm, humid oxygen (42° C to 46° C)[b]
- Obtain IV access
- Infuse warm normal saline (43° C)[b]

What is core temperature?

<30° C

- Continue CPR
- Withhold IV medications
- Limit shocks for VF/VT to 3 maximum
- Transport to hospital

>30° C

- Continue CPR
- Give IV medications as indicated (but at longer than standard intervals)
- Repeat defibrillation for VF/VT as core temperature rises

[a] This may require needle electrodes through the skin.

[b] A few experts think these interventions should be done only in-hospital, especially with minimally trained rescuers.

[c] Active external rewarming methods include electric or charcoal warming devices, hot water bottles, heating pads, radiant heat sources, and warming beds.

[d] Esophageal rewarming tubes are widely used internationally and are expected to become more widely used in the United States.

"Adapted with permission, Journal of the American Medical Association, 1992, Volume 268, *Guidelines for Cardiopulmonary Resuscitation and Emergency Cardiac Care.* Copyright 1992, American Medical Association"

<table>
<tr><td>

Tanya Vander Schmidt

CASE 2

</td><td>

Desperate for the arrival of additional help, you reluctantly break away from Mr. Mueller. Judging from the skis on Mr. Mueller and the position of his body in relation to the avalanche, you think that perhaps the two skiers saw the avalanche and that they had been trying to

</td></tr>
</table>

outski it. You look farther down the slope, thinking Tanya could have reached the safety of those lower trees if she had been able to remain upright. You send Crystal out again, specifically directing her to search down the slope, in the trees. Within 2 minutes she begins her excited bark, and you see her circling and jumping about a dark object under a fallen tree trunk.

You and the two paramedics quickly ski down to check out what Crystal has located and discover the girl. She is unconscious and curled into a ball as if she had been trying to keep warm. There is a sweater draped over her back. Her left leg at the mid-tibia region appears swollen and slightly angulated. The snow around her has been packed down, and several fallen branches have been arranged as a windbreak near her body. It is obvious that she had made efforts to keep warm and protect herself, and that she had been active and moving perhaps for hours before becoming unconscious.

As you begin your examination, you notice that her limbs and joints are not stiff and that you can straighten her out. She is not breathing and there is no pulse.

Would you attempt resuscitation on Tanya, after having decided to not attempt to resuscitate the young man? If so, how would you proceed?

COMMENTS

- Yes, you will initiate a full resuscitation effort on Tanya. Clearly, the circumstances are significantly different as follows:

  - Mr. Mueller was indeed cold and hypothermic, but his cardiac arrest was due to suffocation, not hypothermia.

  - With Ms. Vander Schmidt you have a more classic example of *exposure to cold* leading to progressive loss of function and eventually cardiac arrest.

  - The broken leg represents another factor leading to the exposure hypothermia—she could not move to seek help or get out of the snow.

- You take the following immediate actions (Fig. 14-1):

  - First, you have to begin attempts to *stop further heat loss and begin rewarming.* For *all* hypothermic patients you must take a series of actions oriented toward these two goals.

  - Remove wet, cold, or (in this scenario) snow-covered and icy garments.

  - Protect against further heat loss and wind chill by providing thick insulation underneath and coverings over and around the victims. Constructing a wind-break and physically moving the victim to another, more sheltered location are both appropriate actions.

  - Blankets and other insulating materials begin the process of rewarming the victim, using passive rewarming and mild active rewarming (assuming the blankets will be warmer than the victim).

- Maintain the horizontal position at all times. The vertical position can precipitate cardiovascular collapse and cerebral hypoperfusion because the vasoconstrictive compensatory mechanisms are disrupted by the hypothermia.

- Avoid rough movements and excess activity. This admonition applies to the force and tempo of CPR chest compressions, the technique for endotracheal intubation, even the force of bag-valve-mask ventilations.

- Perform the **Five Quadrads,** in particular, the **Primary-Secondary Survey,** just as you would in all cardiopulmonary emergencies. This approach will be modified in its details as we will see later, but it remains a useful way of providing an organized, complete intervention and organizational approach, as outlined in Figure 14-1.

PRIMARY SURVEY

- **Airway:** Unchanged from regular guidelines
- **Breathing:** Unchanged from regular guidelines
- **Circulation:** Pulse check and begin chest compressions as follows:

  - *Check the pulse again for 15 to 30 seconds.* Check the pulse centrally, either at the carotid or the femoral artery. Use a Doppler stethoscope if available. This is used because peripheral arteries will be vasoconstricted and may not reflect more central cardiac activity.

  - Although some experts have recommended longer pulse checks (≥60 seconds), you are still going to begin CPR if a pulse is detected at the rate of, for example, 4 beats/min (rate if one pulse was detected at 15 seconds).

- The problems at this point are twofold: one, you do not have a monitor; two, you do not know the core temperature.
  - If you did, for example, have a core temperature reading of less than 30° C and a monitor confirming a sinus bradycardia of 6 beats/min, what would you do?
  - Some experts would argue that CPR would precipitate VF and that the benefits of the 6 beats/min would be lost. The hypothermic patient may benefit even from a rate of 6 beats/min, and you may have harmed this patient by starting CPR.
- The correct answer to the preceeding question remains an area of continuing debate. The AHA recommends that CPR be started in the pulseless hypothermic patient. This seems reasonable, given the constraints of an unknown cardiac rhythm and core temperature.
- *Start CPR if no pulse is detected, as follows:*
  - Should you perform CPR at a slower rate, as some experts recommend? For example, some argue that the cold heart has slow diastolic filling and that therefore you need to perform CPR at a slower compression rate. This will allow more time for the ventricles to fill. Others argue that the disturbances from the chest compressions will provoke the onset of VF. Again, the issue is based on speculations about which we lack adequate data.
  - The AHA has adopted the rational position that changes in standard guidelines should not be made in the absence of firm, objective data that such changes are definitely superior. *Perform regular CPR at the standard rate of 80 to 100 compressions per minute.*
- **Defibrillation:** The major change to standard guidelines for defibrillating hypothermic patients is to limit the number of shocks for persistent VF. Perform defibrillation as follows:
  - Often you will be unable to defibrillate the cold, hypothermic heart that is less than 30° C (86° F). A problem looms, however, because the initial emergency resuscitation team will not know the core temperature for the heart identified to be in VF. Thus you will not know whether the victim's heart really is less than 30° C (86° F). This may be a patient with normothermic VF who will respond at once to the direct-current shock.
  - Therefore the AHA recommends up to three shocks for persistent VF, no matter what the core temperature. This is based on the rationale that you have at least given the heart a chance to respond.

- If VF continues after three shocks, withhold further defibrillations and proceed with the other elements of the resuscitation protocols.

SECONDARY SURVEY

- **Airway:** Perform endotracheal intubation. Although it is true that endotracheal intubation may precipitate VF in the hypothermic heart, you have no choice. The nonbreathing victim must have ventilation support. The heart may be beating slowly in the nonbreathing victim. Is that person better off intubated and in VF or not breathing and in a slowly perfusing rhythm? This is a tough call. The approach must be to correct all identified problems (nonbreathing victim and VF) as quickly and effectively as possible.

- **Breathing:** Begin ventilations. You should, however, ventilate with *warm, humidified oxygen at a temperature of 42° to 46° C.* This represents an "active, internal rewarming" technique that you need to learn about. All Emergency Departments and certainly all prehospital response vehicles that may encounter hypothermic patients should have the capability of supplying heated, humidified oxygen. There is controversy on this point as follows:
  - Some experts argue that these active, internal rewarming interventions should only be performed inside the hospital, not in the prehospital setting. While almost all experts recommend heated, humidified oxygen in the prehospital setting, other prehospital techniques for active rewarming can produce complications.
  - The so-called "after-drop phenomenon" or "rewarming shock" produces much of this concern as follows:
    - As hypothermic victims rewarm, vasodilation occurs, so the blood pressure falls ("rewarming shock").
    - The vasodilation causes the cold blood in the extremities, often acidotic and filled with waste products, to return to the body's core ("rewarming acidosis").
    - This cold blood causes a drop in the core temperature ("rewarming temperature after-drop") and may precipitate additional arrhythmias from the acidosis.

- **Circulation:** In the Secondary Survey circulation includes starting an IV line, infusing fluids, monitoring the rhythm, and providing rhythm-appropriate medications. Also, for ease of memory, it should include monitoring the core temperature. In hypothermia and in hypothermic cardiac arrest all of these actions need to be modified as follows:
  - *Infuse normal saline at 42° C to 46° C.* This represents another technique for "active, internal rewarming" and has been the subject of the same debate noted earlier for warm, humidified oxygen. Again most Emergency Departments and advanced prehospital units should have the capability of warming IV infusion solutions.

- ***Monitor the cardiac rhythm.*** For this you may need to use the innovative technique of "needle electrodes" to obtain a true picture of the cardiac electrical activity. This is because the cold, hypoperfused skin either will not hold the adhesive monitor electrodes or will not conduct the electrical signal from the myocardium. Some improvisers have learned to simply take an 18- to 22-gauge needle and stick it through the monitor electrode, deep into the skin or muscles. This may provide the only way to pick up any existing signal from the weak, hypothermic heart.

Rhythm Strip

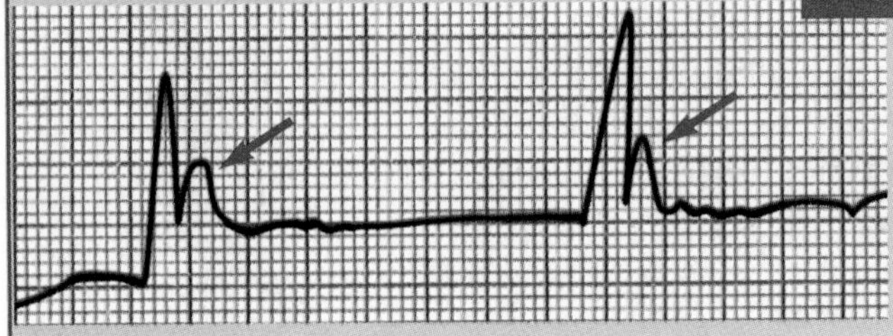

Fig. 14-2: *Rhythm strip showing Osborne or J waves.*

  - ECG changes in hypothermia include Osborne or J waves, T-wave inversion, and prolonged PR, QRS, and QT intervals (Fig. 14-2).
  - Arrhythmias in hypothermia include the following sequence (especially as the core temperature drops below 30° C [86° F]: bradycardia, slow atrial fibrillation, VF, and asystole.

- ***Monitor the core temperature.*** Most glass thermometers read no lower than 34° C (93.2° F). Tympanic membrane thermometers yield a temperature that is closer to the core temperature than does the routine mouth and rectal thermometer. Some tympanic membrane thermometers, however, do not register sufficiently low to indicate all cases of hypothermia. The best technique to use is a high, rectal-probe thermometer. This yields the most accurate measure of core temperature. Certainly all Emergency Departments and all ALS units should be equipped with and have readily available such thermometers.

- NOTE: The Hypothermia Algorithm contains a critical decision point for hypothermic cardiac arrests: whether the temperature is less than 30° C (86° F). This temperature-based decision point determines whether you give IV medications or repeat defibrillations. (You do neither if core temperature is less than 30° C [86° F].

- If the core temperature is greater than 30° C (86° F), give medications at the same dose as standard ACLS protocols. However, the intervals between epinephrine should be at least 5 minutes, rather than 3 minutes.

- In addition, "high-dose" epinephrine should not be administered in hypothermic cardiac arrest. The hypothermic heart may be sensitive to resuscitation medications, particularly as the heart rewarms. In addition, medications may accumulate to levels that will be toxic when rewarming occurs.

- If the core temperature is less than 30° C (86° F), withhold IV medications until rewarming proceeds to greater than 30° C (86° F).

- Some experts have argued that bretylium should be administered early to all victims of severe hypothermia, even those not in cardiac arrest. There are data suggesting that bretylium is particularly effective in treating VF/VT associated with hypothermia. Since bretylium has a long onset of action, the sooner it is administered the sooner it will have an effect. This represents a Class IIb (acceptable, possible helpful) guideline.

- **Differential diagnosis**. When you get to the D (Differential Diagnosis) of the Secondary Survey, you must focus on several other critical aspects of the resuscitation, including the following:

  - ***What rewarming techniques are you going to use?*** As Fig. 14-1 displays, you make the decision about rewarming technique based on the core temperature as follows:

    - Virtually every victim in cardiac arrest resulting from hypothermia will have a core temperature less than 30° C (86° F) because cooling does not stop spontaneous cardiac function until the core temperature drops well below 30° C (86° F).
    - If the core temperature is greater than 30° C (86° F), you must consider whether the cardiac arrest is due to factors other than cardiac cooling.
    - Active internal rewarming will be used for all victims with a core temperature greater than 30°C (86° F). (Techniques are discussed later.)

  - ***Are there other possible causes of this cardiac arrest?*** The most likely "other cause" is a normothermic cardiac arrest that occurred in a cold environment in which the heart simply cooled down after arrest, because of ambient coldness. All the other possible causes (for example, the list given in the Pulseless Electrical Activity [PEA] Algorithm) must not be forgotten.

  - ***Are there associated conditions that may have contributed to this cardiac arrest?*** Often people with hypothermic cardiac arrest have other medical conditions that rendered them unable to regulate their temperature or unable to protect themselves from a cold environment. Some of these possible conditions include the following:

- Drug and alcohol intoxication
- Infectious diseases
- Metabolic or endocrine disorders
- General disability, especially in the elderly
- Acute trauma or injuries
- ***When are you going to transport the patient, and to what level of care?*** Transport the victim as soon as you have completed the Primary-Secondary Survey and

the initial interventions. This means after starting CPR, intubation, IV access, and the first rounds of defibrillation shocks and medications.

- If the core temperature is less than 30° C (86°F) or the victim continues in cardiac arrest at a core temperature greater than 30° C (86° F) transport to a care facility that can perform cardiopulmonary bypass ("heart-lung machine"). This constitutes the definitive rewarming technique.

Tanya Vander Schmidt

CASE 2 Continued

Assisted by your two paramedic colleagues (and the persistent, joyful barking of Crystal), you initiate the following interventions:

- *You place Tanya on the insulated pad that you carry in your backpack.*
- *You initiate basic life support with standard CPR using a pocket face mask and expired air ventilations.*
- *You quickly remove her wet, snow-covered clothes and wrap her in the "space blankets" and two wool blankets carried in your backpacks.*
- *You activate the four portable chemical "hot packs" (wrapped in flannel) and place two against her trunk, under the armpits, and two over her left and right epigastric region. This is a method of starting active external rewarming.*

Four minutes later the search-and-rescue ACLS Snowmobile, alerted by your radio transmission, arrives with two more paramedics and more equipment. They carry a portable monitor-defibrillator, an ALS ventilation kit with oxygen tank, and endotracheal intubation supplies, an IV setup, fluids, and medications. The monitor reveals a slow, idioventricular rhythm of 10 to 12 beats/min, so defibrillation is not needed. No heart tones can be heard with the Doppler stethoscope. You intubate her trachea and attempt to start efforts at a peripheral IV line, but without success.

You radio to the base station that the Cascadia LifeFlight helicopter should be directed to your location. The helicopter was dispatched with your first transmission upon finding the body.

Five minutes later the LifeFlight helicopter arrives with two nurse-paramedics. Their helicopter is equipped for cold weather rescue. They administer warm IV fluids of normal saline at 43° C, at a rate of 500 mL/hour, and add warm, humid 100% oxygen (at 43° C) to the endotracheal tube ventilations. They administer epinephrine 1 mg IV and atropine 0.5 mg IV. They plan to repeat "epi" 1 mg IV every 7 to 8 minutes, depending on the cardiac rhythm. The medical control doctor orders one dose of bretylium at 5 mg/kg.

They carry a portable, battery-operated rectal-probe thermometer, which when inserted reveals a core temperature of 25° C (77° F). The helicopter pilot turns on the heat inside the helicopter to maximum. After quick backboard immobilization, Tanya is lifted onboard the helicopter to begin transportation to the Level 1 Trauma Center Hospital (85 miles away). The lead paramedic radios ahead, alerting the medical center that a hypothermic cardiac arrest patient is en route with ongoing CPR.

What approaches will be used in the medical center when Tanya arrives?

COMMENTS

- When Tanya arrives at the trauma center, resuscitation will continue with active, internal rewarming. A variety of acceptable, effective techniques have been used in the United States and in Europe. These include the following:

  - ***Peritoneal lavage:*** Use potassium-free lavage fluids.

- ***Esophageal rewarming tubes:*** These are closed-circuit tubes that circulate warm solution through soft plastic esophageal tubes. These produce mediastinal "core" rewarming, which many experts think is the most effective, minimally invasive, quickly available technique. Experienced rescue services such as helicopter rescue services in Norway use esophageal tubes in the field and consider them the equivalent of extracorporeal rewarming.

- **Gastric or colonic lavage** with warmed saline. (Use gastric lavage only when the patient's trachea is intubated.)

- **Thoracic cavity lavage:** In this approach, two chest tubes are used to lavage the mediastinum with warmed saline.

- **Bladder lavage with warmed saline:** Use a Foley catheter.

- **Extracorporeal rewarming techniques:** These techniques use the heart-lung bypass equipment employed in cardiac surgery to rapidly perform core rewarming. The records for the lowest known hypothermic recovery (approximately 18° C [65° F] were achieved using the extracorporeal rewarming technique.

- Emergency Departments in the northern United States almost routinely transfer hypothermic cardiac arrest patients to the operating suites for a quick "run" on the cardiopulmonary bypass machine.

- Remember that warm IV fluids and warm, humid oxygen, both supplied at approximately 42° C to 46° C (107.6° F to 114.8° F) are considered active, internal rewarming techniques and can produce a steady, predictable rise in the core temperature.

- NOTE: Virtually all experts have abandoned the out-of-date techniques of hot water immersion. This approach causes vasodilation of the peripheral circulation, producing after-drop shock with central acidosis and refractory cardiac arrhythmias. In addition, this approach interferes with access to the patient for IV lines, medications, chest compressions, monitoring and endotracheal ventilation, and airway control.

Tanya Vander Schmidt

CASE 2 Continued

By the time Tanya arrives at the Emergency Department her core temperature is 28° C (82.4° F). She had one episode of VF that required three shocks and lidocaine 1 mg/kg before conversion to a PEA of a slow junctional escape rhythm of 36 beats/min. A second dose of bretylium at 5 mg/kg was administered. There was no effective circulation with the rhythm. One of the residents suggested that cardiac pacing could be tried, but it was immediately pointed out that pacing for bradycardia in hypothermia is contraindicated because of the tendency to produce VT/VF.

The cardiovascular surgery team took Tanya on to the operating room within 10 minutes of her arrival in the Emergency Department. She was placed on the cardiopulmonary bypass device and perfused so that her core temperature elevated 1° C every 15 minutes. One hour after being placed on the device, at a core temperature of 32° C (89.6° F), she had spontaneous return of cardiac activity that she sustained. She was removed from the pump 20 minutes later with a core temperature of 34° C (89.6° F) with spontaneous circulation at 68 beats/min and a blood pressure of 100/70 mm Hg. She was admitted to the intensive care unit, where she had a stormy course marked by pulmonary edema and adult respiratory distress syndrome.

She had severe frostbite of all 10 toes and eventually required amputation of her left midfoot and her right leg below the knee. She had marked memory loss, personality changes, and depression for months after recovery. One year later she was reported to have recovered almost completely in terms of her mental function and was doing well with a new prosthesis on her right leg. In the summer she hiked up to the scene of her accident and planted a small evergreen tree at the site of Jorritt's death. She was making plans to go skiing that winter.

As you think back on Tanya's ordeal, especially to the period of time she spent lying in the snow with her broken leg, what do you think were the symptoms she displayed as she became progressively more hypothermic?

COMMENTS

- As people cool during cold exposure, they pass through a series of physiologic responses and symptoms that correlate with the core temperature.

- Table 14-1 displays the therapy to employ for hypothermic people who are breathing and have a pulse, as they become progressively more hypothermic. These same levels of core temperature are associated with predictable clinical findings.

| TABLE 14-1 | Hypothermia: Therapy and Clinical Signs and Symptoms Correlated With Core Temperature |

Core Temperature	Signs and Symptoms	Therapy
MILD HYPOTHERMIA (34°C TO 36°C)		
36° C (96.8° F)	Shivering begins. Metabolic rate increases to adjust for heat loss.	Passive or active rewarming (heaters, warm blankets) acceptable.
35° C (95.0° F)	Shivering continues and reaches maximum level.	Protect from further heat loss and wind chill.
34° C (93.2° F)	Extreme subjective coldness; amnesia and dysarthria, but still mentally responsive; adequate blood pressure.	Remove wet, cold garments. May use hot water bottles, other heat sources.
MODERATE HYPOTHERMIA (30°C TO 34°C)		
33° C (91.4° F)	Beginning to show mental confusion; ataxia and apathy; shivering decreases.	Passive rewarming still acceptable. (Continue for all levels of hypothermia.)
32° C (89.6° F)	Consciousness much more clouded; shivering almost stopped; pupils may be dilated.	Active rewarming with external heart sources acceptable, but only on central, truncal areas.
31° C (87.8° F)	Severe peripheral vasoconstriction; blood pressure difficult to obtain.	Active rewarming but of truncal areas only.
30° C (86.0° F)	Muscles increasingly rigid; more loss of consciousness; atrial fibrillation and other dysrhythmias; cardiac output ⅔ of normal.	Active rewarming but of truncal areas only.
SEVERE HYPOTHERMIA (<30°C)		
29° C (85.2° F)	Pulse and respirations slow perceptibly; cardiac arrhythmias become more frequent. Pupils dilate.	Continue passive rewarming; continue active external rewarming; start active internal rewarming as listed below:
28° C (82.4° F)	If irritated from rough movements, heart may fibrillate.	• Warm IV fluid (43° C) • Warm, humid oxygen (42°-46° C)
27° C (80.6° F)	Victim seldom conscious; all voluntary motion stops.	• Above plus, one or more of following: • Peritoneal lavage • Thoracic cavity lavage • Esophageal rewarming tubes • Heart-lung bypass
26° C (78.8° F)	Victim can actually appear dead; deep tendon and skin reflexes and pupillary light reflexes disappear.	All forms of active internal rewarming acceptable.
25° C (77° F)	Heart spontaneously goes into ventricular fibrillation (VF).	Passive rewarming, active external rewarming, plus some form of active internal rewarming.
24° C (75.2° F)	Pulmonary edema, severe hypotension may develop.	Some form of active internal rewarming.
23° C (73.4° F)	VF; greater appearance of death; no corneal or oculocephalic reflexes.	Some form of active internal rewarming.
22° C (71.6° F)	Maximum risk of VF.	Some form of active internal rewarming.
19-20° C (68° F)	Flat EEG; almost invariably asystole.	Some form of active internal rewarming.
18° C (65° F)	Lowest recorded temperature with recovery from accidental hypothermia.	Some form of active internal rewarming.

<table>
<tr><td>

Mabel Lewis

CASE 3

</td><td>

URBAN HYPOTHERMIA

Mabel Lewis is a 72-year-old woman who lives alone. It is the fall of the year when the days are beginning to cool and most people turn on their heat at night. Mabel has adult-onset diabetes controlled by oral

</td></tr>
</table>

hypoglycemic agents. Mabel tends to drink excessively to help alleviate the boredom of having no television. Her power has been cut off for failure to pay her utility bills.

Her neighbors have not seen Mrs. Lewis for the last 3 days and called the police department. When they entered the apartment, they found two extremely hungry cats and Mrs. Lewis, confused, lethargic, and responsive only to deep pain. The ambulance was called, and they have just brought Mrs. Lewis into the Emergency Department, where you are working as a physician.

The nurse obtains the following vital signs: Temperature = 34° C (93.2° F) (rectal); blood pressure = 80/60 mm Hg but weak; Heart rate = 50 beats/min and sinus rhythm (Fig. 14-2); respirations = 12 breaths/min. You notice that her skin feels cool but not clammy; she has urinated on herself. You ask the nurse, "Was her temperature really 34° C (93.2° F)?" and the nurse replies, "Actually, the mercury column seemed to be a little lower than 34° C (93.2° F)."

What are the clues here that Mrs. Lewis might be hypothermic?

COMMENTS

- The major clue in Case 3 is the glass rectal thermometer reading of "34° C." This turns out to be the lowest number etched on standard glass thermometers. Therefore the actual temperature could be much lower.

- Many clinicians would fail to follow up on the following rather obvious clues and risk factors for "urban hypothermia."

CLINICAL CLUES

- Low-reading thermometer
- Lethargy, confusion, incontinence
- Hypotension, difficulty obtaining blood pressure
- Bradycardia with J waves on the ECG
- Cool extremities without diaphoresis

RISK FACTORS

- Elderly patient
- Poor patient who lives alone
- Alcoholism
- Patient too sick and debilitated to take proper care of herself
- Associated chronic medical conditions (the non–insulin-dependent diabetes)
- "Cool" but not cold ambient temperatures

- Your approach would include the standard Emergency Department workup of a patient with confusion, lethargy, and alteration of consciousness.

- However, the hypothermia possibility would need to be pursued with a deep-rectal-probe thermometer.

<table>
<tr><td>

Mabel Lewis

CASE 3 Continued

</td><td>

When the rectal-probe thermometer is obtained, you learn that the rectal core temperature is 29° C. How would you proceed with your evaluation and treatment of Mrs. Lewis?

</td></tr>
</table>

COMMENTS

- The Hypothermia Algorithm (Fig. 14-1) helps us categorize Mrs. Lewis's condition as "severe hypothermia" with her temperature of 29° C (85.2° F). Her symptoms and clinical picture appear consistent with a core temperature of 29° C (85.2° F) (Table 14-1).

- Case 3 is a true hypothermic emergency with the patient at high risk of lethal cardiac dysrhythmias (VF and VT) as well as complete cardiovascular collapse.

- Fig. 14-1 and Table 14-1 outline a treatment approach that would include the standard actions for all hypothermic

patients, as well as passive rewarming and active external rewarming. The major immediate actions to take for Mrs. Lewis are as follows:

- Maintain her in horizontal position without head elevation.

- Start IV infusion of warm (42° C to 46° C [107.6° F to 114.8° F]) normal saline; give at 500 to 1000 mL/hour, but watch for pulmonary edema if pulse rate increases.

- Administer warm, humid oxygen (42° C to 46° C [107.6° F to 114.8° F]).

- Apply active, external rewarming techniques to truncal regions, but not directly against the skin. (Warm bags of IV fluids offer one of the most readily available techniques.)

• In addition, most experts would treat with the usual emergency protocols for patients with altered levels of consciousness, including administration of naloxone, 50% dextrose in water, thiamine, and parenteral vitamins.

Mabel Lewis

CASE 3 Continued

You initiate the actions listed earlier and are considering the use of peritoneal lavage with warm, potassium-free saline. After 30 minutes of relative clinical stability, the rectal-probe thermometer begins to register a steady rise in the temperature. By 60 minutes her core temperature has risen to 31° C (87.8° F) and she is slowly becoming more active, with a blood pressure of 98/70 mm Hg and a heart rate of 55 beats/min.

The initial laboratory values confirm your suspicion of hyperglycemic, hyperosmolar, nonketotic coma with dehydration and mild renal insufficiency. You admit Mrs. Lewis to the intensive care unit, where she makes a slow recovery, eventually being discharged to a local nursing home.

SUMMARY

Hypothermic emergencies and cardiac arrest associated with hypothermia present a number of challenges to the emergency care provider. Proper care of these patients demands a number of important modifications to the Primary-Secondary Survey Approach, as well as some completely unique additions to the ACLS guidelines.

KEY POINTS

UNIQUE GUIDELINES ADDITIONS

• Stop further heat loss.
• Begin rewarming process with the following:
  • Passive external warming
  • Active external warming
  • Active internal warming

PRIMARY SURVEY

• *Airway:* Use warm, humidified oxygen if possible.
• *Breathing:* Perform all ventilations gently and without trauma.
• *Circulation:* Perform pulse check for longer period of time (15 to 30 seconds).

• *Defibrillation:* Limit shocks to three only if VF proves refractory on the first three shocks.

SECONDARY SURVEY

• *Airway:* Perform endotracheal intubation as gently as possible.
• *Breathing:* Ventilate lungs with warm, humidified oxygen at a temperature of 42° C to 46° C (107.6° F to 114.8° F).
• *Circulation:* Several changes from usual secconodary survey approaches as follows:
  • Infuse normal saline at 42° C to 46° C (107.6° F to 114.8° F).
  • Monitor the cardiac rhythm with needle electrodes if necessary.

• Determine the core temperature.
• Withhold IV medications if core temperature is less than 30° C (86° F).
• Space IV medications further apart.
• Avoid high-dose epinephrine.
• Consider routine use of bretylium.
• Avoid pacing.
• *Differential Diagnoses*
  • Initiate appropriate rewarming techniques based on core temperature and the treatment setting (prehospital versus hospital).
  • Consider other possible causes for the arrest.
  • Consider associated conditions that may have contributed to the arrest.
  • Consider early transportation to facility with heart-lung bypass capability.
  • Do not give up too soon.

Cardiac Arrest Associated With Trauma

O V E R V I E W

Cardiac arrest associated with trauma is a "special resuscitation situation." This means you must employ different resuscitation treatment approaches when dealing with victims of trauma. The treatment of cardiac arrest associated with trauma differs in several important ways from the treatment of nontraumatic cardiac arrest. What are these major differences?

- *First, you must always be concerned about additional traumatic injuries, in particular, cervical spine instability and central nervous system damage. In addition, continuing severe hemorrhage must be recognized and controlled if possible.*

- *Second, the causes of compromised airway, breathing, and circulation will be different when associated with trauma. These causes, for example, an upper airway obstructed by acute hemorrhage, will require immediate treatment before the resuscitation effort can continue.*

- *Third, airway problems, compared with cardiovascular problems, play a bigger primary role in traumatic cardiac arrest than in nontraumatic cardiac arrest. Often, compromise of breathing and respiration, for example, from severe head trauma, has produced the cardiac arrest in trauma patients. Attention to airway management, combined with cervical spine stabilization, will be emphasized more in trauma resuscitation.*

- *Fourth, aggressive fluid resuscitation receives more attention in traumatic cardiac arrest than in nontraumatic arrest. Trauma often produces "an empty tank," and it is this empty tank that causes the cardiac arrest rather than a primary pump or rate problem. Resuscitation success depends, in simplistic terms, on refilling this empty tank.*

- *Fifth, in traumatic cardiac arrest the "tank" has become low or empty because the walls are damaged. Intravascular volume has been lost through damaged blood vessels and major organs. This hemorrhage can be stopped only by definitive surgical repair of the injuries. This requires definitive surgical treatment, most often in major trauma centers or the trauma operating room.*

MAJOR CONCEPTS TO MASTER

- Appropriate treatment of cardiac arrest resulting from trauma requires careful attention to several unique concepts not present in cardiac resuscitation as a result of other causes including the following:

  - First, the Five Quadrads and the Primary Survey require some modifications from the Primary Survey used in nontraumatic ACLS. In ACLS you *assess* the victim for the presence or absence of airway, breath-

  ing, and circulation and then *provide* that function (i.e., basic CPR) when missing. In the Trauma ABCDs, however, you look for explicit problems caused by the original trauma. The following problems with ABC must be identified and corrected before proceeding further with the resuscitation:
    - AIRWAY: Could be obstructed by traumatic deformities, blood, teeth, debris, other foreign objects, or tracheal disruption.

- NOTE: *The Airway in the Primary Survey requires careful attention to the possibility of cervical spine injury and immobilization.*

- **Breathing:** The ability to move adequate oxygen into and out of the lungs may be compromised by traumatic injuries such as tension pneumothorax, massive hemothorax, open pneumothorax, and large area of flail chest with pulmonary contusion.

- **Circulation:** Can be ineffective because of cardiac rupture, cardiac tamponade, great vessels injury, or exsanguination.

- **Disability (rather than defibrillation):** In Trauma ABCDs the D of *disability* stands for neurologic status. The patient's neurologic status should be examined for signs of cerebral contusion, intracerebral hemorrhage, and acute subdural or subarachnoid hemorrhage.

- Second, resuscitation of trauma victims requires rapid deployment of advanced airway control and management. This must be done while paying careful attention to cervical spine stabilization and to other injuries that may have occurred with the original trauma. Orotracheal intubation with in-line cervical spine immobilization (not traction!) is the method of choice for securing the airway in suspected cervical spine trauma.

- Third, trauma resuscitation involves aggressive fluid resuscitation. Recall the fifth quadrad in the Five Quadrads: Tank (Volume)/Resistance/Pump/Rate. Cardiac arrest that is due to trauma is *usually* (but not always) secondary to "an empty tank," *sometimes* due to disease or disorder of the "pump," and almost never due to problems with "rate." Consequently, "filling the tank" and "stopping the leakage from the tank" become the major focus of trauma resuscitation. Having said this, however, note the fourth point.

- Fourth, cardiac arrest associated with trauma is not just bleeding to death. In addition to an "empty tank," trauma can lead to cardiac arrest by the following routes in addition to exsanguination:

  - Severe brain injury leading to depressed respirations and cardiac arrest that is due to hypoxia

  - Chest injuries (tension or open pneumothorax, flail chest, hemothorax, tracheobronchial disruption) leading to compromised ventilation and cardiac arrest resulting from hypoxia or hypercarbia

  - Direct injury to vital structures (lungs, heart, aorta)

  - Compromised cardiac output caused by tension pneumothorax or cardiac tamponade

  - Underlying medical problems made worse by the trauma (ischemic heart disease precipitated by fall in hematocrit or cardiac perfusion)

  - Trauma in cold environment that compromises ability to maintain temperature and leads to hypothermic cardiac arrest (for example, fractured leg)

- Fifth, you must be aware of *associated injuries* that occurred with the original trauma. This applies most dramatically to *cervical spine immobilization,* but associated injuries virtually any place on the body may also be present. Few resuscitations from trauma can succeed without careful attention to the cervical spine, to the neurologic system, to pulmonary and cardiac function, and to continuing hemorrhage.

- Sixth, with the tank as the major problem in traumatic resuscitation, there will be a *diminished emphasis on defibrillation and medications.* These interventions do have a role, however, but only in specific subsets of traumatic resuscitations and only at specific stages in those resuscitation attempts.

- Seventh, traumatic cardiac arrest rarely can be treated by ACLS interventions alone. The care provided by ACLS personnel usually falls short of definitive care that requires operating room interventions. This produces a need for rapid alerting of and transport to advanced trauma centers for *definitive operative treatment.* Cardiac arrest associated with trauma has a dismal outcome unless early intraoperative intervention occurs.

  - The preceding situation has led, by 1992, to widespread acceptance that "Load" (first, secure airway, spine, hemorrhage) and then "Go" (start IV lines and give fluids in transport) is the most effective prehospital approach to trauma resuscitation. This is compared to "stay and play" (delay transport until ALS personnel have performed all possible prehospital interventions).

- Eighth, the ACLS provider will also have to distinguish between cardiac arrest *caused* by trauma, and trauma *caused* by cardiac arrest. The clinical picture will often be dominated by the signs of trauma (blood, deformed and disrupted anatomy). In reality the trauma may have been the result of a cardiac arrest of some other origin. The best example of this situation would be the person who has ventricular fibrillation (VF) while driving a car, and then suffers trauma when he or she runs off the highway.

- Ninth, for *prehospital* ACLS providers, *rescuer safety* becomes a concern during the rapid treatment required for traumatic cardiac arrest. Often these resuscitations must occur in harsh environmental conditions such as busy highways, in the rain or snow, or in darkness. The events that caused the trauma often are not far removed from the rescuer. One major rule: Rescuers must always attend to their safety and not become victims themselves.

- Tenth, most trauma that causes cardiac arrest can be *prevented*. Therefore, prevention stands as a major focus in all discussions of the management of the consequences of trauma. This is an eminently reasonable perspective because detailed discussions on how to care for the consequences of trauma become unnecessary when the trauma itself has been prevented.

Critical actions

The critical actions for patients with cardiac arrest associated with trauma are the following:

- Ensure rescuer safety.

- The "big four" of EMS care: Extricate-Stabilize-Resuscitate-Transport.

- Perform the steps of the Primary-Secondary ABCD Survey in the Universal Algorithm (Fig. 15-1), including the following:

  - Perform cervical spine immobilization during the A (Airway) portion of the Primary Survey.

  - Perform CPR when indicated.

  - Properly attach and operate defibrillator and monitor.

  - Recognize the need for and successful performance of endotracheal intubation.

  - Establish IV access.

  - Consider the Differential Diagnoses.

  - Consider Disability.

- Apply the full Five Quadrads to the initial management of traumatic cardiac arrest, as follows:

  - Primary ABCD (modified for traumatic cardiac arrest; see the box on p. 260)

  - Secondary ABCD (modified for traumatic cardiac arrest; see the box on p. 260)

  - Oxygen/IV/Monitor/Fluids

  - Temperature/Blood Pressure/Heart Rate/Respirations

  - Tank (Volume)/Resistance/Pump/Rate

- Initiate appropriate treatment on discovery of any reversible causes of traumatic arrest.

Skills to learn

RECOGNIZE

- Hypovolemia

- Pericardial tamponade

- Tension pneumothorax

- Open pneumothorax

- Flail chest

PERFORM

- IV fluid infusion

- Pericardiocentesis

- Needle decompression of pneumothorax with flutter valve

- Three-sided occlusive dressing

Rhythms to learn

- *Pulseless electrical activity* (PEA), which includes electromechanical dissociation (EMD) plus other rhythms associated with no pulse (Fig. 15-2), as follows:

  - Idioventricular rhythms

  - Pulseless asystolic rhythms

  - Bradyasystolic rhythms

  - Ventricular junctional escape rhythms

  - "Pseudo-EMD"

- *Sinus tachycardia* (sign of hypovolemia)

- *Sinus bradycardia* (hypoventilation, hypoxia signs, or hypovolemia)

- *Ventricular fibrillation/pulseless ventricular tachycardia* (VF/VT)

Medications to learn

- Rapid, massive volume replacement with normal saline, lactated Ringer's solution, and blood and blood products will always be "the medication of first choice" (along with oxygen) for the trauma victim. Never forget this.

- **Epinephrine** and **atropine** are the two other medications recommended in the PEA Algorithm.

- **Norepinephrine** and **dopamine** have indications in hypotension resulting from trauma, but only after virtually complete volume replacement has been achieved.

FIGURE 15-1

Universal Algorithm for Adult Emergency Cardiac Care

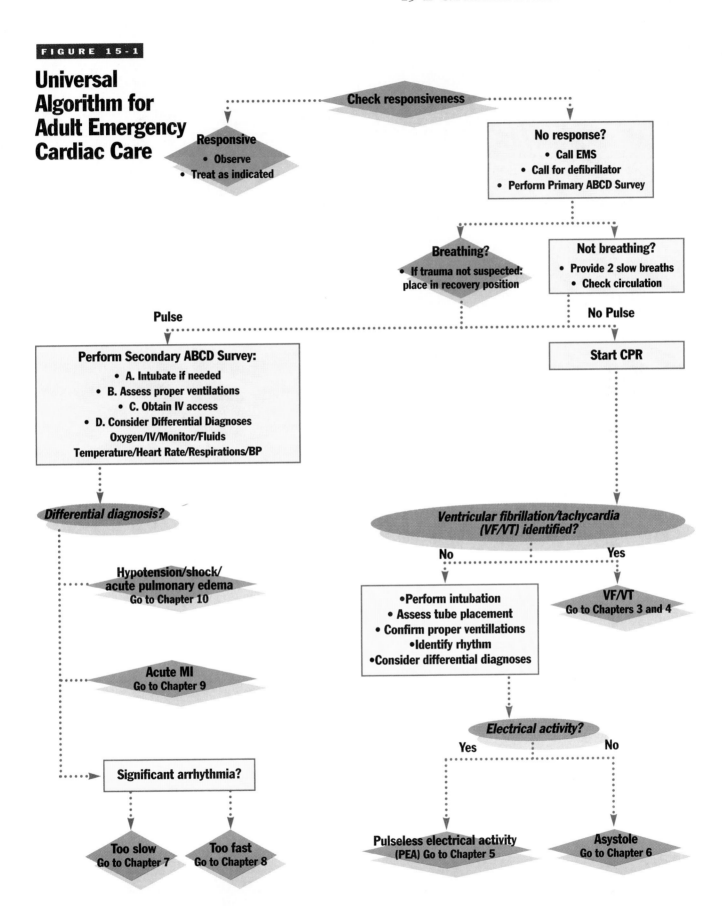

Check responsiveness

Responsive
- Observe
- Treat as indicated

No response?
- Call EMS
- Call for defibrillator
- Perform Primary ABCD Survey

Breathing?
- If trauma not suspected: place in recovery position

Not breathing?
- Provide 2 slow breaths
- Check circulation

Pulse

No Pulse

Perform Secondary ABCD Survey:
- A. Intubate if needed
- B. Assess proper ventilations
- C. Obtain IV access
- D. Consider Differential Diagnoses
Oxygen/IV/Monitor/Fluids
Temperature/Heart Rate/Respirations/BP

Start CPR

Differential diagnosis?

Ventricular fibrillation/tachycardia (VF/VT) identified?

No

Yes

Hypotension/shock/ acute pulmonary edema
Go to Chapter 10

Acute MI
Go to Chapter 9

- Perform intubation
- Assess tube placement
- Confirm proper ventillations
- Identify rhythm
- Consider differential diagnoses

VF/VT
Go to Chapters 3 and 4

Electrical activity?

Yes

No

Significant arrhythmia?

Too slow
Go to Chapter 7

Too fast
Go to Chapter 8

Pulseless electrical activity (PEA) Go to Chapter 5

Asystole
Go to Chapter 6

Adapted with permission, Journal of the American Medical Association, 1992, Volume 268, *Guidelines for Cardiopulmonary Resuscitation and Emergency Cardiac Care*, p. 2216
Copyright © 1992, American Medical Association.

ACLS Primary-Secondary Survey   Modified for Traumatic Cardiac Arrest

PRIMARY ABCDD SURVEY

(note the extra D)

AIRWAY

- *Immobilize cervical spine when indicated (any injury above the clavicles).*
- *Open the airway with jaw thrust–chin lift (avoid head tilt).*
- *Clear upper airway of obstructions (blood, teeth, redundant tissues, debris).*

BREATHING

- *Place oropharyngeal airway.*
- *Provide positive-pressure ventilation using bag-valve-mask ventilation.*
- *Observe for bilateral symmetric chest wall expansion.*
- *Observe for pulmonary mechanical problems (open pneumothorax, flail chest, and so forth).*

CIRCULATION

- *Control hemorrhage.*
- *Check for a pulse.*
- *Perform chest compressions.*
- *Observe for continuing bleeding.*

DEFIBRILLATION

- *Shock VF/VT: This remains appropriate even in cardiac arrest associated with trauma.*

DISABILITY

- *Neurologic injuries may have caused the cardiac arrest because of suppresion of ventilation or cardiovascular collapse on a "central" basis.*
- *If possible, before arrest note the prearrest level of consciousness using the AVPU mneumonic, as follows:*
- *A: Alert to their surroundings?*
- *V: Vocal stimuli evoke appropriate response?*
- *P: Painful stimuli required to evoke a response?*
- *U: Unresponsive to painful stimuli?*
- *Evaluate neurologic function (Glasgow Coma Score) as follows:*
- *Eye movements*
- *Verbal responses*
- *Motor responses*

SECONDARY ABCDDE SURVEY

(note the extra D and E)

AIRWAY

- *Determine the adequacy of the original ventilation and airway techniques.*
- *Perform orotracheal intubation with in-line cervical stabilization, if indicated.*
- *Perform needle or surgical cricothyrotomy, if indicated (inability to intubate the trachea through oral or nasal route, for example, severe maxillofacial trauma).*

BREATHING

- *Confirm that endotracheal tube is placed and working correctly.*
- *Provide positive-pressure ventilations through endotracheal tube.*
- *Assess that chest wall moves with each ventilation.*
- *Listen for bilateral breath sounds at axillae.*
- *Identify the following life-threatening breathing problems:*
  - *Tension pneumothorax*
  - *Open pneumothorax*
  - *Massive hemothorax*
  - *Flail chest*
- *Treat any life-threatening breathing problems when identified, as follows:*
  - *Tracheal intubation (oral or nasal)*
  - *Needle thoracentesis*
  - *Flutter-type valve or three-sided occlusive dressing*
  - *Chest tube thoracostomy*

CIRCULATION

- *Control any severe continuing hemorrhage.*
- *Perform chest compressions.*
- *Obtain IV access with at least two large-bore catheters.*
- *Begin rapid, high-flow fluid resuscitation when indicated (crystalloid, blood and blood products); use at least two large-bore needles and pumps.*
- *Attach monitor leads; identify rhythm and rate.*
- *Administer medications appropriate for the rhythm and vital signs (including treatment for shock).*
- *Look for and treat cardiac tamponade using pericardiocentesis via the subxiphoid route (especially when patients are refractory to other measures).*

DIFFERENTIAL DIAGNOSES/DISABILITY

- *Continue resuscitation phase, as follows:*
  - *Consult with neurosurgery when indicated.*
  - *Insert urinary catheter if there are no contraindications.*
  - *Insert nasogastric tube.*
  - *Continue to reevaluate.*
  - *Arrange interhospital transfer if indicated.*

EXPOSE THE PATIENT COMPLETELY

This provides complete examination and assessment of additional problems.

FIGURE 15-2

Pulseless Electrical Activity (PEA) Algorithm

(see also the box on p.260)

Term "PEA" Includes:
- **Electromechanical dissociation (EMD)**
  - **Pseudo-EMD**
  - **Idioventricular rhythms**
  - **Ventricular escape rhythms**
  - **Bradyasystolic rhythms**
- **Postdefibrillation idioventricular rhythms**
  - **Stabilization of the cervical spine**

Continue BLS Perform Secondary ABCD Survey: • Intubate if needed • Assess ventilations • Obtain IV access	Check for occult blood flow using Doppler ultrasound, echocardiograph, end-tidal CO_2 device Expose patient for complete physical examination

↓

Consider the Differential Diagnoses (possible treatments shown in parentheses):

Five Hs: • Hypovolemia, includes anaphylaxis (volume infusion) • Hypoxia (oxygen and ventilation) • Hypothermia (see Hypothermia Algorithm) • Hyperkalemia, hypokalemia (and other electrolyte abnormalities)[b] • Hydrogen ion (acidosis)	Five Ts: • Tension pneumothorax (needle decompression) • Tamponade = cardiac (percardiocentesis) • Thrombosis = pulmonary (surgery, thrombolytics) • Thrombosis = acute myocardial (thrombolytics; see Chapter 9) • Tablets = drug overdose

↓

• *Epinephrine* 1 mg IV push[a,c] repeat every 3 to 5 minutes

↓

• If rate of electrical activity is slow (<60 beats/min), give atropine 1 mg IV • Repeat every 3 to 5 minutes to a total of 0.03 to 0.04 mg/kg[d]

Class I : Definitely helpful

Class IIa: Acceptable, probably helpful

Class IIb: Acceptable, possibly helpful

Class III: Not indicated, may be harmful

[a] **Sodium bicarbonate** 1 mEq/kg is Class I if patient has known preexisting hyperkalemia.

[b] **Sodium bicarbonate** (1 mEq/kg): Follow these indications:

Class IIa

- If known preexisting bicarbonate-responsive acidosis

- If overdose with tricyclic antidepressants
- To alkalinize the urine in drug overdoses

Class IIb

- If trachea intubated and arrest continues for long intervals
- If circulation restored after prolonged arrest

Class III

- Hypoxic lactic acidosis (unventilated patient)

[c] The recommended dose of **epinephrine** is 1 mg IV push every 3 to 5 minutes. If spontaneous circulation does not return, consider the following Class IIb dosing regimens:

- Intermediate: **Epinephrine** 2 to 5 mg IV push, every 3 to 5 minutes
- Escalating: **Epinephrine** 1 mg to 3 mg to 5 mg IV push, 3 minutes apart
- High: **Epinephrine** 0.1 mg/kg IV push, every 3 to 5 minutes

[d] The shorter atropine dosing interval (3 minutes) is possibly helpful in cardiac arrest (Class IIb).

Adapted with permission, Journal of the American Medical Association, 1992, Volume 268, *Guidelines for Cardiopulmonary Resuscitation and Emergency Cardiac Care*, p. 2219
Copyright © 1992, American Medical Association.

Greg Schiller	BIKE ACCIDENT: HEAD INJURY LEADING TO HYPOXIA AND CARDIAC ARREST
CASE 1	

You are on duty as an urban paramedic when you receive a code green (high priority) dispatch that a bicycle rider has been injured on the Burke-Gilman Bicycle Trail. Greg Schiller is a 52-year-old avid bicyclist training for the Seattle-to-Portland bicycle race. While trying to avoid a jogger, Mr. Schiller swerved and lost control of his bike in the loose gravel on the side of the path. He was traveling at 23 mph and was thrown over the front of the bike, landing on his wrists and then his face.

He was wearing an approved bike helmet but was reported to have been unconscious for "at least 4 minutes" after the accident. When you arrive, you notice that Mr. Schiller is lying completely still on his back, with a dazed look in his eyes. His face is covered with blood from his nose, mouth, and cheeks. He appears to be choking on the blood in his mouth. A bystander remarks, "He has a pulse but he sure is acting out of it!"

How would you and your partner approach the immediate care of Mr. Schiller?

COMMENTS

- Throughout this book we have advocated the Five Quadrads as a valuable conceptual tool to guide your approach to cardiopulmonary emergencies. With some modifications this approach remains useful in cardiac arrest associated with trauma.

- You would approach Mr. Schiller with the familiar Primary-Secondary Survey of ACLS, but modified for traumatic Cardiac Arrest.

- The box on p.260 provides details on the modified Primary-Secondary Survey.

PRIMARY ABCDD SURVEY

- You notice that several things are needed immediately with Mr. Schiller, the most obvious being patency of his airway.

- *Airway with C-spine immobilization:* The Fire Department EMTs arrive almost simultaneously with you and your partner. You request that they prepare to immobilize Mr. Schiller on their full-length backboard, including placement of a rigid cervical spine collar. Mr. Schiller is at high risk for cervical spine injury because of his obvious facial injuries. (Suspect cervical spine trauma with any injury above the clavicles.)

  - You direct one of the EMTs to maintain in-line cervical spine stabilization while you complete your examination and while awaiting the placement of the backboard and the rigid cervical collar.

  - The Primary A (Airway) presents the most immediate problem because the blood running down his throat is already causing him to gag and cough. You are worried that his teeth may be loose enough to threaten aspiration.

  - You put on a pair of heavy-duty latex examination gloves and perform a quick finger-sweep of his mouth. The teeth are loose but not free, and you use the portable, hand-powered suction device to remove 15 mL of blood from the back of his throat.

  - You place an oropharyngeal airway, but you are concerned to observe that he tolerates it without coughing or much gagging. His decreased level of consciousness indicates a depressed sensorium from the head injury.

- *Breathing:* You ask one of the EMTs to begin 100% oxygen through a bag-valve-mask and to gently assist Mr. Schiller with each breath. He appears to be breathing slowly and shallowly, but with symmetric, bilateral chest expansion. There are no obvious chest wall injuries.

- *Circulation:* Mr. Schiller has a weak pulse of 50 beats/min and a blood pressure of 90/60 mm Hg. There are no obvious signs of injury other than the face, and no signs of bleeding from any other location.

- *Defibrillation:* You attach the three-lead monitor from your defibrillator-monitor to Mr. Schiller and confirm a sinus bradycardia at 50 beats/min. Defibrillation is not needed.

- *Disability:* You have been talking to Mr. Schiller as you work, asking him questions about himself and the accident. He does not recognize his surroundings, and he does not respond to your questions with an appropriate answer. Instead he just mumbles incoherently and continuously. Painful stimulation from rubbing your knuckles against his sternum evokes only a vague effort to brush your hand aside. On the Glasgow Coma Scale he scores a disturbingly low total of eight points, as follows:

  - Two points on eye opening (opens only when stimulated)

  - Two points on verbal response (makes incomprehensible sounds, not words)

  - Four points on the motor response (withdraws from painful stimulus)

SECONDARY ABCDDE SURVEY

- A,B, and C pose no immediate problem; however, the DD (Differential Diagnosis/Disability) leads you to think about the mechanism of injury, and more and more you are thinking about significant head injury.

- *Exposure:* You remove the biking jersey and the biking shorts looking for bruising, bleeding, or other signs of trauma. No other injuries are apparent.

- The rest of the Five Quadrads completes the initial assessment, as follows:

  - Temperature = 37.2° C; heart rate = 50 beats/min; blood pressure = 90/60 mm Hg; respirations = 10 breaths/min and shallow

  - Oxygen/IV (perform en route) /Monitor/ Fluids

- Tank (Volume)/Resistance/Pump/Rate: What is the nature of the problem?

  - *Is there a tank problem?* Maybe. There could be slight hypovolemia from the fluid lost during exercise.

  - *Is there a resistance problem?* Maybe. His skin is clammy from the sweat of his exercise, and his fingers are pale.

  - *Is there a pump problem?* Maybe. The blood pressure seems lower than normal, and certainly lower than what you would expect in a healthy man who has just been exercising.

  - *Is there a rate problem?* Maybe. The sinus rate of 50 beats/min seems too low for the blood pressure of 90/60 mm Hg.

Greg Schiller

CASE 1 Continued

Your partner works to help the EMTs place Mr. Schiller on the backboard while at the same time keeping the cervical spine stable in the midline position. You want to "load and go" with Mr. Schiller but your protocols direct one IV access attempt for trauma patients. You attempt to start the IV lines; however, this takes longer than anticipated. You notice that Mr. Schiller has stopped moving or making any sounds. You glance over at the EMT who is "bagging" Mr. Schiller, and he says, "You know, I don't think he is taking any breaths on his own anymore, and I'm not feeling a pulse either."

You quickly place your hand upon the left carotid artery and cannot feel a pulse. "Check his breathing once more." With your hand on the carotid you watch for 15 seconds to see if there are any chest movements. A quick glance at the pupils reveals them to be dilated and minimally responsive to light. The left pupil is much larger than the right. "Okay, he's arrested. Let's start CPR." What has happened here? What are your next actions?

COMMENTS

- At this point the sequence of disease in Mr. Schiller appears clear. He suffered a severe intracranial injury, possibly a brain contusion, or a subdural or epidural bleed.

- Although he regained consciousness from the original concussion, the intracranial bleeding continued, raising the intracranial pressure. These pressure changes led to dysfunction of the brainstem, partial tentorial herniation, asymmetric dilated pupils, and then suppression of respiratory drive. More than 50% of people who die of trauma die as a result of this sequence, which began with the original neurologic injury.

- The hypoventilation produced, first, the bradycardia and cardiac dysfunction; then, probably because of hypoxic acidosis, the heart simply slowed until the pulse was no longer perceptible.

- Your initial actions here are to return to the Primary-Secondary ABCD Survey (modified for the trauma patient).

PRIMARY SURVEY

- **Airway:** Reverify that the airway is open.

- **Breathing:** Continue to supply the bag-valve-mask ventilations while you prepare for orotracheal intubation.

- **Circulation:** The pulse is absent. The monitor shows some wide-complex electrical activity at 12 beats/min.

- **Defibrillation:** Not necessary.

- **Disability:** Neurologic status is a major clinical concern here.

SECONDARY SURVEY

- **Airway:** Perform, as follows, orotracheal intubation at once (Fig.15-3):

  - This will require working around the rigid cervical collar and require having one of the EMTs maintain in-line cervical immobilization.

  - In your system you have started using the new "trach light" lighted stylet technique (Fig. 15-4) to assist with orotracheal intubation when the cervical spine cannot be moved. This new technique (Chapter 2) allows you to slide the endotracheal tube into place, guided by the trach light shining through the tissues of the neck. This prevents struggling with the laryngoscope blade to achieve direct visualization of the cords in a patient whose neck must remain rigid.

- Digital intubation provides yet another useful technique to achieve orotracheal intubation when the neck cannot be moved (Fig. 15-5). This is described in Chapter 2. In this technique the fingers of one hand are used to blindly guide the endotracheal tube into the trachea using fingertip guidance.

- If severe maxillofacial trauma or anatomic distortion prevents intubation through either the oral or nasal route, attempt surgical cricothyroidotomy (Fig. 15-6). This can often provide lifesaving airway maintenance when no other technique is suitable.

- Note carefully that you want "immobilization of the head and neck," and *not* traction on the head.

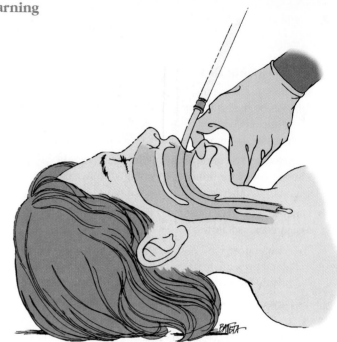

Fig. 15-4: *Lighted stylet intubation.*

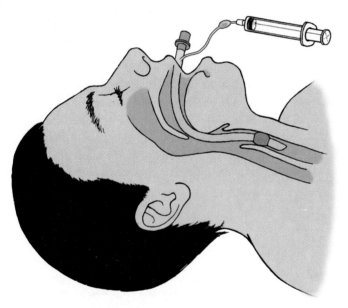

Fig. 15-3: *Orotracheal intubation.*

- **Circulation:** CPR compressions are in progress, and the IV access has been obtained. You order the two medications used in the PEA Algorithm at this point: **epinephrine 1 mg IV push and atropine 1 mg IV push.**

- **Differential Diagnosis and Disability:** Clearly, intracranial disease is playing a major role here. You should call as soon as possible to alert the receiving hospital that you are en route with a patient with a severe head injury, probably an intracranial bleed. This injury has resulted in a hypoxic cardiac arrest; neurosurgical intervention will be needed urgently.

- **Exposure:** You have carefully inspected the patient's entire body for signs of other injuries.

- **Breathing:** Confirm tube placement by five-point auscultation (listening for equal breath sounds, front of chest, left and right; midaxillary line, left and right; midepigastric area for absence of breath sounds) and by using the end-tidal CO_2 detector.

  - Examine once again for any life-threatening breathing problems (tension or open pneumothorax, massive hemothorax, flail chest): none of these are apparent.

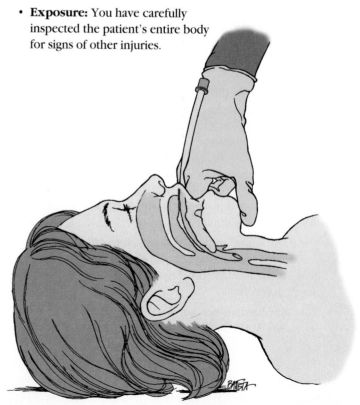

Fig. 15-5: *Digital intubation.*

Greg Schiller

CASE 1 Continued

You continue with hyperventilation of Mr. Schiller's lungs as he is transferred to the ambulance, fully immobilized, on the backboard. One of the EMTs continues with chest compressions. In the ambulance you notice that the heart rate has increased to 50 beats/min and that the carotid pulse has returned. Blood pressure is 110/70 mm Hg.

You contact the medical control physician and report that the cardiac arrest appears to have responded to post-intubation hyperventilation, epinephrine, and atropine. She instructs you to administer mannitol 2 g/kg as a 25% solution over the next 20 minutes.

What are your thoughts about this case? How could you have managed this differently?

COMMENTS

- Since Mr. Schiller responded to good airway management and recovered from his cardiac arrest, you could argue that better and earlier airway management could have prevented the hypoxic arrest. Nevertheless, you had no way of predicting at the start that the head injury was severe. Your management was systematic and logical and followed the recommended sequence of interventions.

- Case 1 is also an excellent example of how cardiac arrests associated with trauma are *not* caused solely by hemorrhage in massively injured victims. Mr. Schiller represents one of the major ways in which good prehospital EMS care saves lives—proper airway maintenance in severely injured patients. In fact, good airway management is probably the major lifesaving intervention in prehospital trauma care.

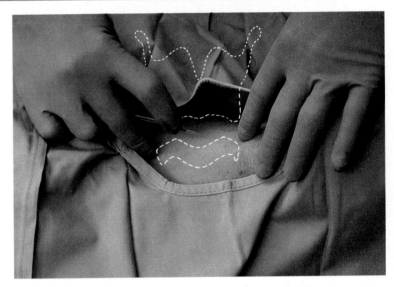

Fig. 15-6: *Cricothyroidotomy.*

Isadora LaSalle

CASE 2

SUICIDE ATTEMPT FROM A BRIDGE:
INJURIES INCOMPATIBLE WITH LIFE

You are a firefighter EMT "cruising your zone" when the 911 dispatcher contacts your unit about a reported "person jumped" from the Aurora bridge. For years this 150-foot drop to the Interlake Channel has been a chosen departure point of depressed, suicidal people. The few who survive the fall to the water usually drown before they are recovered. One widely quoted article confirms occasional "saves" achieved by your EMS system with people who have jumped from this bridge.*

You and your partner arrive in about 2 minutes. You find a large crowd gathered a few feet from the shore. You walk in and out of the shadows cast by the huge expanse of the bridge above you. The roar of the vehicles passing overhead drowns out most of the voices.

The unfortunate woman on the shore missed hitting the deeper water. Instead she landed on the side of her head in about 1 foot of water. The deformed shape of her head and the unnatural angle of her neck are apparent as you approach. The bystanders have dragged her from the shallows to the shore, but they are not touching her.

How would you begin the resuscitation efforts for this woman?

---

*Fortner GS, Oreskovich MR, Copass MK, Carrico CJ: The effects of pre-hospital trauma care on survival from a 50-meter fall. J *Trauma* 23(11):976, 1983.

COMMENTS

- The woman in Case 2 has probably sustained traumatic injuries that are incompatible with life. Most EMS systems have criteria by which resuscitation efforts should not even begin. These usually include the following:
  - Hemicorpectomy
  - Decapitation
  - Total body surface (deep) or full-thickness burns

- Massive, destructive injuries
- Severe blunt trauma without vital signs, pupillary responses, or electrical activity on cardiac monitor
- Rigor mortis or obvious dependent lividity

- Nevertheless, this woman does not fit any of these criteria except severe blunt trauma, and she merits appropriate initial treatment until further information becomes available.
- Again the Primary-Secondary Survey (modified for trauma patients) should be followed.

Isadora LaSalle

CASE 2 Continued

Your initial impressions are dominated by the severe angulation of the neck and the "caved-in" appearance of the side of the woman's head. You hesitate to move her head because of the high probability of cervical trauma. Nevertheless, you determine that the woman is not breathing; the angulation is sufficient to compromise the airway, and there is no pulse.

You put on your examination gloves. You decide to straighten the head back to a neutral position and apply a rigid cervical collar. Under your fingers you can feel a "give" in the skull in the lateral temporoparietal region as you straighten the head. You ask one of the bystanders to run back to the ambulance to get the long backboard.

You check quickly for a pulse, and when none is detected you ask one of the bystanders to begin chest compressions. You instruct your partner to begin bag-valve-mask ventilations with the rigid collar in place while you begin to set up the automated external defibrillator (AED).

What is the purpose of the defibrillator? Why are you attempting this resuscitation?

COMMENTS

- You are now gathering information that will actually allow you to cease efforts on the woman in Case 2. The purpose of the defibrillator is not only to shock VF if it is present, but also to support your search for some sort of electrical activity.

- The chances, by far, are that the woman is in asystole or some other agonal rhythm. By using the defibrillator you are proving that she has lost all electrical activity and has essentially expired.

Isadora LaSalle

CASE 2 Continued

You dry off the woman's torso with a cloth in the defibrillator jump bag. You attach the adhesive defibrillator pads while your partner and the bystander continue with basic CPR.

Your assessment with the AED reveals the complete absence of electrical activity (which you can confirm by looking at the defibrillator screen). "No shock is indicated."

Within 4 minutes the medics arrive and assess the scene at once. "She was in cardiac arrest from the moment we arrived, and we started doing CPR after spinal stabilization. She is in asystole on the monitor. I think she has been dead since she hit the water."

One of the medics checks her pupils and finds them fixed, dilated, and unresponsive to flashlight stimulation. She checks the monitor screen on the AED and confirms the complete absence of electrical activity.

What should be the medics' response at this time?

COMMENTS

- Case 2 is a clinically challenging situation in which common sense should come in to play. Severe, deforming trauma with ongoing CPR for more than 10 minutes, asystole on the cardiac monitor, and fixed and dilated pupils all lead to the conclusion that further resuscitation efforts are futile and inappropriate.

- Prehospital personnel at the level of EMTs are prohibited by law in most states from pronouncing people dead or ceasing resuscitation efforts once started.

- Paramedic-level personnel, however, are usually in direct contact with medical control physicians. In this situation the medical control doctor should be contacted for permission to cease efforts.

Isadora LaSalle

CASE 2 Continued

The Medics do not attempt IV access or orotracheal intubation, but they direct you, the chest compressor, and the airway manager to continue with your efforts.

The lead Medic calls the base station hospital, describing the woman as a suicide victim who jumped from the Aurora bridge. The Medic summarizes the situation: massive traumatic injuries; the victim has been in cardiac arrest for more than 10 minutes; there is confirmed absence of any ventilatory efforts or electrical activity of the heart; there are absent pupil reactions. The medical control doctor concurs with the recommendation and orders the resuscitation efforts to stop.

Should the first arriving personnel have even started resuscitation efforts?

COMMENTS

- The first arriving personnel to this scene, lacking the medical authority to pronounce this woman dead in the field, proceeded with a most appropriate evaluation and initial management.

- This will be a common scenario in the professional career of many BLS and ACLS providers—cardiac arrest in association with trauma in which the injury is incompatible with life.

- These difficult situations are a challenge and must be handled sensitively and compassionately.

Akmed Patel

CASE 3

PENETRATING TRAUMA: PNEUMOTHORAX AND HEMOTHORAX
You are the attending physician in an urban Emergency Department when Akmed Patel, a local taxicab driver, is brought in by the medics. He was stabbed in the left side of his chest with a "sharp, penetrating object" during a robbery attempt. The medics arrived to find him unconscious, not breathing, and without a pulse. They intubated his trachea, started two large-bore IV catheters with the IV lines running wide open and transported him to the Emergency Department with ongoing CPR.

What are the unique features of Mr. Patel's resuscitation?

COMMENTS

- Mr. Patel represents one of the more promising scenarios in resuscitation of cardiac arrest associated with trauma—penetrating chest trauma without massive tissue destruction or significant neurologic injuries. These patients often do well if they are transported to a Level 1 trauma center where definitive care can be provided quickly and efficiently.

- The scenario in Case 3 makes the major point that definitive care for this patient exists in the operating room under the hands of the trauma surgeon.

- The role of the ACLS provider is continued resuscitation, immediate stabilization based on the Primary-Secondary Survey, and the treatment of any immediate, life-threatening problems.

- Here your initial assessment would identify hypovolemia resulting from hemorrhage, an open, "sucking" pneumothorax, and hemorrhagic pneumothorax (hemopneumothorax).

- While final preparations are being made to roll Mr. Patel into the operating room, you have time to do the following:

- Place a flutter valve over the sucking chest wound.

- Insert a chest tube.

- Begin transfusions with prescreened O-negative blood.

- Insert a nasogastric tube.

- Insert a Foley catheter.

- Insert one more 14-gauge IV catheter.

- Obtain a portable chest x-ray.

- Obtain a 12-lead ECG

- The duration of the stay in the Emergency Department for Mr. Patel was 7 minutes and 30 seconds, and he was actually beginning to produce a palpable blood pressure.

- In the operating room a large laceration of his left upper lobe and a small myocardial laceration were repaired. He survived without sequelae, although he did retire from the taxicab profession.

Charles "Slim" Loveridge
CASE 4

VF-INDUCED, SLOW-SPEED MOTOR VEHICLE ACCIDENT
While driving home from your shift as a "Clin Spec Nurse" in the pediatric intensive care unit, you notice the car in front of you swerve several times, leave the road at a slow speed, and strike a small tree. You stop your car and run back to see what is wrong. In the other car is an elderly man slumped over the steering wheel. He struck his face and is bleeding profusely from his nose and mouth. He is not breathing and does not respond to your questions. You check his carotid pulse and it is absent.

What dilemmas does this man pose in terms of a cardiac arrest in association with trauma?

COMMENTS

- You do not know whether Case 4 is a case of severe trauma that led to a cardiac arrest, or whether the man had experienced a sudden cardiac arrhythmia that led to the loss of consciousness and subsequent trauma when he ran off the road.

- The prognosis for the two situations is much different. Collapse from a VF cardiac arrest leading to inadvertent trauma has a far greater possibility of a positive outcome.

- The answer lies in always being systematic and routinely applying the Primary-Secondary Survey Approach.

- In the situation in Case 4 you have to make a decision to move the man from the car without full cervical spine immobilization. Certainly the mechanism of this accident would suggest a high probability of cervical spine injury.

- If the emergency personnel were available, they would rapidly deploy the "short-board extrication" technique (Fig. 15-7), which would allow them to stabilize the head and neck and still provide timely CPR and airway support.

- Nevertheless, a full cardiac arrest demands resuscitation efforts that must be performed even with the risk of cervical spine injury.

- Unless you could hear the ambulance on its way, we would recommend some effort at head and neck stabilization and removal of the man from the vehicle so that basic CPR could be initiated. Death is virtually guaranteed if he is left slumped over in the car, without a pulse and without respiration.

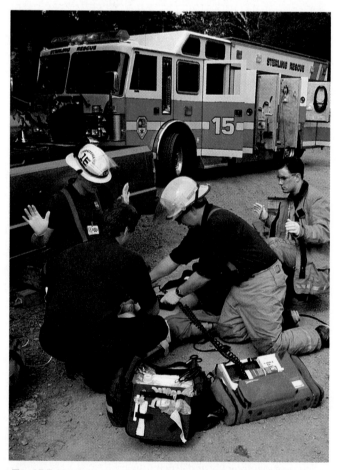

Fig. 15-7: *Ventricular fibrillation (VF) that precipitates trauma should be treated as VF with precautions for trauma.*

SUMMARY

Resuscitation of the person who has had cardiac arrest in association with trauma requires modifications in the Five Quadrads Approach. Learn these modifications. Learn the major challenges that traumatic cardiac arrest presents to the ACLS provider.

- Which came first: the cardiac arrest or the trauma?

- Stabilize the cervical spine and prevent converting a spinal column injury into a spinal cord injury.

- Consider neurologic problems, not just cardiovascular problems.

- Focus more on volume resuscitation and less on defibrillation and medications.

- Know basic techniques for treating associated injuries resulting from the trauma (immediate control of exsanguinating hemorrhage, massive volume replacement, tension pneumothorax decompression, open chest wound stabilization, and decompression of cardiac tamponade).

- Recognize the need for major trauma centers to provide definitive resuscitation care, particularly by having available 24-hour operation rooms, operating room staff, and trauma surgeons.

- Recognize traumatic cardiac arrest patients who have no chance of survival. Rescuer safety (for example, during emergency air evacuation responses or rapid ground transportation) must be considered when treating patients who have virtually no chance of successful, long-term resuscitation.

- Recognize that the real answer lies with prevention of the original trauma.

FILE 16.

Cardiac Arrest Associated With Pregnancy

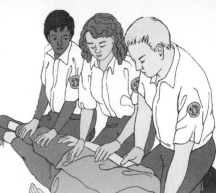

OVERVIEW

Cardiac arrest in the pregnant woman presents a dramatic and challenging emergency. About one in every 30,000 pregnant women will require CPR during her pregnancy. Standard ACLS protocols need to be modified for such resuscitations, and all emergency personnel need to know these modifications.

The cases in this chapter review the immediate resuscitation care of pregnant women who have a cardiac emergency. The unique features to remember about cardiac arrest in the pregnant woman are as follows:

- *Suddenly you must deal with two victims, the mother and the fetus.*
- *Emergency personnel must think about the viability of the fetus.*
- *They must consider the need for emergency cesarean section.*
- *CPR is performed differently (tilt gravid uterus to the left).*

MAJOR CONCEPTS TO MASTER

- Successful resuscitation of the mother offers the best hope for restoration and maintenance of fetal perfusion.
- "Emptying the uterus" for persistent cardiac arrest in the mother offers the best hope for a positive outcome for both the mother and the fetus. Think early about performing an emergency cesarean section (C-section).
- Emergency C-section is indicated as follows:

- When personnel with the appropriate skill and equipment to perform the procedure are involved.
- When mother fails to develop return of spontaneous circulation in five minutes.
- When fetal viability is realistically possible.
- When appropriate facilities and personnel are available to care for the mother and baby after the procedure.
- Know the indications for terminating resuscitation efforts.

THE FIVE QUADRADS IN THE PREGNANT WOMAN

The guiding approach will again be the **Five Quadrad**s. The Five Quadrads Approach provides a systematic, uniform approach that reduces the chances for mistakes and omissions and provides the patient with the best chances of survival.

THE PRIMARY ABCD SURVEY

- CPR is modified in the pregnant woman.
- Perform basic compressions using either a human or mechanical wedge that partially rolls the mother to her left side. This relieves vena caval compression from the gravid uterus thereby permitting blood return to the heart.

- Defibrillation is performed exactly as in the nonpregnant cardiac arrest victim.

THE SECONDARY ABCD SURVEY

- A and B: intubation, and ventilation are performed exactly as in the nonpregnant person.
- C: Administer medications (type and doses) exactly as in the recommended ACLS Guidelines. Previous guidelines recommended reduced doses and longer dosing intervals in the pregnant woman because of concern about drug toxic effects on the fetus. In cardiac arrest, however, it is an irrelevant concern, since immediate resuscitation of the mother should receive the highest priority.

CONTINUED

OXYGEN/IV/MONITOR/FLUIDS
- Unmodified in the pregnant woman.

TEMPERATURE/BLOOD PRESSURE/HEART RATE/RESPIRATIONS
- Unmodified in the pregnant woman.

TANK(VOLUME)/RESISTANCE/PUMP/RATE
- Several features of the pregnant woman's pump, tank, rate, and resistance help her perfuse both herself and her fetus. These same traits cause pregnant women to go into cardiopulmonary crisis more rapidly than other adults.
- Tank (volume) is enlarged and includes the fetus's circulation, including the vast vascular bed of the placenta. The pregnant woman has decreased ability to oxygenate her blood because the diaphragm is pushed up and her large breasts decrease lung expansion during inhalation. Pregnant women have a higher respiratory rate, even at rest, to keep their added blood volume oxygenated. With reduced ventilation the pregnant woman deoxygenates rapidly.
- Pump: With an increased number of circulating red blood cells, more blood volume to pump, and an enlarged network of vessels, the "pump" work of the heart is increased.
- Rate: The heart rate increases to compensate for reduced oxygenation in the greater blood volume.
- Pregnant women can look and feel good and have normal vital signs while the fetus is in distress.

Critical actions

- Apply the Five Quadrads.
- Manage immediately all critical problems found in the Primary Survey.
- Administer all rhythm-appropriate drugs.
- Consider the need to perform emergency C-section.
- Once the decision is made to perform a C-section, do not delay.

Skills to learn

- Learn special CPR techniques for pregnant women.
- Learn how to estimate gestational age in weeks by fundal measurement.
- Know how to initiate actions for emergency C-section in your work setting.

Rhythms to learn

- Pregnant women can have any and all heart rhythms.

Medications to learn

- Resuscitation of the pregnant woman could require any and all of the medications in the *ACLS Formulary*.

Shawndee Brown

CASE 1

PREGNANT WITH GUNSHOT WOUND TO THE HEAD
You are a physician on duty in an inner-city Emergency Department of a large northeastern city. The emergency dispatcher calls to report that the medics are en route to your hospital with the victim of a drive-by shooting. An 18-year-old woman was sitting in the back seat of a parked car with her 2-year-old daughter when "unknown parties" drove by and fired several bullets into the car. The 2-year-old escaped injury. One of the bullets struck the woman in the left thigh and another, in the left side of her skull.

A few minutes later the medics call to report that the woman, who had previously been speaking incoherently, has become unconscious and unresponsive. They report the woman is also 8 months pregnant. As they roll up to the Emergency Department door, one of the medics jumps from the back of the rig, shouting, "She just stopped breathing and she has no pulse!"

What thoughts would you have as you prepare to assume command of this scene? How are cardiac arrests in a pregnant woman handled differently from other arrests?

COMMENTS

- Your first thoughts are, "Oh no, not again!" for this is the third drive-by shooting this month and you are depressed by what is happening with urban violence in your community. Now another innocent victim is probably going to die.
- Second, you realize that at 8 months the fetus is viable and must be considered as the second victim in the resuscitation attempt.
- Third, you know that you are going to need a lot of help in the next few minutes. To the clinic assistant you state the following:

- "Please stat page the OB-GYN resident for an OB emergency in the ED. Tell them to get the OB attending because we may need to perform a C-section."
- "Stat page anesthesiology for the ED."
- "Stat page the pediatric fellow in the newborn nursery."
- "Call the nursing staff in labor and delivery and in the newborn nursery and tell them to bring their equipment for an emergency delivery."

- "Stat page the neurosurgery resident for a gun-shot wound to the head."

- As the medics roll the patient into Room 1 and transfer her to the stretcher, you assign the four tasks of every resuscitation attempt, as follows:
  - Someone at the airway
  - Someone for chest compressions (plus someone to perform uterine displacement)
  - Someone for monitor and defibrillator
  - Someone for IV access and medication delivery

- You direct the clinic assistant not doing chest compressions to get the Cardiff wedge from the labor and delivery suite. Until it arrives, instruct the medical student to stand on the woman's left side and gently pull her gravid uterus to the patient's left. When the student later asks why this was done, you reply as follows:
  - "The gravid uterus can press down on the inferior vena cava and prevent blood return to the heart if the pregnant woman lies flat on her back" (Fig. 16-1).
  - "The Cardiff wedge is a firm backboard that maintains her position at an angle of 30 degrees and provides a firm surface for compression."

- Displacement of the uterus to the left with the wedge

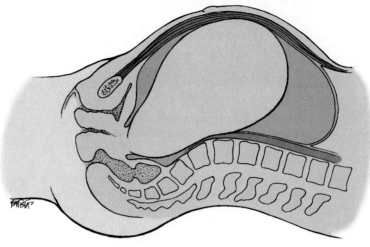

Fig. 16-1: Cross-sectional diagram of body showing gravid uterus's ability to occlude the inferior vena cava.

or with the thighs of rescuers (Fig. 16-2) placed under the victim's back and pelvis will prevent inferior vena cava occlusion.

- If the preceding techniques are not immediately available, you can use manual displacement, as was done in Case 1.

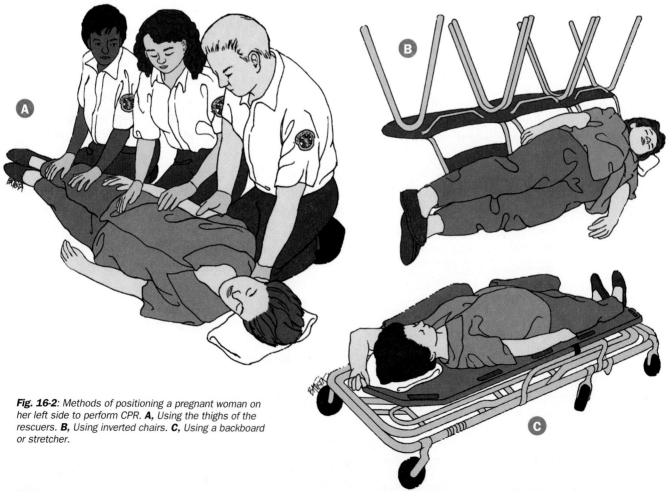

Fig. 16-2: Methods of positioning a pregnant woman on her left side to perform CPR. **A,** Using the thighs of the rescuers. **B,** Using inverted chairs. **C,** Using a backboard or stretcher.

Shawndee Brown

CASE 1 Continued

You observe that although Ms. Brown is on a full-length backboard, her neck has not been stabilized. You ask one of the nurses to apply a stiff neck collar and ask the anesthesiologist, who has just arrived, if she can perform orotracheal intubation with the neck immobilized. With the entrance point of the gunshot wound just above and anterior to the left ear you do not want to perform nasotracheal intubation.

You rapidly review the status of the Primary-Secondary ABCD Survey.

PRIMARY SURVEY

- *Airway: Currently bag-valve-mask ventilations are being provided.*
- *Breathing: The chest is rising bilaterally with each ventilation.*
- *Circulation: Chest compressions are being performed with the uterus pulled to the left.*
- *Defibrillation: Monitor leads display sinus bradycardia at 45 beats/min.*

SECONDARY SURVEY

- *Airway and Breathing: Anesthesiologist is making preparations for endotracheal intubation.*
- *Circulation: The nurses, without being told, have started a second 14-gauge short intracatheter to supplement the IV line started by the medics in the field.*
- *Differential Diagnosis: The sinus bradycardia and the absence of a pulse mean that Shawndee has pulseless electrical activity (PEA). With the only apparent injury being the gunshot wound to the head, you are not sure why Shawndee is in PEA. There has been little blood loss from the head wound or thigh wounds, so hypovolemia is unlikely.*

What interventions would you order now? Would you adjust the doses of any medications to protect the fetus from toxic effects?

COMMENTS

- Before 1992 the ACLS Guidelines for resuscitation of pregnant women recommended decreased medications in resuscitation attempts. Although the intention was to protect the fetus from possible harmful effects, this was misplaced concern: without a viable mother the fetus would never live long enough to have any toxic effects. Therefore the current emphasis has shifted to doing everything possible without hesitation or delay to get back a beating heart in the mother.

- With the arrest rhythm of PEA, administer **e**pinephrine 1 mg IV bolus and atropine 1 mg IV bolus, and start a fluid bolus of 500 mL normal saline to run as fast as possible.

Shawndee Brown

CASE 1 Continued

You look at the large wall clock and realize that 6 minutes have passed since the medics burst through the door announcing that Shawndee has lost her pulse. Her trachea is now intubated, and she has received epinephrine, atropine, and 500 mL normal saline. The heart rate has increased to 55 beats/min, but she remains pulseless without measurable blood pressure. You order a second dose of epinephrine as a 5-mg IV bolus.

The obstetric resident listens over the abdomen with a Doppler stethoscope and states, "The fetal heart tones are slow at 90 per minute, but they sound strong. We are going to have to make a decision soon."

What are elements of decision making at this point in the resuscitation?

COMMENTS

- You have now crossed the recommended "5-minute limit" on standard ACLS resuscitation efforts, yet there has been no restoration of the mother's spontaneous perfusing rhythm. The fetal heart rate is slowing, and soon the baby's chances of living will be severely compromised.

- All the following indications for an emergency C-section are present:
  - Aggressive trial of standard resuscitation efforts have been attempted without success.
  - Resuscitation efforts have not been continued

for a period beyond which chances of mother-fetus viability vanish.

- Baby is well within the range of viability once delivered. Take your paper centimeter tape and measure from the symphasis pubis to the top of the uterus.

The reading in centimeters is comparable to the age of the baby in weeks.

- Trained personnel are available to perform the C-section.
- Trained personnel are available to provide immediate support for the infant.

Shawndee Brown

CASE 1 Continued

The "OB attending" rushes into the room, and you provide him with a quick review of the situation. "I think we need to take the baby now," you state. "Oh, I agree. Let's get on with it at once. I'll assist the resident. Are the pediatricians here? Good." To the anesthesiologist: "Can we proceed?"

Within 2 minutes the physicians deliver a 6-pound infant girl with an immediate Apgar score of 2 and a 3-minute Apgar score of 8. The mother has a return of spontaneous circulation within 2 minutes of delivery of the child via C-section, needing only mechanical ventilation and a dopamine drip.

The mother is transferred from the Emergency Department to the recovery unit, where she gets an emergency cerebral arteriogram. The bullet has produced massive brain damage that is thought to be nonviable. When you go off shift 3 hours later, you learn that the transplant team has been called in to discuss organ donation with Shawndee's family.

How common is this scenario?

COMMENTS

- Traumatic injuries to pregnant women through motor vehicle accidents or the type of violence represented in Case 1, are becoming more and more frequent. This is especially true in our urban Emergency Departments. In fact, post-mortem C-sections—delivery of the child after the mother has been declared dead—are also becoming more common.

- ACLS providers should always be alert to the question of organ donation. Although resuscitation for the sake of organ donation is a controversial and emotional topic, it should not be ignored. Organ donation could be one mechanism to give some meaning to the many lives being tragically cut short by the modern epidemic of violence in our society.

- See Chapter 1 for a detailed list of the criteria for organ donation (Table 1-2).

Karen Haug

CASE 2

EMERGENCY DELIVERY IN EMERGENCY DEPARTMENT WITH AMNIOTIC FLUID EMBOLISM

You are evaluating a 16-year-old woman who complains of severe, cramping abdominal pain. In the course of your evaluation, following a long and fascinating story, it becomes apparent that Ms. Haug is, in fact, pregnant and appears to be far advanced in active labor.

A quick examination reveals her to be too far along for transport to the labor and delivery floor. The infant's head is visible in the birth canal, and some associated bleeding is observed on the side of the vagina. She is allowed to remain in the Emergency Department as arrangements are made for an emergency delivery.

Suddenly, during a full and very painful contraction, Karen stops screaming and appears to slump backward. A quick glance at her face reveals her to be markedly cyanotic with blue lips, gasping breaths, and a marked panicked appearance in her eyes. With one more frightened glance to each side, she abruptly loses consciousness and falls back on the stretcher. The nurse quickly places her hand against the carotid artery in Karen's neck and then with a look of absolute surprise states, "My god, she's in cardiac arrest!"

What do you think has happened here? How would you proceed from this point?

- The unusual and alarming emergency in Case 2 could result in confusion and disorganization among the emergency care providers. You have a young, apparently healthy woman, in the midst of delivering a baby, and all your thoughts are focused on conducting a successful emergency delivery.

- Suddenly you are faced with an even more dramatic challenge—the abrupt, unexpected, even mysterious death of this young woman. This wrenching "changing of gears" could cause you and your team to lose focus and abandon a systematic and organized approach.

- The answer—even if you are mystified by the sudden loss of a pulse and even if you do mentally jump ahead to "Why??"—is *return to the basics*. Review the Five Quadrads, starting with the Primary-Secondary Survey Approach. (NOTE: It is critical to assign four tasks at the same time you are going through the Primary-Secondary Surveys: airway, chest compressions, monitor/defibrillator, IV access and medication.)

PRIMARY SURVEY

- **Airway:** Place in recumbent position; check the head positioning; open the airway. (Assign the airway team member.)

- **Breathing:** Give two breaths: air enters without difficulty; chest rises bilaterally with each breath; this is not an acute, obstructed airway.

- **Circulation:** There is no carotid pulse felt after 10 seconds; call for help; start chest compressions, *but* place Cardiff wedge under back and pelvis or pull the uterus to the patient's left side. (Assign chest compressor team member.)

- **Defibrillation:** Monitor leads display sinus tachycardia at 110 beats/min. (Assign person to ensure accurate monitor display and to defibrillate if needed.)

SECONDARY SURVEY

- **Airway:** Stat page anesthesiologist to the scene, but begin preparations in the room for emergency intubation and ventilation. Use the "FATS" technique to open and maintain the airway (as described in Chapter 2).

- **Breathing:** Use pocket face mask on the wall or use bag-valve-mask setup, hooked to 100% oxygen at 15 mL/min, and start effective ventilation efforts.

- **Circulation:** The nurses have started a 14-gauge short intracatheter in the antecubital vein of each arm. Since this clinical emergency seems like unexplained pulseless electrical activity (PEA), you immediately order epinephrine 1 mg IV and you ask the medication nurse to repeat epinephrine at 5 mg IV bolus in exactly 3 minutes if the mother is still in cardiac arrest. With a rapid rate of 110 beats/min, atropine would not be indicated.

- **Differential Diagnosis:** Now that you have systematically reviewed the Primary-Secondary Survey, you can think for a moment about the cause of this sudden collapse during labor and delivery. The following things come to mind that you derived from the list of possible causes of PEA (Chapter 5):
  - Acute pulmonary embolism
  - Tension pneumothorax
  - Cardiac tamponade
  - Acute myocardial infarction
  - Occult trauma with bleeding and hypovolemia
  - Toxic shock
  - Arrhythmia or congenital or acquired heart disease in the mother
  - Drug reaction, drug overdose, or an acute anaphylactic reaction
  - Cerebrovascular accident
  - Electrolyte abnormality

- None of these possibilities seems to be the obvious cause of the problem. You recall, however, that this case sounds similar to descriptions you have read of amniotic fluid embolism.

- You proceed with diagnostic orders (12-lead ECG, portable chest x-ray, hematocrit, white blood cell count, arterial blood gas studies, and blood tests for electrolytes and bleeding parameters such as prothrombin time, partial thromboplastin time, fibrinogen products, and platelet counts).

- **Vital signs:** Temperature = 37.2° C; blood pressure = not obtainable; respirations = not breathing spontaneously; heart rate = 110 beats/min on the monitor, sinus tachycardia.

- **Oxygen/IV/Monitor/Fluids:** All have been initiated except for the fluids, and you order 500 mL bolus of normal saline.

- **Tank (Volume)/Resistance/Pump/Rate:** What is the nature of the problem?:

  - *Is this a tank problem?* Unclear. You have little evidence of volume loss, although the vaginal bleeding is worrisome; in addition, pregnant women often have intravascular volume depletion near the end of term. Is she vasodilated or vasoconstricted? You have no evidence of shock before the arrest. It is certainly appropriate at this time to push fluids for empirical volume replacement.

  - *Is this a pump problem?* Quite possibly. You know that many of the causes of PEA include processes that would affect the flow of blood into and out of the heart and affect the pumping action of the heart. Pulmonary embolism and amniotic fluid embolism are two possible conditions that could have produced this clinical picture of sudden deterioration. In addition, you know that the gravid uterus, even early in pregnancy, can alter the hemodynamic state severely. While considering whether this is a pump problem, your thoughts turn to the question of emergency C-section or emergency vaginal delivery of the fetus.

- *Is this a rate problem?* No. The rate is sinus tachycardia, appropriate for the acute distress of the patient.

Karen Haug

CASE 2 Continued

You should take pride at how well you have responded to this emergency. Even though you have no idea what caused this sudden death in a young woman in the process of having a baby, you have systematically initiated the first resuscitation efforts. The patient is receiving CPR modified for the pregnant woman. Her trachea is intubated and the lungs are being "bagged" rapidly and well; she has an IV and is receiving fluid replacement and epinephrine. Appropriate diagnostic inquiries such as ECG and chest x-ray are in the process of completion. You have "stat paged" the obstetrics-gynecology service and the pediatrician covering the newborn service. You ask the first arriving obstetric nurse to check for fetal heart tones.

However, after 4 minutes, you still have a woman in apparent full cardiac arrest with the top of the fetal head showing per vagina. How would you proceed at this point?

COMMENTS

- Remember, you always have two victims when a pregnant woman has a cardiac arrest—the mother and the unborn child.

- You have focused on resuscitation of the mother so far, with only a brief request to ask someone to check the fetal heart tones of the infant (the rate was relatively slow at 90 beats/min). You know, however, that perimortem C-section, to save both the mother and the child, has been recommended by the ACLS Guidelines of the AHA, written in collaboration with the American College of Obstetrics and Gynecology.

- You really have no idea how old the baby might be or what his or her chances of living are if delivered. The young woman was unclear and vague about her last menstrual period and the use of birth control.

- Take a measurement from the symphasis pubis to the fundus. The baby's age in weeks is approximate to the number of centimeters for a single fetus.

- You can proceed further here only with collaboration and consultation with the pediatrician and obstetrician. The elements of decision-making to consider are the following:

  - Potential for viability of the child.

  - Ability and experience of the obstetricians.

  - Availability of support for the mother and the child after delivery.

  - Passage of time: If mother's pulse has not been restored in 4 to 5 minutes, the chances of success grow remote. If you are going to move, you must move quickly.

- Be prepared for the mother to regain a pulse after the baby is delivered.

Karen Haug

CASE 2 Continued

The obstetrician examines the mother quickly during continuing CPR efforts and decides that the infant cannot be delivered vaginally in the absence of maternal pushing and uterine contractions.

You ask whether a "crash C-section" could be performed in the labor and delivery suite immediately or will it need to be performed in the Emergency Department. The Emergency Department nurse says, "We have the elevator locked open down the hall. L and D says bring her up at once and we will take her right to C-section!"

You ask the clinic assistant to climb up on the stretcher to straddle the mother and continue chest compressions during the trip to the elevator and into the delivery suite.

Within 2 minutes the entire group moves down the hall to the waiting elevator: defibrillator-monitor, IV infusion pump and stand, anesthesiologist ventilating the lungs through the endotracheal tube; clinic assistant doing chest compression on top of the patient.

CONTINUED

Karen Haug

CASE 2 Continued

After the crash C-section the infant boy weighed only 510 g. Accurate estimates of gestational age could not be obtained from the mother; however, morphologic features suggested a gestational age of 23 weeks. The child lives for about 12 hours in the neonatal intensive care unit (ICU) and dies of respiratory failure caused by lung immaturity.

The mother survived the emergency C-section with some improvement in her hemodynamic state after the delivery. Severe adult respiratory distress syndrome developed, which required a ventilator and continuous positive-pressure ventilations to maintain oxygenation. Disseminated intravascular coagulation also developed, and she had a stormy course for the next 3 days, including intracerebral hemorrhage, renal failure, and hypotension.

Her respiratory failure increased, and it became impossible to adequately ventilate and oxygenate the lungs. After consultation with her single mother and her boyfriend, the ICU team decided not to attempt CPR should she have further deterioration. Over the course of that afternoon she became progressively hypotensive and bradycardic and died.

Does this mean perimortem C-sections should not be performed for pregnant women in cardiac arrest?

COMMENTS

- There are few published articles on the topic of perimortem C-sections. Most studies have been simple case reports or case series with heterogeneous patient mixes. In one series on perimortem C-sections the survival rate for the infants was 15%, and "occasionally" there was restoration of the pulse in a woman who appears dead on clinical observation.

- The general consensus at this time is represented as follows in the guidelines adopted by the AHA and the American College of Obstetrics and Gynecology (ACOG):

- Consider perimortem C-section as a possible way to save the mother and the infant in refractory cardiac arrest.

- Consider it early (within 4 to 5 minutes of the arrest) rather than as a late, last-ditch effort when nothing else works.

- Take into account the viability of the infant.

- Consider the skills of the person who will have to perform the C-section.

- Co nsider whether neonatal hospital care will be adequate.

Sharon O'Dell

CASE 3

ABRUPTIO PLACENTAE

You are a paramedic working in a suburban EMS service. The dispatcher radios an urgent call from a pregnant woman with sudden onset of unrelenting abdominal pain. The woman, Sharon O'Dell, is sitting in a chair, rubbing her distended abdomen.

You get a brief history while obtaining vital signs. She is 38 years old, at 38 weeks of gestation with her first pregnancy. She relates that she has felt great until this evening. A sharp, sudden onset of low abdominal pain has not subsided for 20 minutes. There is no vaginal bleeding, and she was quietly watching TV all evening before the pain.

Her vital signs reveal a blood pressure of 104/68 mm Hg; pulse, 90 beats/min; respirations, 30 breaths/min; her skin color is good, with a pink tinge to her cheeks. She doesn't appear to be in much physical distress but says, "I just feel something is not right about this pain." Ms. O'Dell puts a hand to her cheek and says suddenly, "Hey, the room is spinning!"

You continue your physical examination as your partner hooks up a nasal cannula with oxygen to Ms. O'Dell. He attaches an ECG monitor and starts an IV of normal saline. Physical examination shows a hard, almost rigid abdomen at 38 weeks gestation by fundal measurement. A quick Doppler check for fetal heart tones is futile. During your examination she moans and becomes unconscious.

What is your approach to Ms. O'Dell?

- Begin with **the Five Quadrads**.

PRIMARY ABCD SURVEY

- The Primary Survey defines Ms. O'Dell in full cardiac arrest. Proceed as follows:

  - *Airway:* Open the airway.

  - *Breathing:* Provide two breaths with positive-pressure ventilation.

  - *Circulation:* Give chest compressions modified for the pregnant women (Fig. 16-2, *A-C*). Common techniques for out-of-hospital CPR for pregnant women are the following:

    - Position patient lying supine on a backboard.

    - Tilt the backboard 30 degrees to the left and prop it there (Fig. 16-2, *C*).

    - Simultaneously have someone gently pull the gravid uterus to the left.

    - Bend her left knee slightly to support her weight.

    - Pull her right thigh across the left leg. (This position rotates her abdomen off of the uterus and keeps her C-spine and thorax straight against the board and her uterus tilted away from great vessels.)

    - Give compressions vigorously against the backboard.

    - An alternate technique for unexpected CPR outside the hospital when no backboard is readily available is to roll the woman to her left side against the backs of one or two straight-backed chairs pushed against a wall (Fig.16-2, *B*). This will give a firm 30-degree tilted rigid surface for compressions (Fig. 16-2).

  - *Defibrillation:* Attach defibrillator and assess for presence of VF.

SECONDARY ABCD SURVEY

- *Airway and Breathing* are being provided adequately, although you wonder when the best time to intubate the trachea will be.

- *Circulation:* Chest compressions are administered now by a fireman who arrived to assist you to the hospital.

- *Oxygen/IV/Monitor/Fluids* are all provided. Her ECG rhythm is PEA. En route to the hospital you administer the following:

  - **Epinephrine** 1 mg IV bolus

  - **Atropine** 1 mg IV bolus

  - **Fluid bolus of 500 mL** of normal saline run wide open.

- **Differential diagnosis**

  - All symptoms point toward abruptio placentae as the cause of her collapse. Although initially she did not show extreme distress, Ms. O'Dell was using all her compensatory reserves for herself. The fetus lost perfusion and oxygenation because of the sudden abruptio placentae.

  - Her unremitting pain and stiff abdomen were subtle clues that the placenta had separated from the uterine wall. She was bleeding into the uterus, but not transferring any blood through the placenta to her fetus.

- **Temperature/Blood Pressure/Heart/Rate/Respirations:** Blood pressure is 0; heart rate by monitor, 100 beats/min; respirations are absent; temperature is normal.

- **Tank (Volume)/Resistance/Pump/Rate:** She appears now to be in hypovolemic shock. PEA exists because her pump is empty.

Sharon O'Dell

CASE 3 Continued

You report to the Emergency Department base station: "We are coming in with a full witnessed cardiac arrest of an almost-term pregnant woman. We have CPR in progress for about 2 minutes. She has one IV line with normal saline running wide open, she is not intubated. We suspect an abruptio. Please set up to meet us on the ambulance ramp, for an immediate possible C-section with possible viable fetus."

The Emergency Department assembles the following staff in the resuscitation room:

- ***OB-GYN surgeon*** *prepared for a stat C-section*
- ***Respiratory therapist*** *and intubation equipment*
- ***Pediatrician*** *and neonatal resuscitation equipment*
- ***Labor and Delivery*** *nursing staff with a full setup for an emergency delivery*

About 10 people converge on the ambulance ramp and assist with transporting Ms. O'Dell, with CPR in progress, to Room 1. As a respiratory therapist intubates her trachea, the surgeon performs a brief examination, and confirms an "abruptio" diagnosis. An emergency C-section is completed in 2 minutes. Intubation tube placement is verified as a nurse starts a second IV line.

The neonatal resuscitation team is handed a flaccid, dusky-blue baby covered in meconium. Apgar Score = 0. Vigorous resuscitation efforts get no response from the baby. They move to the room next door, where further resuscitation efforts are unsuccessful.

Continued

Sharon O'Dell

CASE 3 Continued

"Hey! I have a carotid pulse! It's rapid and weak, but definitely there!" says the RN. All eyes turn toward the monitor. "Blood pressure is 80/60!" Her ECG is sinus rhythm at a rate of 110 beats/min. She makes a stormy recovery, regaining her own circulation with the baby's weight removed from her great vessels. Sharon O'Dell is discharged to home 5 days later.

What important lesson does this case teach us about prehospital cardiac arrest of the pregnant woman?

COMMENTS

- Strictly speaking, the woman in Case 3 needed an emergency C-section in the field. Some systems have anecdotal experience of perimortem C-sections of the mother performed in the field. They make good stories but often represent bad decision making. The elements of such decision making have been outlined before: experienced operators, proper equipment, and proper care of the mother and the baby in the immediate post–C-section period. These elements are usually missing in the field and in the back of an ambulance.

- However, the field personnel can certainly recognize the indications for an emergency C-section, as they did in this case. The base hospital must respect the clinical impressions of the field personnel and prepare to perform immediate "ambulance bay" or Emergency Department C-sections.

- No questions could be asked about consent before proceeding with the C-section. The C-section is the procedure of choice in a last-ditch effort to save both the mother and fetus. "Implied consent" is usually assumed in such situations—what a rational person would consent to if she were conscious and awake.

- Since she had the arrest outside the hospital, only a smooth, coordinated effort between prehospital personnel and Emergency Department and surgery saved her from death.

KEY POINTS

SUMMARY

- **Cardiac arrest in the pregnant woman always poses dramatic clinical and emotional challenges. Your first obligation is to the mother, but the fetus must be kept in mind.**

- **Clinicians occasionally have to make decisions in which one victim must be sacrificed to save the other. Clinicians must not become paralyzed by the possible medicolegal conundrums they face. There are no easy answers to dilemmas like these.**

- **In our cases we have not provided firm answers but have simply described some of the factors and some of the guidelines that have to enter into this most challenging of clinical situations.**

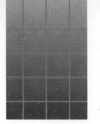

ACLS Formulary

This formulary presents the major drugs used in emergency cardiac care. This is provided for quick reference. ACLS interventions should be considered in the context of four questions:

- ***Why*** *do you give the drug? (mechanism of action)*
- ***When*** *do you give the drug? (indications for use)*
- ***How*** *do you give the drug? (how supplied, how to mix, dose to administer, comments)*
- ***Watch Out!*** *(precautions)*

DRUGS IN THE ACLS FORMULARY:

Adenosine	Dobutamine	Nitroglycerin
Aminophylline	Dopamine	Nitroprusside
Amrinone	Epinephrine	Norepinephrine
Aspirin	Furosemide	Oxygen
Atropine sulfate	Heparin	Procainamide
Beta blockers	Isoproterenol	Sodium bicarbonate
Bretylium tosylate	Lidocaine	Thrombolytic agents
Calcium chloride	Magnesium sulfate	Verapamil
Calcium channel blockers	Morphine sulfate	
Diltiazem	Nifedipine	

Adenosine (Adenocard)

WHY? (Actions)

- Decreases conduction through the atrioventricular (AV) node; thus interrupts reentry pathways.
- Stops both narrow-complex and wide-complex paroxysmal supraventricular tachycardia (PSVT).

WHEN? (Indications)

- First drug to use for hemodynamically stable PSVT.
- Give after vagal maneuvers have failed.
- Also recommended (after lidocaine) for wide-complex PSVT or tachycardias of uncertain origin.

GENERAL TREATMENT SEQUENCE FOR PSVT

- Vagal maneuvers.
- **Adenosine** 6 mg IV push (1- to 3-second injection).
- **Adenosine** 12 mg (may give second 12-mg bolus in 1 to 2 minutes, if required).

GENERAL TREATMENT SEQUENCE FOR WIDE-COMPLEX PSVT OR TACHYCARDIAS OF UNCERTAIN ORIGIN

- Lidocaine 1 to 1.5 mg/kg IV.
- Lidocaine 0.5 to 0.75 mg/kg IV.
- Adenosine 6 mg IV push (1- to 3-second injection).
- Adenosine 12 mg (repeat in 1 to 2 minutes if needed).
- Procainamide 20 to 30 mg/min.

HOW?

SUPPLIED

- 3 mg/mL in 2-mL vial = total of 6 mg.

DOSE

- 6 to 12 mg IV bolus push over 1 to 3 seconds.

TECHNIQUE

- Use proper administration or will seldom succeed.
- Have a properly functioning IV with large-gauge needle.
- Supplemental oxygen through nasal prongs.
- Have lidocaine, atropine, and a monitor-defibrillator immediately available.
- Check that defibrillator gel or pads are present.
- Place the patient flat in bed, in slight head-down position.
- Tell patient he or she may feel facial flushing, shortness of breath, chest pressure, headache, nausea, or other odd sensations.
- Start strip-chart recorder on the monitor.
- Administer adenosine 6 mg by rapid (1 to 3 seconds) IV push.
- Run the IV wide open after the push; elevate extremity.

- Observe for change in rhythm in 10 to 15 seconds; most conversions occur in less than 30 seconds.
- Give second dose (12 mg IV) after 1 to 2 minutes in the same rapid manner.
- Give third dose (12 mg IV) as above if needed.

WATCH OUT! (Precautions)

- With conversion, patient may display several seconds of asystole followed by resumption of normal sinus rhythm. Can result in syncopal symptoms.
- Move to verapamil if the complex remains narrow and the blood pressure remains acceptable.
- Drug interactions: methylxanthines (larger adenosine doses may be needed); dipyridamole (smaller doses of adenosine needed or avoid completely); carbamazine (higher degress of heart block may occur).
- Be alert for clinical instability or deterioration.

Aminophylline (Amoline, Phyllocontin, Somophyllin, Truphylline)

WHY? (Actions)

- Acts as a bronchodilator, relaxing bronchial smooth muscle.
- Increases myocardial contractility and heart rate.

WHEN? (Indications)

- Third-line agent for acute pulmonary edema.
- Use only when wheezing and severe bronchospasm accompany acute pulmonary edema ("cardiac asthma").

HOW?

SUPPLIED

- 25 mg/mL in 10-mL vials (total of 250 mg).
- 50 mg/mL in 10-mL vials (total of 500 mg).

MIX

- Mix in 250 mg to 1 g in 250 mL of 5% dextrose in water (D_5W) or normal saline (NS).

DOSE

- Loading dose of 5 mg/kg given over 30 to 45 minutes.
- Follow with infusion of 0.5 to 0.7 mg/kg per hour.

WATCH OUT! (Precautions)

- Do not mix with other drugs; do not exceed a 500-mg loading dose.
- May cause ventricular tachycardia (VT), seizures, hypotension, nausea and vomiting, and anxiety.
- Avoid aminophylline in patients with PSVT or acute arrhythmias associated with ischemic heart disease.

Amrinone (Inocor)

WHY? (Actions)

- Increases cardiac output through increased contractility (strong inotropic effect).
- Causes vasodilation.
- Lowers myocardial oxygen demand by decreasing wall tension.

WHEN? (Indications)

- A third-line agent to use for persons with severe congestive heart failure.
- An adjunctive agent to use in patients who have not responded to diuretics, vasodilators, and conventional inotropic agents.

HOW?

SUPPLIED

- 5 mg/mL in 20-mL vial; 100 mg per vial.

MIX

- Administer as supplied, or dilute in 0.4% or 0.9% saline solution to a maximum concentration of 3 mg/mL (750 mg/250 mL).

DOSE

- 0.75 mg/kg given over 10 to 15 minutes. Follow by infusion of 5 to 15 µg/kg per minute.
- Give via infusion pump.
- Titrate to effect.
- Administer with hemodynamic monitoring if possible.

WATCH OUT! (Precautions)

- Do not mix with other drugs or dextrose solutions.
- Can precipitate tachyarrhythmias and hypotension.
- May increase myocardial ischemia.
- Avoid extravasation.

Aspirin

WHY? (Actions)

- Blocks formation of thromboxane A_2.
- Thromboxane A_2 causes platelets to aggregate and arteries to constrict.
- These actions will have the following effects:
  - Reduce overall mortality from acute myocardial infarction (AMI).
  - Reduce nonfatal reinfarction.
  - Reduce nonfatal stroke.

WHEN? (Indications)

- Give as soon as possible to all patients with new pain suggesting an active, AMI.
- Give within minutes of arrival.
- Should be given routinely in all EMS systems or Emergency Departments caring for potential AMI patients.

HOW?

DOSE

- 160- to 325-mg tablet taken by mouth as soon as possible.
- Most EMS systems have paramedics administer aspirin in the prehospital setting.
- Emergency Departments should keep containers of aspirin in treatment rooms to allow immediate administration.

WATCH OUT! (Precautions)

- Relatively contraindicated in patients with active ulcer disease or asthma.
- Contraindicated in patients with known hypersensitivity to aspirin.
- Higher doses may interfere with prostacyclin production and hence interfere with benefits.

Atropine sulfate

WHY? (Actions)

- Acts as a parasympatholytic drug, a vagolytic drug, and an anticholinergic drug.
- Benefits conditions with excess vagal activity.
- Increases sinus node automaticity and AV conduction when suppressed by abnormal parasympathetic or vagal discharges.
- Works at the sinus and AV node only; little effect on infranodal lesions.
- Not effective for asystolic conditions that lack a vagal component.

WHEN? (Indications)

FOR SYMPTOMATIC BRADYCARDIAS

- Use when the bradycardia causes the signs and symptoms. Atropine works on the "rate" portion of the cardiovascular quadrad when you have symptomatic bradycardia.
- *Sinus bradycardia*: Patient must be symptomatic from the bradycardia.
- *First-degree AV block:* Patient must be symptomatic from the bradycardia.
- *Type I, second-degree heart block (Mobitz type I):* Highly effective, since Mobitz type I is almost always caused by excessive parasympathetic discharge.

- *Type II, second-degree heart block (Mobitz type II):* Helpful if QRS complexes are narrow; less helpful with broad complexes (infranodal blocks).
- *Third-degree heart block:* Appropriate to use as the Bradycardia Algorithm recommends. However, atropine rarely increases rate in these patients because disease exists at an anatomic level where atropine has no effect.

FOR CARDIAC ARREST

- Second agent to use after epinephrine for asystolic or bradycardiac arrhythmia plus slow pulseless electrical activity (PEA) cardiac arrest.
- Give early in the arrest.

HOW ?

SUPPLIED

- 0.1 mg/mL in 10-mL preloaded syringe (total = 1 mg).
- 0.1 mg/mL in 1-mL vial for endotracheal tube administration.

DOSE

For Cardiac Arrest

- Asystole or PEA: Give first dose 1.0 mg; repeat every 3 to 5 minutes to a maximum dose of 0.03 to 0.04 mg/kg.
- Give the higher doses and shorter dosing intervals when the clinical situation is more severe. For example, in full asystolic cardiac arrest give 1.0 mg every 3 minutes; in mildly symptomatic bradycardia give 0.5 mg every 5 minutes.
- Endotracheal drug administration: Remember "ALE" for atropine-lidocaine-epinephrine. Double the dose (1 to 2 mg), and dilute it in 10 mL of sterile water or NS.

For Bradycardia

- First dose is 0.5 to 1.0 mg.
- Repeat every 3 to 5 minutes up to a total of 0.03 to 0.04 mg/kg.
- End point for atropine is clinical response: Do not give repeat doses if the heart rate has responded well.
- If patient does not respond satisfactorily to 0.04 mg/kg, move to next interventions in the sequence (pacing, dopamine, epinephrine, isoproterenol).

WATCH OUT! (Precautions)

- Do not give doses lower than 0.5 mg. Can produce slowing of heart rate rather than speeding it up. (Prepare to perform pacing.)
- Can increase the heart rate too much and produce an unwanted tachycardia.
- Postatropine tachycardia can precipitate ventricular fibrillation (VF) or VT.
- In patients with coronary artery or ischemic heart disease, can increase their angina and ischemic chest pain.
- Atropine, as an anticholinergic agent, can precipitate the anticholinergic syndrome that occurs in overdose of such agents: delirium ("mad as a hatter"), decreased salivation ("dry as a bone"), flushed, hot skin ("red as a beet"), blurred vision ("blind as a bat").
- Avoid in hypothermia.

Beta blockers

- Atenolol (Tenormin)
- Esmolol (Brevibloc)
- Metoprolol (Lopressor)
- Propranolol (Inderal)

WHY? (Actions);

- Decrease automaticity and arrhythmias.
- Lower heart rate by reducing sinus node discharge.
- Lower blood pressure.
- Lower myocardial contractility.
- Block catecholamine stimulation.
- Reduce myocardial oxygen consumption.
- "Salvage" myocardium and reduce overall infarct size.

WHEN? (Indications)

- Give to all AMI (anterior) patients with evidence of excess sympathetic activity (elevated heart rate and blood pressure).
- Give to all patients with large MIs treated early, within 6 hours of pain.
- Give to patients with refractory chest pain or tachycardias resulting from excessive sympathetic tone (e.g., PSVT, atrial fibrillation, or atrial flutter).

HOW? (Dose)

- Several different beta blocker "recipes" for AMI patients are described in this section.

ATENOLOL (Tenormin)

- *Supplied:* 0.5 mg/mL in 10-mL ampule; total = 5 mg.
- *Dose:* give 5 mg IV infusion (over 5 minutes). Wait 10 minutes, then give second dose of 5 mg IV (over 5 minutes). If tolerated, can begin 50 mg by mouth (PO), then give 50 mg twice a day (bid).

ESMOLOL (Brevibloc)

- *Supplied:* 10 mg/mL in 10-mL single-dose ampule = 100 mg.
- *Dose:* Give 500 µg/kg over 1 minute, followed by infusion starting at 50 µg/kg per minute infused over 4 minutes. Esmolol has a short half-life (less than 10 minutes).

METOPROLOL (Lopressor)

- *Supplied:* Either 1- or 5-mL ampules = 1- or 5-mg, total.
- *Dose:* Give 5 mg IV infusions (slow), 5 mg IV every 2 minutes (three doses) to a total of 15 mg; then 50 mg PO every 6 hours for 48 hours. (Begin 15 minutes after last IV dose, then 100 mg PO.)
- Metoprolol possesses the advantage of a short half-life (30 minutes). If it lowers the blood pressure or slows the heart rate too much, the infusion can be stopped and the effects will soon fade away.

PROPRANOLOL (Inderal)

- *Supplied:* 1 mg/mL in 1-mL ampule, or 4 mg/mL in 5-mL vial; total = 20 mg.
- *Dose:* Give 1 mg IV (slow) every 5 minutes to a total of 5 mg. Repeat a second dose after 2 minutes if needed.

WATCH OUT! (Precautions)

- Start IV beta blockers with caution.

- Do not give after IV verapamil or diltiazem.

- Be alert for myocardial depression. Administering beta blockers to patients with AMI may have significant side effects.

- Be aware that the following conditions can become worse with beta blockers:

  - Congestive heart failure or pulmonary edema.

  - Bronchospasm or history of asthma.

  - Bradycardia (less than 50 to 60 beats/min), especially with second- or third-degree block.

  - Hypotension (blood pressure less than 100 mm Hg systolic).

Bretylium tosylate (Bretylol)

WHY? (Actions)

- Acts as ventricular antiarrhythmic and adrenergic blocker.

- Increases fibrillation threshold (the point at which the myocardium fibrillates).

- Adrenergic (alpha) blockade can produce severe hypotension. (This effect places bretylium in a second-line position behind lidocaine in the VF/VT algorithm.)

WHEN? (Indications)

- Refractory malignant ventricular arrhythmias (VF/VT).

- Use as follows:

  - When VF/VT persists, despite epinephrine, shock, lidocaine.

  - When VT continues after maximum doses of lidocaine.

  - In recurrent VT, despite lidocaine and procainamide.

  - As first antiarrhythmic for hypothermic VF.

HOW?

SUPPLIED

- 50 mg/mL in prefilled 10-mL syringes or vials (total = 500 mg).

DOSE

For Cardiac Arrest Patients

- 5 mg/kg rapid IV push. Follow in 30 to 60 seconds with defibrillation.

- Repeat in 5 minutes at 10 mg/kg.

- May continue to repeat at 5- to 30-minute intervals to maximum dose of 30 to 35 mg/kg.

TECHNIQUE

- If you get return of circulation, start a continuous infusion at 1 to 2 mg/min.

- Bretylium may require several minutes for the antifibrillatory properties to take effect.

- Do not delay shocks after administering the medication.

For Stable VT Patients:

- 5 to 10 mg/kg over 8 to 10 minutes. Wait 10 to 30 minutes

before next dose.

- Maximum total of 30 mg/kg over 24 hours.

- Maintenance infusion: 1 to 2 mg/min.

WATCH OUT! (Precautions)

- For nausea, vomiting, and postural hypotension.

Calcium chloride

WHY? (Actions)

- Increases myocardial contractility.

- Stabilizes the myocardial toxic condition from hypocalcemia associated with cardiac arrhythmias.

WHEN? (Indications)

- For known hyperkalemia, hypocalcemia, hypermagnesemia, toxic effects of calcium channel blockers.

- For preventing hypotension before giving IV calcium channel blockers.

HOW?

SUPPLIED

- 100 mg/mL in 10-mL vial for a total of 1 g (272 mg calcium) in a 10% solution.

MIX

- Use NS; precipitates when mixed with sodium bicarbonate.

DOSE

- For hyperkalemia and calcium channel blocker overdose: give 5 to 10 mL IV.

- For prophylactic pretreatment before IV calcium channel blockers: Give 2 mL.

WATCH OUT! (Precautions)

- Do not use routinely for cardiac arrest; use only for the conditions noted earlier.

- Use with extreme caution in persons taking digitalis compounds.

Calcium channel blockers

- See separate section on each of the following agents:

  - Diltiazem

  - Verapamil

  - Nifedipine

WHY? (Actions)

- The three major calcium channel blockers used in emergency care (verapamil, nifedipine, and diltiazem) vary in their strength of effect in the following areas:

  - Negative inotrope effect (decrease strength of contraction of the heart). This is a negative consequence of the calcium channel blockers and one that has to be observed carefully.

- Vasodilation (lowers the blood pressure). **Nifedipine** acts as the more powerful arterial dilator; therefore it is used for hypertensive urgencies. However, poor control of this response makes it relatively contraindicated in AMI.
  - Conduction. Slows conduction through the AV node (antiarrhythymic for supraventricular arrhythmias): **Verapamil,** a potent AV nodal depressor is used commonly for PSVTs. Diltiazem also is a potent AV nodal depressor and therefore is commonly used for rate control in atrial fibrillation and atrial flutter. **Diltiazem** does not cause the blood pressure drop that the other two agents cause.
- Theoretically, this group of drugs should improve outcomes following AMI. The drugs produce an overall reduction in ischemia and size of infarction by means of the following actions:
  - Dilate coronary arteries.
  - Dilate peripheral arteries.
  - Depress AV and sinoatrial nodal activity.
  - Increase flow to ischemic areas.
  - Slow heart rate.
  - Reduce afterload.

Diltiazem (Cardizem)

WHY? (Actions)

- Slows conduction through the sinoatrial and AV node; thus slows ventricular response to the stimuli of rapid atrial fibrillation and atrial flutter.

WHEN? (Indications)

- Give to control ventricular rate in atrial fibrillation or atrial flutter with a rapid response.
- Use after adenosine to eliminate PSVT with narrow QRS complex and adequate blood pressure.
- Unstable angina (Class I recommendation).
- Postinfarction angina (should be combined with nitrates) (Class IIb recommendation).
- Consider for persistant chest pain when no relief from IV nitrates.
- Consider as cardioprotective agent in non-Q-wave infarction (Class IIa recommendation). Diltiazem is the only calcium channel blocker used for cardioprotective effects in AMI. The others produce too much depression of myocardial function. The AHA, however, does not recommend the routine use of calcium channel blockers in the initial management of AMI.

HOW?
SUPPLIED

- 5 mg/mL in 5- or 10-mL vial (total = 25 or 50 mg).

DOSE

- Diltiazem 0.25 mg/kg IV over 2 minutes; repeat as needed in 15 minutes at 0.35 mg/kg (20 to 25 mg over 2 minutes) (for conversion of atrial fibrillation and atrial flutter).
- Maintenance infusion: 15 to 20 mg/hour titrated to heart rate.
- IV diltiazem is used primarily for ventricular rate control in atrial fibrillation and atrial flutter. Conversion to normal sinus rhythm often occurs.
- Diltiazem 30 to 60 mg PO three or four times a day (for cardioprotective effects).

WATCH OUT! (Precautions)

- Do not use for wide-complex QRS tachycardias of uncertain origin.
- Hypotension.
- Bradycardia.
- Decreased left ventricular contractility.
- Avoid in patients with any signs of left ventricular failure or dysfunction (shortness of breath, fatigue, limited exercise capacity, rales, pulmonary congestion on chest x-ray). These patients could get much worse.
- Do not use with IV beta blockers.

Dobutamine (Dubutrex)

WHY? (Actions)

- Increases contractility of the heart.
- Mild peripheral vasodilation (decreases afterload).

WHEN? (Indications)

- Use for pump problems such as pulmonary edema and congestive heart failure.
- Especially useful for pump failure when blood pressure is greater than or equal to 90 to 100 mm Hg and there are no signs of shock.

HOW?
SUPPLIED

- 12.5 mg/mL in 20-mL vial; total = 250 mg.

MIX

- Dilute 500 to 1000 mg (40 to 80 mL) in 250 mL of NS or D_5W.

DOSE

- Infusion rate is usually between 2 and 20 µg/kg per minute.
- Titrate so that heart rate does not increase greater than 10% of baseline.
- Requires hemodynamic monitoring for optimal use.

WATCH OUT! (Precautions)

- Causes hypotension at higher doses due to vasodilation.
- Tachycardias and ventricular arrhythmias may occur.

Dopamine (Dopastat, Intropin)

WHY? (Actions)

- A sympathomimetic, natural catecholamine. Depending on dose, dopamine stimulates different adrenergic receptors. The different receptors produce different effects: increased renal output; increased cardiac contractility; increased blood pressure.

- Works on the "tank" portion (producing vasoconstriction and a smaller tank) and on the "pump" portion (leading to stronger cardiac action).

WHEN ? (Indications)

Four main indications:

1. Symptomatic bradycardia in patients with hypotension/hypoperfusion: To use dopamine to raise the blood pressure in hypotensive bradycardic patients, make sure that the patient has a "full tank" and is not hypovolemic. If patient is hypovolemic, dopamine will achieve only minimal effectiveness.

2. Symptomatic hypotension in patients without hypovolemia. Recommended to treat hypotension with signs and symptoms of shock when the systolic blood pressure is 70 to 100 mm Hg. Most commonly, the symptomatic hypotension is due to bradycardia (not hypovolemia) and dopamine is highly effective.

3. Post resuscitation hypotension. Use dopamine in vasopressor doses (10 to 20 µg/kg/min) to treat (transient *hyper*tension is the goal).

4. Cardiogenic shock, cardiac failure. Should be combined with vasodilators (nitroglycerin and nitroprusside) to reduce preload and improve cardiac output. The vasodilators antagonize the arterial and venous constriction caused by the dopamine.

HOW?

SUPPLIED

- 5-mL ampules at 40 mg/mL (total = 200 mg) or 160 mg/mL (total = 800 mg)

MIX

- Either 400 mg or 800 mg in 250 mL of NS, LR, or D_5W

DOSE

Select the dose of dopamine based on the effects you are trying to achieve:

- *Low-dose dopamine (1 to 5 µg/kg per minute)* so-called "renal doses." These doses produce a dopaminergic effect that dilates the renal, mesenteric, and cerebral blood vessels. This increases renal output. Do not use this lower dose in patients you are treating for symptomatic bradycardia.

- *Moderate-dose dopamine (5 to 10 µg/kg per minute)* so-called "cardiac doses." These doses produce beta-1 and alpha-adrenergic effects that increase cardiac contractility, and cardiac output, and raise blood pressure. This is the dose to start with for patients with symptomatic bradycardia.

- *High-dose dopamine (10 to 20 µg/kg per minute)* has been called "vasopressor doses." Here the alpha-adrenergic effects produce strong arterial and venous vasoconstriction that raises the blood pressure. You would use these doses in patients with low blood pressure and signs and symptoms that suggest clinical shock. (Combine with volume replacement.)

- *Norepinephrine doses (more than 20 µg/kg per minute.)* At doses this high you get the profound vasoconstrictive effects of norepinephrine.

WATCH OUT! (Precautions)

- Do not mix with sodium bicarbonate or any alkaline solution as this will inactivate dopamine.

- Taper gradually (over several hours) to avoid a sudden drop in blood pressure.

- Reduce the dose to one-tenth the usual dose in people taking monoamine oxidase inhibitors.

- Watch for excessive increases in heart rate (may induce supraventricular and ventricular arrhythmias).

- May induce angina and ischemic changes in people with severe coronary artery disease.

- May cause tissue necrosis and sloughing, if local skin infiltration occurs.

- May aggravate pulmonary congestion in people with heart failure.

- MAO inhibitors (Eutonyl, Parnate, Nardil) will potentiate the effects of dopamine.

- Patients taking dilantin may experience excessive hypotension with dopamine.

- Patients with pheochromocytoma may experience hypertensive crisis when given dopamine.

Epinephrine (Adrenalin)

WHY? (Actions)

- A catecholamine (sympathomimetic) with alpha- and beta-adrenergic action.

- The drug of choice for patients in cardiac arrest. No medication is known to do a better job of increasing blood flow to the brain and heart.

- Raises blood pressure by constricting the peripheral blood vessels (pressor effect). The vasoconstrictive actions improve coronary and cerebral blood flow and increase the chance for survival.

- In bradycardic patients, epinephrine increases the heart rate by increasing electrical activity in the myocardium and the intrinsic cardiac automaticity (chronotropic effects); also increases myocardial oxygen consumption.

HOW?

SUPPLIED

- Preloaded 10-mL syringe at 1 mg/10 mL.
- Glass ampule at 1 mg/mL .
- Multidose vial, 30 mL at 1 mg/mL .

MIX

- 1 mg (1 mL of a 1:1000 solution) to 500 mL of NS or D_5W. Gives concentration of 2 μg/mL.
- 30 mg (30 mL of a 1:1000 solution) to 250 mL of NS or D_5W to run at 100 mL/hour (again titrating to hemodynamic effects).
- Sodium bicarbonate and epinephrine must not be mixed in the same IV line.

DOSE

Cardiac Arrest Doses

Recommended dose is 1 mg IV push every 3 to 5 minutes. If this dose does not convert the ECG, one of the other Class IIb dosing regimens can be used as follows:

- Intermediate: Epinephrine 2 to 5 mg IV push, every 3 to 5 minutes.
- Escalating: Epinephrine 1 mg to 3 mg to 5 mg IV push, 3 minutes apart.
- High: Epinephrine 0.1 mg/kg IV push, every 3 to 5 minutes.

Symptomatic Bradycardia Doses

- Start IV infusion at 1 μg/min. Mix 1 mg (1:1000) in 500 mL NS; infuse at 1 to 5 mL/min. Titrate to blood pressure and heart rate, usually 2 to 10 mg/min.

Endotracheal Epinephrine Dose and Administration

- Draw up 2 to 2.5 mg of epinephrine from either glass 1-mL ampules (1 mg/mL) or from a multidose 30-mL vial (1mg/mL). Use a 10-mL or larger syringe.
- Add NS to a total volume of 10 mL.
- Ventilate lungs using the resuscitation bag several times.
- Remove the bag from the end of the endotracheal tube.
- Insert a long through-the-needle catheter deep into the endotracheal tube.
- Cease chest compressions.
- Quickly inject the 2 to 2.5 mg (in the saline) down the catheter.
- May follow with an additional 10 mL of NS to flush the drug deeper into the lungs.
- Rapidly attach the ventilation bag and ventilate lungs three or four times in quick succession.
- OR: Use a heparin lock in the following manner: attach heparin lock to a 20 gauge needle through the wall of the endotracheal tube. Administer the medication with ventilations to help aerosolize the drug further into the lungs for better absorption.

WATCH OUT! (Precautions)

- Epinephrine, by raising the blood pressure and increasing the heart rate, can precipitate myocardial ischemia, increasing angina and chest pain.
- Be particularly careful, since by definition people with symptomatic bradycardia who need epinephrine are people with a diseased myocardium, usually coronary artery disease.
- Watch out for the increase in myocardial oxygen demand. Even small doses of epinephrine (20 μg/min or 0.3 μg/kg per minute) can elevate the blood pressure and induce or exacerbate ventricular ectopy and VT or VF.
- Patients who are taking digitalis are much more likely to have toxic side effects from epinephrine.

Furosemide (Lasix)

WHY? (Actions)

- Reduces preload on the heart as follows:
  - By decreasing venous tone and thus increasing venous capacitance; this causes a fall in left ventricular filling pressure.
  - By producing a marked diuresis several minutes later; this reduces the intravascular volume and thus the left ventricular filling pressures.
- Corrects *tank* problems, primarily by making the "tank" (intravascular volume) bigger with the increase in venous capacitance and then making the volume in the tank smaller (with the diuresis).

WHEN? (Indications)

- For adjunctive therapy of acute pulmonary edema in patients with systolic blood pressures greater than 90 to 100 mm Hg.
- Hypertensive emergencies and urgencies.
- Hypercalcemia (severe).

HOW?

SUPPLIED

- 10 mg/mL in ampules, vials, syringes of 2 mL, 4 mL, and 10 mL.

DOSE

- 0.5 to 1.0 mg/kg over 1 to 2 minutes.
- If no response in 10 to 15 minutes, double the dose to 2 mg/kg and give slowly over 1 to 2 minutes.
- Administer an initial dose twice the daily oral dose if patient is already taking oral furosemide.

- Use higher doses if patient has massive fluid retention or renal insufficiency, or both.

WATCH OUT! (Precautions)

- Can produce hyponatremia, hypokalemia, hypovolemia, hyperuricemia, tinnitus.
- Follow urinary output.
- Monitor blood pressure, electrolyte, blood urea nitrogen, creatinine, and uric acid levels.

Heparin

WHY? (Actions)

- Prevents recurrence of thrombosis.
- Prevents mural thrombus formation in patients with a large, anterior AMI.

WHEN? (Indications)

- Current practice is to use heparin with only one thrombolytic agent, alteplase, recombinant (TPA) since studies have not supported value of heparin with streptokinase. Options are as follows:

  - Option 1: Use at same time as thrombolytic agent. (This is most common practice.)
  - Option 2: Use on completion of thrombolytic infusion.
  - Option 3: Use heparin empirically in patients with large, anterior acute MIs without thrombolytics to prevent mural thrombi. Many clinicians use echocardiography to determine which patients should get heparin: if echocardiography shows large hypokinetic area of the ventricles, give heparin.
  - Option 4: Use empirically in patients with unstable angina.

HOW?

- Begin heparin immediately with rt-PA.
- Initial bolus IV dose: 80 international units (IU)/kg.
- Continue: 18 IU/kg per hour (round to the nearest 50 IU).
- Then adjust as follows to maintain activated partial thromboplastin time: (aPTT) at 1.5 to 2.0 times the control values:

  - Target range for aPTT after first 24 hours = 60 to 85 seconds (may vary with laboratory).
  - Value for aPTT should be checked at 6, 12, 18, and 24 hours.
  - If aPTT is less than or equal to 60 seconds at 24 hours, rebolus with 20 IU/kg heparin; increase infusion to 3 IU/kg per hour; recheck aPTT in 2 hours.

- Almost all patients receiving thrombolytics should receive **aspirin** 160 to 325 mg along with the heparin.
- Drug reversal if necessary: Protamine 25 mg slow IV infusion over 10 minutes or longer. (Calculate dose as 1 mg protamine per 100 IU heparin remaining in the patient; heparin plasma half-life = 60 minutes.)

WATCH OUT! (Precautions)

Heparin has the same contraindications as thrombolytic therapy, as follows:

- Active bleeding.
- Recent intracranial, intraspinal, or eye surgery.
- Severe hypertension.
- Bleeding tendencies.
- Gastrointestinal tract bleeding.

Isoproterenol (Isuprel)

WHY? (Actions)

- A pure beta-adrenergic agent; synthetic sympathomimetic amine.
- Causes increased strength of cardiac contractions, increased heart rate, but peripheral vasodilation and venous pooling.

WHEN? (Indications)

- Third-line agent for temporarily increasing the heart rate in patients with symptomatic bradycardia.
- Use only after atropine, transcutaneous pacing, or dopamine, and epinephrine infusion have failed.
- Most experts now prefer other chronotropic and inotropic agents (dopamine, dobutamine, and amrinone). Often beneficial for denervated (transplanted) hearts.
- Another second-line indication is to achieve "pharmacologic overdrive pacing" of patients in the VT known as "torsades de pointes." Attempt only after infusion of magnesium sulfate has failed.

HOW?

SUPPLIED

- 1 mg/mL in 1-mL vial; 1 mg in 5 mL vial.

MIX

- Mix 1 mg in 250 to 500 mL NS, lactated Ringer's solution (LR), LR, or D_5W
- Use a volumetric infusion pump to carefully control the flow.

DOSE

- Infuse initially at low doses of 2 µg/min.
- Limit the dose to 2 to 10 µg/min.
- Gradually titrate up to achieve a heart rate of 60 to 70 beats/min.
- When using isoproterenol to "break" torsades de pointes, titrate the dose to achieve an increase in heart rate that suppresses the VT.

WATCH OUT! (Precautions)

- Do not use during cardiac arrest. The vasodilatory actions reduce coronary perfusion pressure and may increase mortality. This is a Class III (harmful) use of the agent.

- Avoid isoproterenol in patients with ischemic heart disease; may increase the heart rate and myocardial oxygen requirements so that disastrous myocardial ischemia results.
- The effects on symptomatic bradycardia patients with coronary artery disease also may be catastrophic—they get severe myocardial ischemia and worsening hypotension and can even have full cardiac arrest.
- Bradycardic patients may respond to isoproterenol with severely symptomatic tachycardia, VT, VF, and full cardiac arrest.
- Avoid isoproterenol in patients with possible toxic effects of digitalis.

Lidocaine (Xylocaine)

WHY? (Actions)

- Increases the amount of current needed to cause fibrillation (raises "fibrillation threshold"); decreases the amount of current needed for defibrillation (lowers the "defibrillation threshold").
- Decreases excitability in ischemic tissue.
- Suppresses ventricular irritability.

WHEN? (Indications)
RECOMMENDED
Cardiac Arrest Resulting From VF/VT

- Administer after initial defibrillation shocks, intubation, and epinephrine.
- First antiarrhythmic to use for refractory VF/VT.

Stable, perfusing VT.

AMI patients with new-onset *symptomatic* ventricular ectopy.

NOT RECOMMENDED

- Routine *prophylactic* lidocaine to prevent VF/VT for AMI patients.
- *Prophylactic* lidocaine before thrombolytic therapy.
- Routine treatment of "warning arrhythmias" in AMI, as follows:
    - Six or more premature ventricular contractions (PVCs) per minute.
    - Closely coupled PVCs.
    - R on T (PVC on T wave).
    - PVCs in pairs.
    - PVCs in runs (short bursts of three or more).
    - Multifocal PVCs.

HOW?
SUPPLIED

- Preloaded 5-mL syringe with 20 mg/mL; total = 100 mg.
- Also in 5-mL vial of 10 mg/mL; total = 50 mg.

DOSE
Cardiac Arrest Resulting From VF/VT

- First dose: 1.0 to 1.5 mg/kg IV push.
- Repeat: Bolus in 3 to 5 minutes to a maximum dose of 3 mg/kg.
- Repeat: 0.5 mg/kg boluses may be given, but no more often than every 8 to 10 minutes.
- NOTE: Some clinicians prefer to use 1.5 mg/kg as the maximum dose for lidocaine, and this is acceptable.
- Continue: If circulation returns, start a continuous infusion at 2 to 4 mg/min.

Stable Perfusing VT

- Bolus: 1 to 1.5 mg/kg IV.
- Repeat: at 0.5 to 0.75 mg/kg every 5 to 10 minutes.
- Total: 3 mg/kg.
- Continue: 2 to 4 mg/min or 30 to 50 mg/kg per minute.

WATCH OUT! (Precautions)

- Watch for signs of lidocaine intoxication (seizures, respiratory compromise) in patients who regain circulation after the use of higher doses of lidocaine. The clinical signs of lidocaine intoxication are related to the nervous system and include the following:
    - Paresthesias
    - Dizziness
    - Slurred speech
    - Drowsiness
    - Altered consciousness
    - Decreased hearing
    - Muscle twitching
    - Seizures
    - Respiratory arrest
- *Use lower doses and longer intervals* for patients who will not metabolize lidocaine well and who may end up with toxic effects. These include the following:
    - Elderly (over 70 years of age).
    - Those with liver failure.
    - Those with heart failure.
    - Those with small body size.
    - Those with bradycardias.
    - Those with conduction disturbances.

Magnesium sulfate

WHY? (Actions)

- Known association between magnesium deficiency, arrhythmias, and sudden death.
- Provides antiarrhythmic effects.

- Improves electrical stability in the heart.
- Reduces coronary artery spasm.

WHEN? (Indications)

- In cardiac arrest that is due to VF/VT, give magnesium to patients with known or clinically suspected low magnesium levels (hypomagnesemia). Class IIA (acceptable, probably helpful).

- Suspect magnesium deficiency in patients with poor dietary intake and habits and chronic diseases (alcoholism, renal failure, chronic gastrointestinal tract problems associated with malabsorption).

- Torsades de pointes: Magnesium is the treatment of choice in this form of VF/VT.

- Use magnesium to *treat* known or *suspected* magnesium deficiency in patients with AMI.

- Magnesium is acceptable as a *prophylactic* antiarrhymic in AMI (Class IIa).

HOW?

SUPPLIED

- 2- and 10-mL glass ampules of 50% $MgSO_4$ = 1 and 5 g.
- Preloaded 10-mL syringe for a total of 5 g/10 mL.

MIX

- 2 to 4 mL of a 50% solution diluted in 10 mL of D_5W.

DOSE

- Refractory VF/VT cardiac arrest with known or suspected hypomagnesemia: 1 to 2 g (2 to 4 mL of 50% $MgSO_4$) IV push.

- Torsades de pointes pattern of VF/VT: 1 to 2 g IV (2 to 4 ml of 50% $MgSO_4$) over 1 to 2 minutes. (Even higher doses, up to 5 to 10 g, may be needed to control the torsades de pointes.)

- AMI prophylaxis: 1 to 2 g (2 to 4 mL of 50% $MgSO_4$) diluted in 100 mL of NS, over 5 to 60 minutes. Follow with 0.5 to 2.0 g/hour up to 24 hours.

- Continue infusion for 24 hours at 0.5 to 1.0 g/hour if magnesium deficiency is documented after resuscitation.

WATCH OUT! (Precautions)

- Toxic effects are rare.
- Side effects include flushing, sweating, mild bradycardia, hypotension, and hyporeflexia.
- Signs of excessive serum magnesium levels are diarrhea, depressed reflexes, paralysis, circulatory collapse, and respiratory weakness.
- Patients with renal failure: Adjust later doses.

Morphine sulfate

WHY (Actions)

FOR POSSIBLE AMI:

- Reduces pain of ischemia.
- Reduces anxiety.
- Increases venous capacitance.
- Decreases systemic vascular resistance.
- Reduces oxygen demands on the heart.
- Lessens ischemia and infarct extension.

WHEN (Indications)

- Continuing chest pain.
- Evidence of vascular congestion (acute pulmonary edema).

HOW?

SUPPLIED

- 2 to 10 mg/mL in 1-mL syringe.

MIX:

- Direct IV injection.

DOSE

- 2 to 5 mg IV. Give 1 mg/min every 5 minutes for 30 minutes.
- Goal is to eliminate the pain while watching for excessive blood pressure drop or respiratory depression.

WATCH OUT! (Precautions)

- Keep blood pressure above 90 mm Hg systolic.
- Use cautiously, if at all, with hypovolemia.
- Watch for fall in blood pressure, especially with the following:
  - Volume-depleted patients
  - Patients with increased systemic resistance
  - Patients receiving beta blockers
- Use Trendelenburg's position as first response to moderate-to-severe blood pressure drops. (Use caution in obese patients.)
- Depression of ventilation. (Use naloxone 0.4 to 2.0 mg IV to reverse respiratory depression.)
- Nausea and vomiting (common).
- Bradycardia.
- Itching and bronchospasm (uncommon).

Nifedipine (Adalat, Procardia)

WHY? (Actions)

- Smooth muscle vasodilator; most potent vasodilator of the calcium antagonists.
- Improves diastolic relaxation of ventricles.

WHEN? (Indications)

- Hypertensive urgencies. (For hypertensive emergencies use IV nitroprusside or intravenous nitroglycerin.)

HOW?

SUPPLIED

- 10- and 20-mg capsules.
- Capsules can be punched with needle; patients then "bite and swallow" for sublingual administration.

DOSE

- 10 to 20 mg PO or sublingual; repeat 1 to 2 times every 30 minutes.

WATCH OUT! (Precautions)

- Hypotension.
- Bradycardia.
- Decreased left ventricular contractility, especially in patients taking beta blockers.
- Avoid in patients with signs of left ventricular failure or dysfunction.

Nitroglycerin (Nitrobid, Nitrostat, Tridil)

WHY? (Actions)

- Dilates venous capacitance vessels.
- Inhibits venous return to the heart (reduces preload).
- Decreases systemic vascular resistance and facilitates cardiac emptying (reduces afterload).
- Decreases myocardial oxygen consumption.
- Dilates coronary arteries.

WHEN? (Indications)

- Chest pain of suspected cardiac origin.
- Unstable angina (change in angina pattern).
- Acute pulmonary edema (especially with blood pressure elevated above 100 mm Hg systolic).
- Congestive heart failure.
- Hypertensive crisis or urgency with chest pain.
- Elevated blood pressure in setting of AMI (especially with signs of left ventricular failure).
- Helps correct "tank" problems by making the "tank" (intravascular volume) bigger.
- Most clinicians now consider nitroglycerin to be the most effective agent used for acute pulmonary edema.
- Many physicians administer routine nitroglycerin infusions to people with high suspicion of AMI. This is controversial.

HOW?

SUPPLIED

- Sublingual tablets: 0.3, 0.4, and 0.6 mg.
- Spray: 0.4 mg per dose.
- Ampules: 5 mg in 10 mL, 8 mg in 10 mL, 10 mg in 10 mL.
- Vials: 25 mg in 5 mL, 50 mg in 10 mL, 100 mg in 10 mL.

MIX

- 50 mg in 250 mL of D_5W or NS to give 200 µg/mL.
- IV infusion is route of choice for emergencies; allows precise control of dose and greater predictability of effect.

DOSE

- IV infusion: infuse at 10 to 20 µg/min. Titrate to effect; increase by 5 to 10 µg/min every 5 to 10 minutes. Use IV infusion sets provided by the manufacturer. Do not mix with other drugs.
- Spray inhaler: Spray for 0.5 to 1.0 seconds; repeat every 5 minutes.
- Sublingual: One or two 0.4-mg tablets. Repeat every 5 minutes if systolic blood pressure is greater than 90 to 100 mm Hg.
- Paste: apply 1 to 2 inch strip. Spread into thin layer with backing paper (less preferable).
- Limit to systolic blood pressure drop of 10% if patient is normotensive (e.g., 120 to 110 mm Hg systolic); 30% if patient is initially hypertensive (e.g., 180 to 120 mm Hg systolic).

WATCH OUT! (Precautions)

- Nitroglycerin will lower the blood pressure; therefore use with caution in patients with systolic blood pressures less than 100 mm Hg.
- Avoid dropping the blood pressure below 90 mm Hg.
- If the patient with evidence of AMI is hypertensive, limit the blood pressure drop to 30% of original levels.
- If the patient with evidence of AMI is normotensive, limit the blood pressure drop to 10% of original levels.
- Watch for headache, excessive drop in blood pressure, syncope, and tachycardia.
- Instruct patient to sit or lie down.

Nitroprusside (Nipride)

WHY? (Actions)

- Acts as potent peripheral vasodilator.
- Reduces blood pressure by reducing arterial resistance.
- Reduces blood pressure by increasing venous capacitance.
- For heart failure, increases cardiac output by increasing stroke volume and reducing arterial resistance.

WHEN? (Indications)

- Hypertensive emergencies.
- Heart failure and acute pulmonary edema (reduces afterload).
- Acute mitral or aortic valve regurgitation (reduces afterload).
- Drug of second choice in treating congestive heart failure and acute pulmonary edema in patients with coronary artery disease. (Nitroglycerin is drug of first choice because of improved coronary blood flow.)

HOW?

SUPPLIED

- 10 mg/mL in 5-mL vial; total = 50 mg.

MIX

- 50 or 100 mg in 250 mL D_5W.
- Extremely sensitive to light. (Cover drug with opaque material.)

DOSE

- Begin at 0.1 µg/kg per minute, and titrate upward every 3 to 5 minutes to desired effect (up to 5 µg/kg per minute).
- Use an infusion pump.

WATCH OUT! (Precautions)

- Effects occur within 1 to 2 minutes.
- Can lower the blood pressure severely, causing stroke, infarction, or cardiac ischemia.
- Must use with hemodynamic monitoring for optimal safety.
- Reduces coronary artery perfusion to ischemic myocardium; therefore do not use when patients with acute pulmonary edema also have coronary artery disease and myocardial ischemia.

Norepinephrine (Levophed)

WHY? (Actions)

- Potent alpha effects of arterial and venous vasoconstriction.
- Stimulates heart (beta$_1$ effects) but not lungs (beta$_2$ effects).
- Raises blood pressure without increasing heart rate.

WHEN? (Indications)

- Cardiogenic shock.
- Significant hypotension (blood pressure less than 70 mm Hg).
- Used as a last choice for treatment of ischemic heart disease and shock.

HOW?

SUPPPLIED

- 4 mg (1 mg/mL) in 4-mL ampule.

MIX

- 4 mg in 250 mL D_5W or D_5NS. (Avoid NS alone.)

DOSE

- 0.5 to 1.0 µg/min.
- Titrate to clinical effect; up to 30 µg/min.
- Monitor cardiac output.
- Use large vein to decrease risk of extravasation.
- Administer via an infusion pump with piggyback setup.

WATCH OUT! (Precautions)

- Increases myocardial oxygen consumption.
- Use with caution in setting of acute ischemia.
- Extravasation may cause tissue necrosis (local subcutaneous injection of phentolamine Regitine may decrease tissue injury).
- Keep at hand: Atropine (to reverse reflex bradycardic effects); phentolamine 5 mg IV (for increased vasopressor effects); propranolol (for arrhythmias).

Oxygen

WHY? (Actions)

- Essential for cellular metabolism and survival.
- First drug to use for respiratory compromise.

WHEN? (Indications)

- Use in any suspected cardiopulmonary emergency.
- Use with any complaints of shortness of breath.
- Use for any patient complaining of chest pain.
- Use for any suspected hypoxemia.

HOW?

SUPPLIED

- Deliver at 100% concentration from portable tanks, or from wall-mounted sources through delivery devices.
- Various delivery devices give the following percentages of oxygen:

DEVICE	FLOW RATE (L/MIN)	OXYGEN DELIVERED (%)
Nonrebreather mask	8-12	80-95
Partial rebreather mask	6-10	35-60
Venturi mask	4-8	24-40
Simple face mask	5	60
Nasal cannula	1-6	24-44

WATCH OUT! (Precautions)

- Do not withhold oxygen from anyone who might need it.
- Observe closely when using on the rare patient dependent on hypoxic respiratory drive. (Be prepared to ventilate patient's lungs.)

Procainamide (Pronestyl)

WHY? (Actions)

- Supresses cardiac automaticity and ventricular ectopy.

- Slows intraventricular conduction, which can lead to bidirectional block.

- This bidirectional block may terminate reentrant arrhythmias in supraventricular tachycardias.

WHEN? (Indications)

- Third-line agent to use for persistent VF/VT (after lidocaine and bretylium).

- Use for "stuttering" codes when patients in unstable condition are "in and out" of cardiac arrest. These interposed periods of perfusion allow time for procainamide administration.

- Useful for tachycardias in patients who are not in full cardiac arrest, both VT and supraventricular tachycardia, especially atrial fibrilliation with rapid rate in Wolff-Parkinson-White syndrome. This is a second- or third-line agent.

HOW?

SUPPLIED

- 100 mg/mL in 10-mL vial; total of 1 g.

- 500 mg/mL in 2-mL vial; total of 1 g.

DOSE

For Non-cardiac Arrest Tachycardia

- 20 to 30 mg/min, to a total dose of 17 mg/kg. (For example, a 70 kg person would receive 1.2 g, requiring 40 to 60 minutes to administer.) Use the following end points:

  - The arrhythmia is suppressed.

  - Hypotension becomes excessive.

  - QRS complex become widened by 50% of its original width.

  - Loading dose has been administered (17 mg/kg).

For Cardiac Arrest

  - 17 mg/kg as loading dose over 15 to 30 minutes, followed with a pressor agent such as norepinephrine or dopamine. (This is the authors' recommendation, not a specific AHA recommendation.)

  - Start a continuous infusion at 1 to 4 mg/min (mix 1 g in 250 mL or 2 g in 500 mL to equal 4 mg/mL) if procainamide suppresses the arrhythmia.

WATCH OUT! (Precautions)

- Observe the ECG monitor closely, and measure the blood pressure when administering procainamide, especially when using rapid infusion rates.

- Can produce strong vasodilatory effects and negative inotropic effects.

- Can widen the QRS complex and lengthen baseline PR and QT intervals.

- These effects lead to AV conduction problems such as heart blocks and cardiac arrest.

- Be particularly cautious when patients have low potassium or magnesium levels.

Sodium bicarbonate

WHY? (Actions)

- Acts as a buffer agent administered to neutralize hydrogen ions.

WHEN? (Indications)

- Ventilation with endotracheal intubation provides the major treatment of acidosis associated with cardiac emergencies.

Class I Intervention (Definitely Helpful)

- Known, preexisting hyperkalemia.

Class IIa (Acceptable, Probably Helpful)

- Cardiac arrest associated with overdose of tricyclic antidepressants.

- Cardiac arrest associated with preexisting bicarbonate-responsive acidosis.

Class IIb (Acceptable, Possibly Helpful)

- Patient remains in cardiac arrest, despite successful intubation and effective ventilations and chest compressions.

- Patient achieves return of spontaneous circulation after a long arrest interval.

Class III (Not Acceptable, Harmful)

- Patient is in cardiac arrest, and lungs are not effectively ventilated. Unless there is some other specific indication, bicarbonate should not be administered to a patient who does not have endotracheal intubation.

HOW?

SUPPLIED

- 50-mL preloaded syringe (8.4% sodium bicarbonate at 50 mEq/50 mL).

DOSE

- 1 mEq/kg IV bolus.

- Repeat ½ dose every 10 minutes or per arterial blood gas levels.

WATCH OUT! (Precautions)

- Do not give sodium bicarbonate to patients with hypoxic lactic acidosis, such as occurs in extended cardic arrests.

- Treatment of the acidosis of cardiac arrest includes ventilation and restoration of normal circulation. The best "buffer therapy" we possess is good CPR.

- Sodium bicarbonate can produce a variety of side effects, including the following:
  - Mixed venous intracellular acidosis.
  - Hyperosmolality.
  - Hypernatremia.
  - Metabolic alkalosis.
  - Acute hypokalemia.

Thrombolytic agents: Alteplase (tissue plasminogen activator), streptokinase, anistreplase

WHY? (Actions)

- So-called "clot busters," thrombolytic agents dissolve acute thrombi that may be occluding cardiac arteries.
- Agents activate plasminogen to the proteolytic enzyme plasmin.
- Activated plasmin then degrades fibrinogen and fibrin clot (clot lysis).

WHEN? (Indications)

- Major indication: AMI with active ECG signs of continuing injury. "Continuing injury" is displayed by ST-segment elevations in two or more contiguous leads. New left bundle branch block also can benefit from thrombolytic therapy.
- *ECG criteria* (measure ST deviation 0.04 seconds after the J point; PR segment is baseline) are as follows:
  - Anterior leads (V_1 to V_4): Two contiguous leads with ST-segment elevation of 2 mm or more.
  - Inferior leads (leads II, III, and aV_F): Two contiguous leads with ST-segment elevation of 1 mm or more.
- In addition, to ECG criteria, the "story" must be right for an Acute MI, and the patient must lack contraindications to thrombolytic therapy.
- Therefore, thrombolytic therapy is indicated when the answers to the following four questions are appropriate:
  - Is the history (pain) consistent with AMI?
  - Is the ECG consistent with acute injury (ST-segment elevations)?
  - Does the patient have any absolute contraindications to thrombolytic therapy?
  - Does the patient have any relative contraindications to thrombolytic therapy?
- Thrombolytic therapy is most beneficial for anterior and multiple location infarcts.
- Thrombolytic therapy is most beneficial, if the patient's chest pain duration is greater than 12 hours. It may help for chest pain that lasts less than 12 hours, if the pain is intermittent or ST elevation persists.
- Absolute age limits have not been defined. Thrombolytic therapy should not be withheld from anyone simply on the basis of the patient being "too old" or "too young."

ABSOLUTE CONTRAINDICATIONS

- Active internal bleeding
- Suspected aortic dissection
- Known traumatic CPR (fractured ribs, fractured sternum, hemothorax, pneumothorax)
- Severe persistent hypertension despite pain relief and initial drugs (>180 systolic or >110 diastolic)
- Recent head trauma or known intracranial neoplasm
- History of CVA in past 6 months
- Pregnancy

RELATIVE CONTRAINDICATIONS

- Recent trauma or major surgery in the past 2 months
- Initial BP >180 systolic or >110 diastolic that is controlled by medical treatment
- Active peptic ulcer or guaiac-positive stools
- History of CVA, tumor, injury, or brain surgery
- Known bleeding disorder or current use of warfarin
- Significant liver dysfunction or renal failure
- Prior exposure to streptokinase or anistreplase during the preceding 12 months
- Known cancer or illness with possible thoracic, abdominal, or intracranial abnormalities
- Prolonged CPR without known trauma (> 15 to 20 minutes, especially with endotracheal intubation)

HOW?

STREPTOKINASE (Streptase, Kabikinase)

- 1.5 million units in a 1-hour infusion
- Dilute in 50 mL of D_5W
- Heparin is not necessary

Adjunctive therapy:

- Aspirin 160 mg po. Give as soon as possible.
- Metoprolol (Lopressor) 5 mg IV every 2 minutes $\times$ 3 doses; then 50 mg po q6hours $\times$ 48 hours (begin 15 minutes after last IV dose then 100 mg po BID).

ALTEPLASE (recombinant tissue plasminogen activator; rtPA; Activase)

Accelerated infusion (1.5 hour):

- Give 15-mg bolus over 1 to 2 minutes
- Then 0.75 mg/kg over next 30 minutes (not to exceed 50 mg)
- Then decrease to 0.50 mg/kg over the next 60 minutes (not to exceed 35 mg)
- Total dose $\leq$ 100 mg

Three-hour infusion:

- Give 60 mg IV in first hour (initial 6 to 10 mg is given IV push)

- Then 20 mg/hour for 2 additional hours
- Total dose ≤100 mg

Adjunctive therapy:

- Aspirin 160 mg po. Give as soon as possible.
- Begin **heparin** immediately with rt-PA.
- Initial heparin bolus IV dose: 80 international units/kg.
- Continue: heparin 18 IU/kg/hour (round to the nearest 50 IU), then
- Adjust to maintain activated Partial Thromboplastin (aPTT) Time 1.5 to 2.0 times the control values.
  - Target range for aPTT after first 24 hours = 60 to 85 seconds (may vary with laboratory).
  - aPTT should be checked at 6, 12, 18, and 24 hours.
  - If aPTT is ≤60 seconds at 24 hours, rebolus with 20 IU/kg heparin; increase infusion to 3 IU/kg/hour; recheck aPTT in 2 hours.
- **Metoprolol** (Lopressor) 5 mg IV every 2 minutes ×3 doses; then 50 mg po q6hours × 48 hours. (Begin 15 minutes after last IV dose then 100 mg po BID.)

ANISTREPLASE (APSAC; anisoylated plasminogen-streptokinase activator complex)

- 30 U IV over 2 to 5 minutes
- Aspirin 160 mg po as soon as possible

WATCH OUT! (Precautions)

- Allergic reacions: give diphenhydramine 50 mg IV plus methylprednisolone 125 mg IV
- Internal or central nervous system bleeding: stop thrombolytic; reverse heparin with protamine 25 mg IV. Consider cryoprecipitates, platelets, or fresh frozen plasma.
- Thrombolytics have a limited role in patients with the combination of AMI and cardiogenic shock. Cardiogenic shock in the setting of an AMI is an indication for emergency angioplasty and inter-aortic balloon pumping.

Verapamil (Calan, Isoptin)

WHY? (Actions)

- A potent slower of conduction through the AV node.
- Relatively strong vasodilator and negative inotrope.

WHEN? (Indications)

- Use for narrow-complex supraventricular tachycardias (PSVT) that have not responded to vagal maneuvers and at least two correctly administered doses of adenosine.
- Use only if the PSVT remains narrow and the patient is not hypotensive.
- Can convert wide-complex tachycardias that are supraventricular in origin. Use verapamil if the blood pressure is normal or elevated and the wide complex tachycardia is known with certainty to be PSVT. Some experts, however, argue that you can only confirm this diagnosis by means of electrophysiologic stimulation testing.

HOW?

SUPPLIED

- 2.5 mg/ml in 2-, 4-, and 5-mL vials; total equals 5, 10, and 12.5 mg.

DOSE

- Use 2.5 to 5 mg IV given over 1 to 2 minutes.
- A second dose of 5 to 10 mg can be given in 15 to 30 minutes if the PSVT persists or recurs, and if the blood pressure remains acceptable.

WATCH OUT! (Precautions)

- The Tachycardia Algorithm asks the following questions before using verapamil for persistent PSVT after adenosine:
  - First, is the complex still narrow? *Never* use verapamil if the supraventricular complex is wide.
  - Second, does the blood pressure remain reasonably normal? If the answer to either of these questions is "no," do not use verapamil. *Never* use verapamil if the blood pressure is low or unstable.
- Administration of verapamil to a patient with VT can be a *lethal error*. Patients in VT who are in stable condition usually have achieved that "stability" by maximum myocardial contractility and vasoconstriction. Verapamil, as a vasodilator, can cause decompensation and hemodynamic collapse.
- In addition, verapamil can accelerate the heart rate even further and decrease the blood pressure in all patients, but especially in patients with the Wolff-Parkinson-White syndrome. *Do not give verapamil to patients with a wide-complex tachycardia unless the tachycardiar is known with certainty to be of supraventricula origin.*
- Give smaller amounts (2 to 4 mg) over longer periods of time (3 to 4 minutes) for the elderly or when the blood pressure is in the lower range of normal.
- Verapamil often produces a significant decrease in blood pressure that can be reversed with calcium chloride 0.5 to 1.0 g given slowly IV.
- Many clinicians *pretreat* patients with an IV infusion of calcium chloride over 5 to 10 minutes before administration of verapamil. Do this for patients with questionable hemodynamic suitability for verapamil.
- If hemodynamic compromise develops *and the PSVT continues,* immediately perform cardioversion.
- A helpful rule: *Always* treat wide-complex tachycardias of uncertain type as if the rhythm is VT.
- There are several clinical situations where you should *not* use verapamil, or at least use it with extreme caution. These include the following:

- Patients with low blood pressure.

- Patients with wide-complex tachycardias.

- Patients who have recently been given IV beta blockers.

- Patients who routinely take oral beta blockers.

- Patients with Wolff-Parkinson-White syndrome plus atrial fibrillation.

- Patients with sick sinus syndrome.

- Patients with AV block without a pacemaker.

- **Paroxysmal Supraventricular Tachycardia**

- General treatment sequence is as follows:

  - Vagal maneuvers.

  - **Adenosine** 6 mg.

  - **Adenosine** 12 mg (may repeat once in 1 to 2 minutes.)

  - **Verapamil** 2.5 to 5 mg (if complex width is narrow and blood pressure is normal).

  - **Verapamil** 5 to 10 mg.

  - As a vagal maneuver carotid sinus pressure is contraindicated in patients with carotid bruits; avoid ice water immersion in patients with ischemic heart disease.

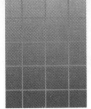

Appendix A
Automated Defibrillators: Operator's Checklist

Automated Defibrillators: Operator's Shift Checklist

Date _____ Shift _____ Location _____

Mfr/Model No. _____ Serial No. or Facility ID No. _____

At the beginning of each shift, inspect the unit. Indicate whether all requirements have been met. Note any corrective actions taken. Sign the form.

	OK as Found	Corrective Action/ Remarks
1. Defibrillator Unit Clean, no spills, clear of objects on top, casing intact		
2. Cables/Connectors a. Inspect for cracks, broken wire, or damage b. Connectors engage securely and are not damaged*		

3. Supplies
a. Two sets of pads in sealed   f. Monitoring electrodes*
   packages, within expiration date*   g. Spare charged battery*
b. Hand towel   h. Adequate ECG paper*
c. Scissors   i. Manual override module, key,
d. Razor   or card*
e. Alcohol wipes*   j. Cassette tape, memory module,
         and/or event card plus spares*		

4. Power Supply
a. Battery-powered units
  (1) Verify fully charged battery in place
  (2) Spare charged battery available
  (3) Follow appropriate battery rotation schedule per
       manufacturer's recommendations
b. AC/battery backup units
  (1) Plugged into live outlet to maintain battery charge
  (2) Test on battery power and reconnect to line power		

5. Indicators*/ECG Display a. Remove cassette tape, memory module, and/or event card* b. Power-on display c. Self-test OK d. Monitor display functional* e. "Service" message display off* f. Battery charging; low battery light off* g. Correct time displayed; set with dispatch center		
6. ECG Recorder* a. Adequate ECG paper b. Recorder prints		
7. Charge/Display Cycle a. Disconnect AC plug – battery backup units* b. Attach to simulator c. Detects, charges, and delivers shock for VF d. Responds correctly to nonshockable rhythms e. Manual override functional* f. Detach from simulator g. Replace cassette tape, module, and/or memory card *		
8. Pacemaker* a. Pacer output cable intact b. Pacer pads present (set of two) c. Inspect per manufacturer's operational guidelines		
Major Problem(s) Identified **(Out of Service)**		

*Applicable only if the unit has this supply or capability

Signature _____

Appendix B
Manual Defibrillators: Operator's Checklist

Defibrillation

Manual Defibrillators: Operator's Shift Checklist

Date _____ Shift _____ Location _____

Mfr/Model No. _____ Serial No. or Facility ID No. _____

At the beginning of each shift, inspect the unit. Indicate whether all requirements have been met. Note any corrective actions taken. Sign the form.

	OK as Found	Corrective Action/ Remarks
1. Defibrillator Unit Clean, no spills, clear of objects on top, casing intact		
2. Paddles (including pediatric adapters)* a. Clean, not pitted b. Release from housing easily c. If internal paddles are included, verify their availability in a sterile package. Periodically inspect as with external paddles.		
3. Cables/Connectors a. Inspect for cracks, broken wire, or damage b. Connectors engage securely and are not damaged		
4. Supplies a. Two sets of pads in sealed packages, within expiration date* f. Razor g. Spare ECG paper b. Monitoring electrodes h. Spare charged battery available* c. Alcohol wipes i. Cassette tape* d. Hand towel j. Gel or other conductive medium e. Scissors present and stored properly*		

5. Power Supply
a. Battery-powered units
   (1) Verify fully charged battery in place
   (2) Spare charged battery available
   (3) Follow appropriate battery rotation schedule per manufacturer's recommendations
b. AC/battery backup units
   (1) Plugged into live outlet to maintain battery
   (2) Test on battery power and reconnect to line power		

6. Indicators/ECG Display a. Power-on display b. Self-test OK* c. Monitor display functional d. "Service" message display off e. Battery charging; low battery light off* f. Correct time displayed; set with dispatch center*		
7. ECG Recorder a. Adequate ECG paper b. Recorder prints		
8. Charge-Display Cycle for Paddle or Adhesive Pad Defibrillation a. Disconnect AC plug – battery backup units b. Charge to manufacturer's recommended test energy level c. Charge indicators working d. Discharge per manufacturer's instructions e. Reconnect line power		
9. Pacemaker* a. Pacer output cable intact b. Pacer pads present (set of two) c. Inspect per manufacturer's operational guidelines		
Major Problem(s) Identified **(Out of Service)**		

*Applicable only if the unit has this supply or capability

Signature _____

Index

B

L

M